Fitness through Aerobics

Ninth Edition

JAN GALEN BISHOP
Central Connecticut State University

PEARSON

Boston   Columbus   Indianapolis   New York   San Francisco   Upper Saddle River
Amsterdam   Cape Town   Dubai   London   Madrid   Milan   Munich   Paris   Montréal   Toronto
Delhi   Mexico City   São Paulo   Sydney   Hong Kong   Seoul   Singapore   Taipei   Tokyo

Executive Editor: Sandra Lindelof
Development Manager: Barbara Yien
Editorial Manager: Susan Malloy
Editorial Assistant: Briana Verdugo
Managing Editor: Deborah Cogan
Editorial Project Manager: Carol Traver/Azimuth Publisher Services
Production Project Manager: Dorothy Cox
Production Management and Composition: PreMediaGlobal
Cover Designer: Tandem Creative, Inc.
Cover Photographs: (top) Kris Hanke/Getty Images; (bottom) Andresr Imaging/Shutterstock
Manufacturing Buyer: Stacey Weinberger
Marketing Manager: Neena Bali

All photos copyrighted by the author or Pearson Education, Inc. except for fig. 9.8 by MartinBaraud/Getty Images.

Library of Congress Cataloging-in-Publication Data is available on request from the Library of Congress.

ISBN-13: 978-0-321-88452-7
ISBN-10: 0-321-88452-3
1 2 3 4 5 6 7 8 9 10 —EBM— 17 16 15 14 13

Contents

---

* Note: All worksheets are available online at www.pearsonhighered.com/bishopaerobics. Selected worksheets are also available as indicated at the end of the book.

Preface

The nine editions of this book chronicle the growth of group fitness. The first edition was written as Jackie Sorensen, inspired by Ken Cooper's ideas of aerobic fitness, set dance steps to music, and Judy Shepard-Misset quickly followed with Jazzercise. Aerobic dance exploded with popularity, especially among women. As the movement spread, there was a need for more resistance during the body toning exercises, opening the door for exercise bands in the 2nd edition. The 3rd edition placed aerobic exercise within the wellness context. Also at this time, an injured and rehabbing Gin Miller recognized that stepping up and down on a bench could be used for more than rehab and brought us step aerobics, which helped make "aerobic" classes more popular as a coed activity. Aerobic-exercise styles and methods exploded: low-impact, middle-impact, non-impact, funk, Latin, double benching, aqua benching...the 4th edition tried to do them all justice. By the 5th edition, aerobic group training had jumped off the dance floor and onto cardio equipment, with group cycling leading the way but also including elliptical, treadmill, and rowing classes. The martial arts also kicked and punched their way onto the aerobic scene, working to music and appealing to a whole new group of people. Interest in more muscular fitness began to grow. Dumbbell exercises graced the 5th edition, stability balls, the 6th edition, and body bars, the 7th edition. Pilates, yoga, and the mind-body connection were also gaining popularity in the United States during this time. The 8th edition took notice of fitness technology, adding information on pedometers and heart rate monitors. Now the 9th edition arrives in time to share with the reader the current trends embracing functional fitness, cross training, high-intensity interval training, and fusion classes. Amazingly, what started simply as "aerobic dance" is now "group fitness" and enjoyed in its many forms by millions of people worldwide.

As classes continue to thrive with new and veteran exercisers, this enthusiasm for group fitness has created a delightful dilemma. People who have never exercised before or who have had limited instruction in exercise are asking all kinds of questions about aerobics and muscular fitness. Instructors are faced with educating a gymnasium filled with people in an environment that demands movement and motivating music, not talk. A good instructor can educate as the class proceeds but is often severely limited by time and acoustics. This book was written to provide a solution. Students can read through vital information outside class; instructors can quickly clarify, reinforce, and supplement the information during class; and everyone has time to enjoy a full aerobic workout.

Therefore, the goal of the ninth edition of *Fitness Through Aerobics* is to provide the group fitness participant with important information on the four health-related components of physical fitness: cardiorespiratory fitness, muscular fitness, flexibility, and body composition. Knowledge presented in this book will enhance the participants' ability to (1) understand the important relationship between regular exercise, health, and wellness, (2) perform exercises correctly, (3) maximize the training effect of exercise, and (4) take control of planning and setting forth on a lifetime fitness plan.

NEW TO THIS EDITION

Group fitness classes continue to grow in exciting ways, including the use of a wide variety of equipment, innovative choreography, and motivating styles. To keep pace, many updates, additions, and improvements have been made to the ninth edition. Three of these changes affect the whole book and many more enrich individual chapters:

- One of the global changes is to fully embrace the group fitness movement in both language and content (including a new chapter), while still retaining coverage of the rhythmic aerobics that led the way and continue to be popular in a variety of forms.
- A second big change, at the request of instructors, is the addition of Commonly Asked Questions to more chapters.
- The third book-wide change is the fresh new look of updated and new photographs throughout.

CHAPTER-SPECIFIC CHANGES

- A brand new chapter, Chapter 9, Group Fitness Exercise, includes coverage of cardio machines (especially cycling), martial arts (kickboxing), functional training, cross training, military style training (i.e. Bootcamp), high-intensity interval training (HIIT), and water aerobics.
- Chapter 7, Flexibility, now features diagrams of the muscles being stretched for all the flexibility exercises.
- A new website (www.pearsonhighered.com/bishopaerobics) offers over 40 videos that demonstrate proper techniques for resistance training and flexibility exercises. The videos can also be accessed using the QR codes located within the book.
- All of the book's worksheets are now available online at www.pearsonhighered.com/bishopaerobics so that students can easily access them. Selected worksheets also appear at the end of the book.
- Chapter 12, The Mind-Body Connection, offers increased coverage of yoga with accompanying photographs.
- Updated exercise physiology information now appears in Chapters 1 and 4.
- The OMNI Scales for rating perceived exertion during both cardiorespiratory and muscular work have been added to Chapters 4 and 10.
- A quick reference table (Table 4.1) that compares methods of estimating exercise intensity is now available in Chapter 4.
- New posture-enhancing activities, a guide for how to sit properly at a desk, and updated information on back care have been added to Chapter 6. Balance equipment is also introduced.
- An updated section on rest intervals and intensity monitoring of muscular fitness training has been added to Chapter 10.
- New exercises have been added, including stretches for the latissimus dorsi (back) and anterior tibialis (shin) in Chapter 7, and muscular strength exercises including high and low seated row and external rotation in Chapter 11. Nutrition information has been updated, including MyPlate (replacing My Pyramid) and recommendations from the American Dietary Guidelines, 2010 (replacing those from 2005).
- Information on the prevention of injuries that reflects the broader focus on group fitness has been added in Chapter 14.

CHAPTER ORGANIZATION AND DESCRIPTIONS

The text opens with a discussion of wellness and how exercise, particularly group fitness exercise, can enhance personal wellness. Chapter 1 explains the importance of a lifetime habit of exercise, including the benefits of exercise to achieve mental, social, emotional, spiritual, and physical wellness. Guidelines, including the most recent 2008 Physical Activity Guidelines, are presented with a historical perspective to enhance understanding of why there are more than one set of guidelines and the implications for goal setting. The chapter concludes with a discussion of the many short- and long-range effects and benefits of exercise on the systems of the body.

Chapter 2 addresses the issue of tailoring "one-size-fits-all" exercise programs to meet individuals' needs. Guidelines are provided for conditions such as asthma, back and joint pain, pregnancy, diabetes, and obesity—conditions that may require an individual to adjust his or her exercise plan.

Chapter 3 covers foundational information about fitness components and exercise principles—information that is applied to aerobic fitness in Chapter 4, and again later in the book to flexibility and muscular fitness.

Chapter 4 focuses on how to set and monitor aerobic exercise intensity. This chapter also thoroughly examines the different guidelines for exercise in an effort to clarify the variety of published recommendations. The discussion provides guidance in interpreting the different guidelines to help the student design a personalized exercise program.

Chapter 5 takes the next step to show the reader how to establish specific and attainable exercise goals. Logging worksheets for aerobic, muscular fitness workouts and pedometer counts are provided online to make tracking goals easy.

Chapters 6 through 11 delve into the specifics of exercise technique using numerous photographs and detailed descriptions of exercises. Chapter 6 discusses postures important both in daily activities and in exercise performance. Alignment and back care are an integral part of this chapter, complete with self-tests for alignment and an introduction to core training. Chapter 7 educates students on how to stretch, warm up, develop flexibility, and cool down. Dynamic warm-ups and flexibility are discussed in addition to more traditional static stretching. A variety of rhythmic aerobics approaches are discussed in Chapter 8, including low-, high-, combination-, and moderate-impact, circuit, interval, and step aerobics. One section discusses how choreography is set to music. Understanding how music is organized and how the steps are set to it will enable students to work with rhythmic movement more easily. Basic information to help students choreograph their own songs when instructors give them the opportunity is palso included.

Chapter 9 focuses on group fitness beyond the aerobic dance styles. Here the reader is introduced to the basics for group cycling, and the martial arts (kickboxing) and military (Bootcamp) approaches to group fitness. Also included is a discussion of the concepts that underlie functional training, cross training, and high-intensity training (HIT). The chapter closes with information on water aerobics including how to adjust heart rate monitoring for this activity.

Chapters 10 and 11 focus on muscular fitness and how to add resistance to body weight exercises. Chapter 10 applies the fitness components and principles of exercise to muscular strength and endurance. Chapter 11 is filled with detailed descriptions of exercises and includes explanations of techniques, photographs, and icons highlighting the muscles used in each exercise. Those exercises that work the same muscle or muscle group are presented together. This allows students to see how they can challenge muscles using different positions and forms of resistance such as dumbbells, barbells, bands, and stability balls.

At this point, three important concepts have been addressed: (1) why exercise is important, (2) how best to optimize your benefits from exercise, and (3) how to exercise safely and effectively. Chapter 12 takes the next step by exploring the connection between the body and the mind and includes discussions on stress and strategies for managing stress. Yoga and Pilates, two popular forms of group exercise, are introduced in this chapter, along with several techniques for relaxation and mental rehearsal.

Chapter 13 adds the crucial element of nutrition. Many exercisers list at least one goal that has to do with weight control. This chapter explains how exercise and diet are linked and how to use the power of both to obtain the results you want.

Chapter 14 provides information on how to stay injury free when participating in exercise. The chapter emphasizes injury prevention, focusing on common injuries and their symptoms. This knowledge will help prompt early detection and promote a speedier recovery if a problem should develop.

The final chapter (Chapter 15) encourages the reader to look beyond the immediate college course, take a fitness-for-life approach, and plan how and where to exercise in the future.

Each chapter opens with an overview and closes with a summary, a list of knowledge tips, review questions, and pertinent references. A section containing commonly asked questions, coupled with answers, is included at the close of most chapters. Key words, highlighted in bold throughout the book, are defined in a glossary at the back. Tear-out worksheets that allow the reader to apply the information presented in the chapters are located at the back of the book, with additional worksheets available online. Printed worksheets include fitness tests such as a timed run and step test, flexibility tests, and healthy weight calculations. These printed worksheets are also available online, along with all of the worksheets that previously appeared in the book, including a fitness log, a pedometer log, nutrition awareness logs, and a health and fitness log. New online worksheets include a guide to yoga styles and safety instructions for martial arts group exercise.

Appendices at the end of the book include an illustrated guide to muscles of the body, information on clothing and equipment, and Internet resources.

The information in this book is a synthesis of my experiences teaching at colleges, private clubs, instructor training/certification workshops, and conventions, plus knowledge and ideas I have gathered from instructors, professors, professional organizations, and, perhaps most important, students. These pages contain what I believe is the most pertinent, up-to-date information available. My hope is that this book will enable readers to more fully realize their exercise dreams.

ACKNOWLEDGMENTS

As the ninth edition emerges, I am struck by how many exceptional people have dedicated their talents to making this book an ever-evolving success over many years. Let me lead off by thanking the most recent team, including Susan Malloy, Editorial Manager, who inspired me to work hard (and more quickly!) with her cheerful encouragement and Carol Traver, at Azimuth Publisher Services, whose practiced and careful eye have put all the details in place. I would like to continue to thank the individuals who came before this team; it is upon their work that we build, and I thank all of you. Even though my book has long left the capable hands of the GSP staff, I'd like to express a continued debt of gratitude to Gay Pauley and Colette Kelly for seeing me through three and a half editions and for taking me into their hearts as a friend. I would also like to thank the Allyn & Bacon staff, who picked up and ran with the improved fourth edition. A special nod to Marret Kauffner, who added just the right touches and dealt beautifully with my eccentricities. Fifth edition appreciation goes to Benjamin Cummings' Susan Teahan, Wendy Earl, Anna Reynolds Trabucco, Cecelia Morales, and especially to Leslie Austin, who managed to chuckle every time I added another headache to her ace production efforts. Continued thanks to Sandy Lindelof, Emily Portwood, Dorothy Cox, and the production team at EPS. The ninth edition is built on their excellent work on the eighth.

Valuable information has been provided in the form of reviews by colleagues and professional advisors. I couldn't have done it without Jennifer Morley (artistic director at Figments Dance Ensemble), who provided my Pilates education; my Central Connecticut State University colleagues, Catherine Fellows, MS, who inspired and assisted in developing the improved yoga section; Jason Melnyk, PhD., who reviewed the new chapter on group fitness; David Harackiewicz, PhD., who reviewed the nutrition chapter; Sean Walsh, PhD., Jason Sawyer, PhD., Frank Frangione, PhD., Peter Morano, M.S., and Susan Smith, M.S., for fielding all my anatomy and physiology questions; and Patricia Gaedeke for keeping me up-to-date with trends in group fitness both on campus and in the clubs. Thank you to Ruth Sova, MS (founder and president of the Aquatic Therapy and Rehabilitation Institute, Inc.) and Kristie Romley (University of Arizona) for my education in water aerobics. Thank you to the reviewers for this edition for all of their helpful comments and advice: Glenna G. Bower (University of Southern Indiana), Lisa Brashier (Lone Star College), Marcos B. Briano (University of Southern California), Amanda Rachel Brown (Blinn College), and Shawnee Jones-Bonnette (Del Mar College).

Photographs bring the information alive; my thanks to the generous, kind, and very talented photographer Marc-Yves Regis I. I would also like to acknowledge the work of previous edition photographers, many of whose photographs continue to appear in this edition: David Mager and his assistant, Elbaliz Mendez; Lisa Lake; Tony Neste; William G. Nelson and his assistant, Christopher St. Johns; Bob Pangrazi; and John Dice. Thanks also to Dave Neurath, whose illustration appears in the instructor's guide. A special thank you also to owners Jack Banks and Paul Carson for allowing us to shoot some of our photographs for previous editions at their Malibu Fitness & Powerhouse Gym in Farmington, CT.

Pictured in this book are some very special people—my models. You all have so effectively brought the information in this book alive: Stephanie Douglas, Thiago Bitencourt, Anna Ausanio, Noah Bishop, Champagne Goldston, April Adorno, Jennifer DelSanto, Tracy Anderson, Matheus Bitencourt, Robert Harris, Omaris Journet, Chanhdy Ly Dan Matthews, Shanley Fitzgerald, Cassie Stewart, Katie Wartonick, Ashley M. Hill, Doug Semenuk, Robert Kucharski, Sherrie Santangelo, Patricia Gaedeke, Amanda Lang, Jennifer Morley, Sean Callahan, Amanda K. Hilson, Anne M. Charter, Heather Snyder, Larry Holmes Jr., Eileen Sachs, Ashley Smith, Steven Cook, Brittany L. Auld, Kyle Dailey Joanna Hollenback, Rebecca Rhodes, James Braswell, Jim Wal-czyk, Jessica Aman, Dara Elena Johnson, Teri So Dame, Patrick Decker, Ed Duclos, Richard Bishop, and our youngest models, Noah Ramon Bishop, Olivia Jean Bishop, and Marie Louisa Bishop.

Finally, I'd like to thank those closest to me—my neighbors, friends, and family—who have seen me through countless deadlines. Thank you, Dad, for encouraging me with a passion for healthy living; Mother, for your kitchen-counter editing and countless years of good advice; sister Melissa Bennie for your artistic eye and original shoe drawing; brothers Robert, Timur, and Derrick, who helped shape my active childhood; husband Rich for your loving support and unwavering faith in me; and my three teenagers, Noah, Olivia and Marie, for exercising my heart so well every day.

Jan Galen Bishop
Associate Professor
Central Connecticut State University

To my family, Rich, Noah, Marie, and Olivia,
for the love and magic they bring to my life.

1

Aerobics, Wellness, and You!

"The only thing that ever sat its way to success was a hen."

SARAH BROWN

- What is aerobics?
- Why is doing aerobics important? What are the benefits?
- What is a wellness lifestyle, and how do I achieve it?
- What should I expect an aerobic dance exercise class to be like?

AEROBICS

"Aerobics" has been a word for only 44 years, but in its short history it has become a household term that has dramatically reshaped the public's approach to fitness. The adjective "aerobic" is much older and, according to *Merriam-Webster's Collegiate Dictionary,* 11th edition, means "living, active, or occurring only in the presence of oxygen." You and I are aerobic. We take in and use oxygen in combination with carbohydrates and fats to produce energy. In 1968, Dr. Kenneth Cooper, a researcher and flight surgeon for the U.S. Air Force, put the "s" on the end of the adjective "aerobic" and defined his new noun **aerobics** as any physical activity that requires oxygen for a prolonged period of time. Such activities, he argued, cause a training effect that will improve the pulmonary and cardiovascular systems—the key to good fitness. When Cooper published his little book, titled *Aerobics,* he began what has become a lifetime conversation with the public about the benefits of aerobic exercise. Cooper's research over the past 35 years—as well as that of many other notable researchers—has linked aerobic fitness to numerous health benefits and spurred many of us to think about exercise as preventive medicine and a way to a more fulfilling life.

Prior to the aerobics movement, physical fitness was often thought of in terms of muscle development. Individuals performed calisthenics, isometrics, and weight training. Jack Lalanne used television to lead millions in a series of calisthenics. Sports, particularly team sports, were also popular, primarily among young men. The idea of **aerobic exercise,** defined as any large-muscle, continuous, rhythmic activity, completely changed the focus. People who wanted health-related fitness started taking up aerobics-based activities such as jogging, cross-country skiing, rowing, cycling, and swimming.

The aerobics revolution, and evolution, was off and running—literally. At the same time as thousands took to the pavement to run, Jacki Sorensen, an Air Force wife stationed in Puerto Rico, was asked to develop a fitness television program for other Air Force wives at the base. Her background was in dance, but she was also familiar with Cooper's Air Force Aerobics Program. Based on her own fitness from dance and Cooper's concepts of aerobic fitness, she developed a set of vigorous dance routines set to lively music and gave birth to aerobic dancing. It became very popular, particularly among women. When she returned to the mainland in 1971 and started promoting her program, Jacki Sorensen started one of the most popular fitness movements ever seen. At one point it was estimated that over 24 million people were participating in aerobic dance, although the exact numbers are not known. Although it was never meant to refer to only one kind of aerobic exercise, in the 1970s and 1980s, the word "aerobics" for many, especially women, became synonymous with aerobic dance.

Since aerobic dance was developed, it has been shaped and changed by many innovative and creative instructors. Judi Sheppard Missett used her dance background in the early 1970s to develop Jazzercise. Gin Miller added step aerobics to the mix in the late 1980s. High-, low-, and nonimpact styles influenced by jazz, hip-hop, Latin American dance, modern dance,

1

boxing, kick boxing and other martial arts, yoga, and many other styles of movement emerged. Step instructors got creative and used two steps at a time (double step) and even put them in the pool (aqua-step). The wide varieties of aerobic exercise classes available today are popularly referred to under the umbrella term "group fitness." **Group fitness** is any type of exercise led by an instructor and performed together by a class (group) of people. This includes activities that are aerobic or muscle developing in nature and still others that have been designed to accomplish both—to cross train. Group fitness "cardio" workouts with equipment include spinning (stationary bicycles), trekking (treadmills), rowing (rowing machines), and stepping (elliptical or stair steppers). One common element among the various group fitness activities is strongly motivating music.

Because the group setting is so important to motivation and having fun, instructors are challenged to lead an aerobic workout that fits the needs of a group of individuals who in many cases encompass a wide range of fitness levels. One of the best ways to meet this challenge is to educate participants on how to make movements easier or more challenging, so that they can perform a workout at their own fitness level. A good instructor will flow from one level to another, demonstrating different intensities and modifications of exercises. For example, in step aerobics more fit participants can challenge themselves with higher steps, while others use lower steps (or even no steps). Power moves and arm work can also add intensity. To individualize the workout in spinning (cycling), more advanced students can increase pedal resistance or speed to simulate challenging terrain, while beginners can maintain a more level ride.

The wide variety of styles in aerobic fitness classes keeps the activity fresh and exciting and enables people of all ages and fitness levels to join in the fun. Innovative instructors and exercise-smart participants are riding the wave of wellness … and aerobic group exercise is one of the popular ways they are doing it. Welcome back if you are experienced; welcome aboard if you are a newcomer!

WELLNESS AND YOU

You are the heart of the aerobics program. Your needs, your goals, your preferences—in short, your wellness—are what should determine your workout. And it can, if you take an active role in designing your fitness plan. How? By combining what you know about yourself with the expertise of the instructor. If you take a "one size fits all" program and tailor it to fit your needs, you will be more motivated to stay with your program and reach your goals.

In the 1960s and 1970s, rapid advancements in medicine lulled people into believing that they could lead any kind of life and medical science would bail them out if they became sick or injured. Individuals allowed the primary responsibility for their health to shift to doctors and other health care professionals; a "here I am, doctor—cure me" attitude evolved. But medicine is not a cure-all. Each year millions of people in the United States die prematurely from heart disease, cancer, stroke, and tobacco-related illnesses.

The good news is that you can substantially lower your risk of disease and premature death by adopting healthy lifestyle habits. Behaviors such as eating a low-fat, nutrient-rich diet, getting enough rest, managing stress, and exercising regularly put prevention on the front line and allow medicine to be an effective second line of defense. These are all things each of us can do for ourselves.

In the 1980s the idea of taking responsibility for your own well-being became the cornerstone of what is now popularly known as the **wellness** movement. There are two main tenets of wellness: (1) that you take control of your personal well-being by adopting and maintaining healthy lifestyle habits; and (2) that to be completely well, you must be more than physically healthy; you must also be socially, emotionally, mentally, and spiritually healthy. (Some definitions include occupational and environmental wellness.) The following metaphor, the balloon theory, describes how the wellness concept works.

THE BALLOON THEORY

Imagine that you are standing on the ground holding on to five balloons.[1] Each balloon represents a part of you—the emotional, mental, social, spiritual, and physical parts. Your five balloons can inflate or deflate with helium, depending on what is happening in your life. Most of the time, the balloons have some helium in them, and you are pulled upward. A big date may have your social balloon tugging you to the stratosphere, whereas breaking up with someone could temporarily deflate it, sending you back toward earth. Your mental health balloon may be inflated by a compliment from a professor, whereas financial problems could affect your emotional balloon.

Because all the balloons are connected, any upward or downward motion of one balloon will create a pulling effect on the others. If, for example, you abuse your physical health through sleep deprivation,

---

1. Portions of this section also appear in J. G. Bishop and S. G. Aldana, *Step Up to Wellness: A Stage-Based Approach.* Copyright © 1999 by Allyn & Bacon. Reprinted by permission of Pearson Education, Inc.

poor diet, chronic injury, or drugs, you will also be affected mentally, emotionally, socially, and spiritually. Similarly, prolonged or intense mental and emotional stress can result in physical ailments such as headaches or stomach upset. The reverse is also true. People with good social relationships have, on the average, longer, healthier lives.

Although all the balloons that encompass your life are loosely tied together, you do have control in that you can deliberately choose to deflate a balloon. Occasionally it may be good to let a balloon deflate while you attend to something else. For example, some religions celebrate holy days by fasting. The spiritual benefits of such rites may outweigh any temporary loss in physical nourishment. Caring for a sick child, parent, or sibling, or helping a friend in crisis may detract from your ability to progress academically, but fulfilling this social role as a good friend or family member may be more important during critical times. These swings are okay as long as they do not come one right after another and no one balloon is neglected for a prolonged period. If you lead a fairly balanced life and consciously decide when to alter the balance, you will have the reserve needed to handle surprises and emergencies, and the energy to take advantage of opportunities. In new situations, such as entering college or starting a new job, everything can look important, and it takes a little time to sort out priorities and find a balance. Problems occur most often when an imbalance lasts too long or the sacrifice is too large.

Learning to manage your balloons (your life) and taking responsibility for decisions that affect you describes a "wellness lifestyle." Consistent wellness lifestyle habits fill the balloons even when a sudden disturbance occurs. For example, individuals can lean on their spiritual faith, family, and friends when faced with a traumatic experience. This helps them stay emotionally and mentally stable; the spiritual and social balloons lift the others, thus preventing a total loss of self. There may be times when all your balloons are deflating. Sometimes this is the result of poor personal choices. Substance abuse, for example, can plummet you into disaster. In these cases, seeking help from friends, clergy, or physicians or other health care professionals may be necessary to get your balloons back in the air. You will weather lows better if you have built a good wellness network around you.

Occasionally, you will find that everything in your life is going just right. All the balloons are filled to their maximum, and it feels good. Take a deep, satisfying, relaxing breath, and admire the world around you. You are feeling very "well" indeed! These moments are to be savored. However, if you consider anything short of this a failure, then most of your life will

be judged as such. Life is full of changes, and living a "well" life is not about having all the balloons filled all the time. Living a well life means keeping a positive attitude as you manage your balloons and successfully handle the changes that come your way.

Wellness does not imply that you are free of disease, disability, or other limitations. It does imply a proactive stance. People with a wellness attitude take actions to maximize their potential; they do not allow their limitations to control them. We are surrounded by inspirational people who do just that. For example, boxer Muhammad Ali, his muscles weakened by Parkinson's disease, garnered the admiration of millions across the world as he fought for control over his shaking arm to hold high the Olympic torch and light the cauldron for the 1996 Olympic Games. Each day, actor Michael J. Fox shows us how to embrace life and work while living with the same disease. And what an inspiration Congresswoman Gabrielle "Gabby" Giffords has been. She has kept our nation in awe as she has fought back from being shot in the head, relearning how to speak and how to walk, with each step showing us the power of determination and spirit, while her husband, astronaut Mark Kelly, shares with us the power of a loving relationship. If you need any more inspiration, watch some of our Wounded Warriors compete in sports atop artificial limbs or in fast-moving wheelchairs! Wellness is a state of mind and a process, not an outcome. Well people tend to be hardy; they see the good in life and strive for that. Each of us has a story. The question is whether your story is your excuse or your motivation to make change and live well. In addition to the famous people mentioned above, there are many inspirational people around us—you, or perhaps the person next to you in class is such a person.

MAKING CHANGES

Establishing and maintaining a new lifestyle habit is not always easy, and exercise is no exception. Researchers have been trying to figure out why some people successfully change and others do not. James Prochaska, John Norcross, and Carlo DiClemente and colleagues pioneered what is now known as the Transtheoretical Model of Change, sometimes known as the Stages of Change Model, and made us rethink what we know about how people change their behaviors. For years, behavior change programs assumed that everyone would benefit from the same action plan. Unfortunately, most of the people who attended programs (such as those for smoking cessation) failed to stay with the plan or failed to maintain the new behavior after the formal program ended. These types of programs can be effective, but only when you are

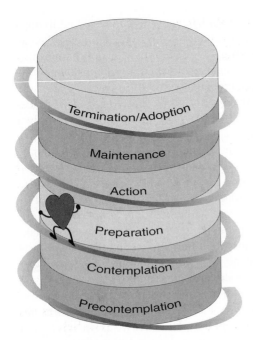

Figure 1.1 Stages of change.

- goal setting
- developing an individualized plan
- identifying and overcoming barriers to continued exercise (including how to restart in the event you stop exercising)
- finding and using sources of motivation
- measuring and evaluating your progress and goals

So in terms of exercise, you are already an action taker, a maintainer, or adopter—terrific! Even if this is the first regular exercise program you have attempted, you have made great progress just by signing up: You have moved from preparation to action. By establishing a lifestyle that includes aerobic exercise, you are practicing preventive medicine and enhancing the quality of your life. The focus of this book is to help you do this in a safe, effective, and fun manner so that you will want to maintain and reap the many benefits of this wellness behavior all your life. Worksheet 1.1, available online at www.pearsonhighered.com/bishopaerobics, provides a health and fitness log that you can fill out and provide to your instructor, if desired.

ready. The Stages of Change Model originally described change as a five-stage process. A sixth stage has since been added. In the first stage, precontemplation, people are not even interested in change; in the second, contemplation, they are thinking about it; in the third, preparation, they are taking tentative steps toward making change (maybe experimenting a little); in the fourth, action, they are carrying out a plan; in the fifth, maintenance, they are sustaining the new behavior; and in the sixth, termination/adoption, they have made the behavior a habit and maintained it for 5 or more years.

The Transtheoretical Model of Change proposes strategies for each of the stages. While there is overlap, the change strategies for one stage are different from the strategies for other stages. Precontemplators, for example, need strategies that help them see the value of changing, not action plans they haven't "bought into" yet. Programs that target change strategies to "where people are at" are more successful. As you can see in Figure 1.1, a person moves in an upward spiral through the stages. It is possible to skip a stage or slide backward, but in general the strategies help you move up the spiral toward permanent change.

Because you have signed up for a group fitness course, you have already taken a step from preparation into action. You may even be a maintainer or behavior adopter. The strategies in this text are aimed at helping you in your present stage. These strategies include the following:

EXERCISE AND WELLNESS

Some people would have you believe that exercise is nothing but a sweaty, hair-messing, laundry-producing time-eater. But those of us who exercise regularly know that it is an energy-giving, life-prolonging, stress-reducing, socially fun thing to do—well worth a little sweat and laundry. Unfortunately, many of the people who start an exercise program don't stick with it long enough to feel the benefits that keep the veterans coming back. Aerobic exercise has obvious physical fitness benefits, which will be detailed in the next section. But it can also have a positive impact on mental, emotional, social, and spiritual wellness.

MENTAL BOOST

Exercise can lift your spirits. Aerobic exercise in particular can help lower anxiety and lift depression. The production of endorphins, hormones that act as natural painkillers and mood elevators, increases with regular aerobic exercise. Endorphins are believed to cause the euphoric feeling or "runner's high" that people feel after exercise. The runner's high is not limited to runners or to running; any aerobic activity can produce it. However, it usually takes 6 to 8 weeks of regular exercise training before you experience it; unfortunately, many people have dropped out of their program before this time. People who exercise enough to experience this feeling are motivated to continue exercising because of it. So while your initial motivation to exercise may be to look good, your motivation to continue may well become to feel good.

INCREASED PRODUCTIVITY

Businesses and insurance companies are now well aware that employees are more productive and absent less often when they exercise regularly. People who exercise will tell you that they feel refreshed and ready to tackle problems again after their workout. Solutions or creative ideas may even come to you while you are being physically active. When I was in college, during finals week a group of us would gather at 10:00 P.M. for a short, refreshing run. That may not be your preferred time or activity, but the point is that a little exercise, even during crunch times, can clear your mind and help you to be more productive.

GREATER SELF-ESTEEM

As people begin to look and feel better physically, they also tend to feel better about themselves. An improved self-image can make you more confident and self-assured, qualities that are nice to have when meeting people, dating, and interviewing for a job.

STRESS-BUSTER

Aerobic exercise also provides an opportunity to exercise out some of the worries and tensions of the day. It is a great release valve for stress. Some classes build in a few minutes of progressive relaxation at the end, a technique that can be used in a number of settings once you have learned it. A lot of people enjoy a group exercise class because of the upbeat music that accompanies it. Music can be motivating, releasing, and energizing.

SOCIAL OPPORTUNITY

An aerobic exercise class is also a wonderful low-stress way to meet other active, energetic people. It can provide a social connection that might otherwise be lost in a busy day—something that may become more important when you graduate from college and have fewer opportunities to meet people. Having friends or family exercise with you is another way to build social time and fitness into your day.

MIND-BODY CONNECTION

More people are becoming attuned to the connection between the body and the mind. Exercising the body can have a positive effect on the mind, and tending the mind can have a positive effect on physical well-being. Yoga and pilates are two forms of exercise that help people focus on this connection. Exercise can help clear your mind of daily concerns and allow deeper thoughts and meanings to emerge. During and after exercise you may feel more centered, refocused, and more able to concentrate. Although yoga is not a religion, it provides many people with a spiritual link to wellness.

HEALTH PROMOTION

Exercise results in numerous other benefits, including improved immune function, better sleep, injury prevention, and a more efficient metabolism. Teamed with a good diet, it helps control body fat, gives you energy, and helps you look and feel your best.

DISEASE PREVENTION

The number one killer of adults in the United States is heart disease. There are seven major risk factors for coronary heart disease (CHD) and stroke:

- smoking
- hypertension
- high blood cholesterol
- physical inactivity
- heredity
- gender
- increasing age

Exercise has long been considered good for your health. But when the American Heart Association added inactivity to the list of major heart disease risk factors, exercise became recognized as a serious member of the wellness team. In our high-tech world of remote controls and computers, it is important to get up and move. Individuals with poor fitness levels have an 8 times higher risk of death due to cardiovascular disease and a 5 times higher probability of dying from cancer (the second leading cause of death) than do persons who have good or excellent levels of fitness. Any amount of exercise helps cut the risk of breast cancer.

Exercise also has a positive effect on some other major risk factors: smoking, elevated blood cholesterol, and hypertension (high blood pressure), and the contributory risk factors obesity and diabetes. As you will read in more detail shortly, regular aerobic exercise helps prevent plaque from adhering to the arteries and lowers blood pressure. In addition to reducing heart disease risk, this helps prevent strokes, the fourth leading cause of death. An active lifestyle also helps maintain a healthy body weight, which, in turn, lowers the risk of developing obesity and diabetes. Exercise may also help stop cancer by aiding people in their attempts to stop smoking (or never start). Because it is difficult to smoke and exercise at the same time, exercise is a good substitute activity during periods of craving. Exercise may also help prevent weight gain and/or offset some of the extra calories a smoker might eat after quitting. Exercise can also help offset or relieve stress. Although it isn't a panacea, exercise is one of the most positive things you can do for your health.

HOW MUCH EXERCISE IS ENOUGH?

A recurring question in exercise research is, How much is enough? The answer depends on your personal goals. Are you interested in improving health? Physical fitness? Both? And to what level? Moderate-intensity physical activities can enable you to achieve substantial health-related gains, and more vigorous exercise will allow you to achieve greater health benefits and higher levels of physical fitness. You may have heard several different guidelines for how much, and how hard, you should exercise. It is easy to be confused. Here is an abbreviated explanation of why there is more than one set of guidelines.

In the 1970s, the question was examined in terms of how much exercise (training) would result in certain performance capabilities. For example, what kind of training do I need to improve my cardiorespiratory endurance so that I can run faster and longer? One of the leading organizations in exercise science, the American College of Sports Medicine (ACSM) formed a committee to review the available research to help grapple with this "dose-response" question. ACSM published its first set of exercise guidelines for healthy adults in a book in 1975 and in summary format as a position paper in 1978. Every 4 to 5 years, the ACSM has revisited the research and updated its guidelines. Their book, ACSM's *Guidelines for Exercise Testing and Prescription*, is in its 8th edition (2010), and the most recent position statement was released in 2011. The early guideline that recommended 20 to 60 minutes of continuous vigorous aerobic intensity three to five times a week was for many people the "gold standard" for a long time, and as you will see, it still has a place in the newest guidelines. Muscular fitness and body composition have also been addressed through the years.

As the wellness movement began in earnest, the research focus widened, creating a second line of inquiry. Rather than just exploring how much exercise is needed *to get fit*, researchers now began asking, How much physical activity is needed *to get healthy*? Evidence of the link between moderate-intensity physical activity and the prevention of heart disease was documented. The new message is that you no longer have to run for 20 minutes; you can do a brisk walk instead and garner many of the health benefits once thought attainable only through vigorous exercise. But remember that you need to engage in this moderate level of activity often. In 1995, the Centers for Disease Control and Prevention (CDC) and ACSM made a new recommendation that most U.S. adults should accumulate 30 minutes or more of moderate-intensity physical activity on most, and preferably all, days of the week. In 1996, the Surgeon General's Report on Physical Activity, the American Heart Association, and the National Institutes of Health all published similar guidelines. The news was out that everyday physical chores, shoveling snow, walking the dog, or gardening could yield health benefits. Even three 10-minute bouts could be effective. The goal was to move a growing number of sedentary Americans into health-enhancing levels of physical activity. The ACSM adjusted its 1998 position statement to include lower-intensity recommendations for low-fit individuals and by 2000 was endorsing daily moderate activity for health promotion.

Just as everyone was becoming familiar with this guideline, the Institute of Medicine (IOM) published a report in which they claimed that 30 minutes of moderate exercise was insufficient to maintain body weight in adults in a desired range. In 2002, they recommended that individuals complete 60 minutes of moderately intense physical activity each day. Suddenly the press was telling everyone to double their exercise minutes.

In 2004, Steven Blair, Michael LaMonte, and Milton Nichaman published an article tracing the evolution of physical activity recommendations. After an in-depth look at how each set of guidelines had been established, they suggested a careful blending of the recommendations for health-related physical activity. They recommended that individuals who were having trouble controlling their weight after meeting the 30 minutes per day of moderate-intensity physical activity and consuming an appropriate number of calories perform additional exercise or make additional caloric restrictions to reach energy balance and minimize the likelihood of further weight gain. They also recommended that individuals who were weight stable and meeting the physical activity guideline of 30 minutes a day consider building up to 60 minutes a day in order to receive additional health benefits.

Four years later, a comprehensive review of the research was undertaken by an external committee appointed by the director of the U.S. Department of Health and Human Services (USDHHS). From the committee's report, along with input from government agencies and the public, the *2008 Physical Activity*

Guidelines for Americans was born. These guidelines are not much different than the previous ones except that the emphasis is on total accumulation of minutes of activity a week versus a certain amount per day. As an example, scientific evidence does not allow researchers to say that the health benefits are any different for 5 days with 30 minutes of activity each day and 3 days with 50 minutes of activity each day. Thus you are free to accumulate the time in a variety of ways.

The *2008 Physical Activity Guidelines for Americans* (USDHHS) focuses on the volume of physical activity a person needs to receive health benefits. In brief, the recommendation for adults is to accumulate 150 minutes of moderate-intensity aerobic physical activity a week, or 75 minutes of vigorous-intensity aerobic physical activity a week, or an appropriate combination of the two. In addition, muscle-strengthening activities should be performed two or more days a week.

Separate guidelines are available for children and adolescents, older adults, and special populations. Visit the website at www.health.gov/paguidelines for a complete listing of the U.S. Department of Health and Human Services *2008 Physical Activity Guidelines for Americans.*

The 2011 ACSM position statement, *Quantity and Quality of Exercise for Developing and Maintaining Cardiorespiratory, Musculoskeletal, and Neuromotor Fitness in Apparently Healthy Adults: Guidance for Prescribing Exercise*, embraces the 2008 USDHHS guidelines and includes more in-depth coverage of the frequency, intensity, time, type, volume, pattern, and progression of exercise. The ACSM guidelines are more scientific as they are written for professionals who will be prescribing exercise while the 2008 USDHHS guidelines are written for the general public. Recommendations drawn from both of these sources for cardiorespiratory (aerobic), muscular (resistance) and flexibility exercises are discussed in more detail in the chapters devoted to these topics.

More research needs to be done. There are still many questions, especially in regard to the connection between exercise and weight management. There is also a need for more information on exercise programming for special populations and different age groups. As we learn more, we can adjust and fine-tune individual workouts. Watch for new developments, but make sure they are being reported by credible sources.

How you use the guidelines and the level of physical activity you choose will depend on your goals. Goals can be health-related (weight management and disease prevention) or performance-related (for sport or competition). In Chapter 4, you will have the opportunity to use the guidelines (ACSM and USDHHS) to determine the proper intensity and duration of aerobic exercise to meet your goals. You should also keep in mind that although the USDHHS guidelines focus on activity for health enhancement, there are many other reasons to be physically active, including having fun with friends, engaging in the thrill of a game or sport, enjoying the outdoors, and improving your appearance.

THE PHYSIOLOGICAL BENEFITS OF EXERCISE

The remainder of this chapter is about how exercise promotes physical health. It is about how the body works and how exercise works on the body. Why do you need to know this? Because this information can help you take primary responsibility for your health. You can choose the benefits that are important to you and make sure that the exercises that result in those benefits are included in your exercise program. With a basic understanding of exercise physiology, you can talk with professionals on a more knowledgeable level, ask intelligent questions, and evaluate the quality of instruction you are receiving. Plus, if you understand how something works and believe that it is important, it is easier to stick with it. As you tangle up your feet on a new aerobic step or are challenged by a new overload, you will be able to fill your head with positive thoughts such as how your heart is getting stronger and healthier, fat is disappearing, and toned muscles are emerging.

The human body is intricately engineered and fantastically coordinated. At this very moment, inside you, millions of chemical reactions are occurring, brain signals are flying along nerve pathways, muscles are contracting and relaxing to maintain your posture against gravity, and food is being digested and converted to energy. All these things and many more are happening simultaneously, routinely, and without conscious thought. Each body system—cardiovascular, muscular, respiratory, and others (see the Benefits of Physical Activity box)—is influenced by exercise. Each system is affected in a manner specific to the kind of exercise performed. Aerobic group exercise emphasizes improvement of the metabolic, cardiovascular, respiratory, and muscular systems.

At rest, the body is in a state of balance called **homeostasis,** in which energy is being produced at the same rate that it is being used. When you begin to exercise, your body uses energy faster than it is being produced. In an attempt to restore homeostasis, you breathe faster, your heart rate increases, your energy production increases, and you sweat more to dissipate heat. All these changes help you establish homeostasis at a higher level of energy production and utilization. When you stop exercising, the energy output decreases and your body adjusts once again. The changes involved in maintaining homeostasis are called short-term, or acute, adaptations.

Something that disturbs homeostasis and causes the body to make changes is called a stressor. Exercise is a stressor. When the body is stressed repeatedly over time, long-term, or chronic, adaptations take place. The right amount of stress causes healthy changes. Too much stress results in unhealthy changes. For example, taking an aerobic dance exercise class 3 to 5 times a week will increase your cardiorespiratory efficiency and tone your muscles. Taking two classes every day may lead to overuse injuries such as tendinitis and stress fractures. In the following chapters, you will learn how to set up a program with the amount of stress needed to maximize your long-term benefits. The following discussion examines the systems of the body most affected by participation in group fitness classes and discusses the long-term benefits of exercise for each system.

THE METABOLIC SYSTEMS

The metabolic systems, often referred to as the energy systems, convert food into energy. The food you eat is broken down through various chemical pathways with the purpose of producing **adenosine triphosphate (ATP),** which is a high-energy phosphate molecule. When ATP is split apart, it releases energy that the cells in your body can use. Muscle cells use ATP to fuel contraction, and movement is possible as long as ATP is available. (Nonavailability of ATP results in rigor mortis.) It is extremely important, then, to have ways to resynthesize ATP when it has been broken down for energy.

There are two types of metabolic systems: aerobic and anaerobic. The type, intensity, and duration of activity you are engaged in determine how much energy is produced by each system. It is important to note that activities are not purely aerobic or anaerobic. When an activity is referred to as aerobic, that means the energy for movement is predominantly, but not exclusively, supplied by the aerobic system. When you perform exercises that emphasize the aerobic system, you get a different kind of conditioning than when you emphasize the anaerobic system. Familiarity with these systems can help you select activities that will lead toward your fitness goals.

ANAEROBIC METABOLISM

Anaerobic means "without oxygen."[2] During short, intense bursts of activity, such as running up a flight of stairs, the body cannot meet the muscles' demand for oxygen. For this situation, the body is equipped with two energy-producing systems that do not depend on oxygen: the phosphagen (ATP-PCr) and glycolytic systems. These **anaerobic systems** are rapid sources of ATP for short periods of time. In a sense, the cells are making energy while they hold their breath.

PHOSPHAGEN (ATP-PCR) SYSTEM The most rapid anaerobic system is called the **phosphagen (ATP-PCr) system.** This form of stored energy is used to get you going at the beginning of exercise, especially if you start quickly. It also allows you to leap out of your seat when someone yells "Free concert tickets!" Small amounts of high-energy phosphagens are stored directly in the muscle cell. As ATP is broken down, the high-energy phosphagens build it back up. The muscle can store only enough high-energy phosphagens to produce ATP for 1 to 6 seconds of activity. Training this system is important only if you want to participate in sports such as weight lifting or sprinting. The lactic acid and aerobic systems are much more important to lifetime fitness. As the phosphagen system is depleted, the lactic acid system takes over as the main energy producer.

GLYCOLYTIC SYSTEM The **glycolytic system** (also known as **anaerobic glycolysis**) produces ATP by breaking down carbohydrate (glucose) without oxygen. Along with energy, **lactic acid** and heat are produced. If the anaerobic activity is intense enough, the lactic acid builds up and makes the muscle feel heavy and "burn." The buildup of lactic acid is associated with muscle exhaustion.

When you stop exercising or drop to a lower intensity, the concentration of lactic acid decreases. The excess heat is dissipated through sweat. You breathe hard after an anaerobic bout of exercise because your body requires oxygen to clear up the lactic acid and to return the cardiorespiratory system to homeostasis.

Activities that depend on the anaerobic metabolism for energy are usually short, intense, and powerful. Predominantly anaerobic activities last for less than a minute. Sprints and strength-training exercises are examples of anaerobic exercises. Many exercises are partly anaerobic and partly aerobic. The glycolytic system also plays a major role in intense activities that last for 1 to 3 minutes. People like Bonnie Blair, an Olympic gold medalist in speed skating, who can perform well in a middle-distance event, must be in excellent condition both anaerobically and aerobically.

A number of exercise benefits are associated with anaerobic training. The most important are muscular strength and endurance and cardiorespiratory fitness. The latter is achieved using interval training, which involves a series of short intense bouts of exercise, such as

---

2. Portions of this section also appear in J. G. Bishop and S. G. Aldana, *Step Up to Wellness: A Stage-Based Approach*, pp. 35–6. Copyright © 1999 by Allyn & Bacon. Reprinted by permission of Pearson Education, Inc.

BENEFITS OF PHYSICAL ACTIVITY

SKELETAL SYSTEM

- Increases bone density and strength
- Helps prevent osteoporosis (brittle bones)
- Helps maintain good bone alignment, which is especially important to the spine

CARDIOVASCULAR SYSTEM

- Decreases blood pressure
- Decreases blood cholesterol. Increases high-density lipoprotein (HDL)
- Decreases risk of cardiovascular disease
- Decreases resting heart rate (workload on the heart)
- Increases cardiac muscle strength
- Increases the number of capillaries
- Increases systemic and coronary circulation
- Increases blood/oxygen exchange to muscles
- Increases aerobic capacity
- Increases stroke volume (the amount of blood the heart ejects in one beat)
- Increases the functional capacity of asthmatics

RESPIRATORY SYSTEM

- Increases lung capacity
- Increases blood/oxygen exchange in the lungs
- Increases waste removal efficiency (carbon dioxide, or CO_2)
- Raises threshold for asthma-induced symptoms

MUSCULAR SYSTEM

- Increases muscular efficiency and coordination (neuromuscular benefit)

- Increases strength and/or endurance
- Increases muscle size (more so in men than women)
- Increases the ability of the muscles to use oxygen
- Increases fiber length (flexibility)

REPRODUCTIVE SYSTEM

- May enhance sexual pleasure because of increased muscular flexibility, endurance, and control
- May result in an improved ability to cope during delivery
- May result in a speedier recovery after giving birth

NERVOUS SYSTEM

- In combination with the muscular system, increases muscular efficiency and coordination
- May increase motor skill

OTHER

- Increases regular digestion and excretion
- Improves sleep quality
- Decreases risk of breast and colon cancer
- Decreases risk of non-insulin-dependent diabetes
- Improves the body's ability to use insulin
- Decreases body fat; improves body composition

PSYCHOLOGICAL BENEFITS

- Improves self-image, self-concept
- Decreases stress
- May decrease depression and anxiety
- Increases endorphins, sense of well-being
- May provide a means for increasing socialization

Source: J. G. Bishop and S. G. Aldana, *Step Up to Wellness: A Stage-Based Approach.* Copyright © 1999 by Allyn & Bacon. Reprinted by permission of Pearson Education, Inc.

sprints. Only short breaks are allowed between bouts. Since anaerobic training increases tolerance to lactic acid, someone in good anaerobic condition can sustain high-intensity activity longer than someone who is not.

AEROBIC METABOLISM

Aerobic means "with oxygen." To exercise aerobically means to do activity that is fueled by a metabolic system that uses oxygen to produce energy (ATP). The anaerobic systems can produce energy quickly, but they can't sustain the supply needed for aerobic endurance activities, which last longer. Hence there is a need for a third system—the **oxidative system.** Both carbohydrate and fat can be "oxidized" to produce energy.

When carbohydrates are being broken down, the process is called **aerobic glycolysis.** This process begins in the same way as anaerobic glycolysis.

Carbohydrate metabolism produces energy (ATP), water, heat, carbon dioxide, and pyruvic acid. When no oxygen is available, the pyruvic acid becomes lactic acid; but when oxygen is available, the process continues. Pyruvic acid converts to acetyl CoA, which is then used to produce a lot of ATP. (Remember the Krebs cycle from biology class!) Meanwhile, the carbon dioxide is transported to the lungs and exhaled, while the heat and water are released primarily through sweat.

The oxidative system also uses fat for fuel, but only when it is in the form of fatty acids. Fatty acids from food are found in the bloodstream. Fatty acids in the blood also come from the breakdown of triglycerides pulled into the bloodstream from stored adipose tissue. When blood fat is used for energy, the process is called **fatty acid oxidation.** Triglycerides stored in the muscle can also provide fatty acids, and when they are used to produce energy, the process is called **beta oxidation.** Although these processes produce energy more slowly, fat metabolism has the capability to produce a rich and long-lasting supply of energy.

The intensity of exercise impacts the amount of carbohydrate and fat being burned. Low-intensity aerobic activity, such as sitting and reading or taking a leisurely walk, is fueled primarily by fat, with a little help from carbohydrates and phosphagens. Moderate-intensity activities, such as a level-terrain bicycle ride or a brisk walk, are fueled fairly evenly by carbohydrate and fat. A high-intensity exercise, such as sprinting to class, is fueled primarily by carbohydrates with initial help from the phosphagen (ATP-PCr) system and a little help from fats. Protein metabolism plays only a small part in energy production, as long as the individual is well nourished. The fastest energy systems, as mentioned earlier, are the anaerobic systems.

You actually burn the highest *percentage* of fat while at rest or during low-intensity activity, but because you aren't burning very many calories overall, this is not very helpful for weight loss. Exercising at a higher intensity will burn a lower *percentage* of fat but a *higher number* of calories, which can equate to burning more fat. Plus, fit people can mobilize the burning of fat more quickly than unfit individuals—a nice bonus! (These topics are discussed in more detail in Chapter 13.)

Activities that depend on aerobic metabolism for energy are prolonged rhythmic activities using large-muscle groups. Examples of aerobic exercise include walking, jogging, biking, swimming, snow-shoeing, and aerobic dance. Many sport activities, such as basketball, field hockey and tennis, also depend on the oxidative system for energy.

The Cardiovascular System

To understand the cardiovascular system (heart, blood vessels, and blood) better, picture it as an elaborate grocery delivery and garbage removal system. The blood loads oxygen at the lungs, travels down the roadways of the arteries, and delivers it to the doorsteps of the cells. The cells take in the oxygen and other nutrients they need and unload waste products such as carbon dioxide into the blood. The blood then travels back toward the heart through the veins, unloading the waste products at the appropriate dump sites such as the lungs, liver, and kidneys. The heart is the pump that drives the whole system.

The speed of oxygen delivery and waste removal is controlled by the heart. When you start to exercise, your muscle cells call for more oxygen. Your heart picks up its pace so that oxygenated blood is moved to your cells more quickly. After exercise, your heart rate declines rapidly for 1 minute and then declines more slowly as your body reestablishes homeostasis (balance). During recovery, by-products such as lactic acid are removed or converted into other chemical forms. The more efficient your cardiovascular system, the more quickly the heart rate returns to a resting value.

The average healthy heart has a resting rate of 60 to 80 beats per minute (bpm). The amount of blood the heart ejects with one beat is called the **stroke volume.** The **cardiac output** is the amount of blood pumped out of the heart in 1 minute. Increasing either the heart rate or the stroke volume will increase the cardiac output. When you exercise, both the stroke volume and the heart rate increase, but the heart rate increases much more dramatically. Stroke volume increases to about 40% to 60% of maximum output; after that the increase in cardiac output is due to the heart rate. If the heart beats very fast, the stroke volume actually decreases because the chambers of the heart don't have enough time to completely fill.

Blood pressure is the pressure exerted by the blood against the walls of the arteries. When the heart is filling, the pressure in the arteries is fairly low. This is called the **diastolic pressure.** When the heart contracts, blood is forced out into the arteries, thus increasing the pressure of the blood against the arterial walls. This is called the **systolic pressure.** The body is infused with oxygen-rich blood during systole. Blood pressure is expressed as a fraction, with systolic pressure on top and diastolic pressure on the bottom. Resting blood pressure readings less than 120/80 are considered normal. Above that are three levels: prehypertension, Stage 1, and Stage 2. The fraction 140/90 represents the threshold for Stage 1 hypertension.

When you exercise, your blood pressure rises because your heart contracts more often and pushes higher volumes of blood into your arteries. Healthy arteries stretch and can handle the extra blood flow without any problem. Blood pressure stays in a healthy range even with the added stress of exercise. To appreciate the ability of the arteries, imagine an airport or train station with hallways that can expand at prime time to accommodate the extra travelers. Diseases that harden the arteries (**arteriosclerosis**) or cause plaque buildup that narrows the arteries (**atherosclerosis**) cause the blood pressure to rise. Diseased arteries cannot withstand the same amount of stress as healthy arteries, so diseased arteries can severely limit your activity level.

Large arteries starting near the heart branch off into smaller and smaller arteries. The blood in the smallest arteries, called **capillaries,** delivers oxygen to the cells. The blood in the heart does not supply the heart with oxygen. Instead, small arteries that branch off the main artery near the heart take oxygen to the heart cells. These arteries are called **coronary arteries.** The heart is nourished with oxygen-rich blood during diastole through these coronary arteries.

Both aerobic and anaerobic exercise can improve cardiovascular fitness. However, to achieve cardiovascular fitness with anaerobic training, you must train at very high intensities. All-out efforts for short amounts of time are alternated with short rest periods. Many people find this kind of exercise difficult. In addition, it is too intense for beginners and most older individuals. The more moderate intensity and continuous nature of aerobic conditioning seem to be more comfortable for most people. A discussion of the many health benefits of aerobic exercise follows.

BENEFITS OF EXERCISING THE CARDIOVASCULAR SYSTEM

The heart muscle becomes stronger with exercise. Like the skeletal muscles, the cardiac (heart) muscle can improve in strength. It increases a little in thickness and contracts with greater force. The stroke volume also increases, which means the heart can pump more blood with each beat or the same amount of blood with fewer beats. As a result, the resting heart rate (the rate at which the heart beats to sustain the body at rest) decreases. A few beats less per minute saves the heart a lot of beating over a lifetime.

The resting heart rate is influenced not only by the stroke volume, but also by other efficiency improvements in the circulatory system and by genetics. Some people inherit and maintain low resting heart rates regardless of activity level. The average person who trains aerobically will experience a decline in resting heart rate; again because of genetics, however, some

people will experience a greater decline than others who have undergone the same level of training. It is quite common for highly trained endurance athletes to have healthy resting heart rates in the 50s, 40s or even 30s. Some of these athletes, however, have resting heart rates that are more in line with those of average individuals. So although a lower resting heart rate is a sign of improved cardiac function for most people, individual differences do play a role.

Exercise improves the ability of the cardiovascular system to deliver oxygen to the muscles. The ability of the blood to pick up and transport oxygen to the cells improves. The cells also improve in their ability to extract oxygen from the blood. The more oxygen you can supply to your cells and the more efficient your muscle cells become at using it, the longer you can exercise.

A trained individual can exercise longer and with less fatigue than an untrained individual. Think of two people in the same aerobics class working out at the same pace. The one in better shape is working out at a lower percentage of his or her maximum heart rate or aerobic capacity. In addition, the fit individual will enter into fatty acid oxidation more quickly than the unfit person.

Aerobic exercise also causes an increase in the number and size of mitochondria. Think of mitochondria as power plants located in the muscle cells. All aerobically generated energy is produced in the mitochondria. The mitochondria are more able to utilize fat as an energy source during exercise because the number of mitochondrial enzymes increases)

Imagine, for a moment, a city with only one main freeway. As rush hour hits, the freeway becomes congested. When an accident occurs, it stops traffic. Some cars head for the surface streets, but if these streets are inadequate, they too quickly get congested. However, if a city has a well-developed highway system and plenty of surface streets, traffic moves with ease even during peak hours.

Exercise increases the number of capillaries (surface streets) and, through cholesterol regulation, it helps keep the arteries (highways) clear. An increase in the number of capillaries means better oxygen/carbon dioxide exchange at the cellular level. It also means that when an artery becomes blocked, blood flow can be diverted to other healthy branches. This ability to divert blood flow is extremely important in the coronary network of arteries. Coronary circulation improves with endurance exercise: This helps prevent heart attacks.

Aerobic exercise increases the level of HDL (high-density lipoproteins) in your blood. HDL helps carry fat out of the bloodstream, which helps prevent it from forming plaque along the arterial walls. Plaque formation narrows arteries, thus restricting blood flow, raising blood pressure, and limiting stress-free activity. See the discussion on cholesterol in Chapter 13.

Evidence also indicates that exercise helps minimize the risk of having a heart attack and improves your chances of survival if you do have one. Improved cardiovascular fitness can also reduce stress-induced tension, alleviate depression for some individuals, and provide an overall sense of well-being.

THE RESPIRATORY SYSTEM

The respiratory system and the cardiovascular system work together to deliver oxygen to the cells. When you breathe in, you draw oxygen through the trachea and down the bronchial tubes into the lungs. The bronchi branch repeatedly and eventually become small alveolar ducts. At the ends of these ducts are numerous alveoli and alveolar sacs. It is between these alveoli and the tiny arteries and veins that oxygen and carbon dioxide are exchanged.

BENEFITS OF EXERCISING THE RESPIRATORY SYSTEM

Cardiorespiratory endurance exercises strengthen the respiratory muscles and increase the amount of air you can breathe into and out of your lungs (pulmonary ventilation). More surface area of the lung also becomes available for the exchange of oxygen and carbon dioxide. Each red blood cell has the capacity to carry one molecule of oxygen, yet blood is almost never 100% saturated. The blood moves by the lungs too quickly to load all the red blood cells with oxygen. Endurance training, however, can improve the blood's ability to load and unload oxygen.

THE SKELETAL SYSTEM

Each of the 206 bones in the human skeleton is a living entity. The bones you see when you look at a skeleton are dead. They give you a good idea of the shape and placement of living bones, but they do not represent live bone any more than the steak on your plate represents the living flesh of a cow. Living bones generate new bone tissue and repair and maintain healthy bone structure. Blood circulates through the bone tissue delivering nutrients.

BENEFITS OF EXERCISING THE SKELETAL SYSTEM

When you are active (walking, jumping, aerobic dancing, etc.), you stress your bones. The bones adapt by becoming stronger and more dense. Exercise helps prevent osteoporosis, a disease that causes bones to become porous and brittle. Osteoporosis is most common among postmenopausal women and is often the cause of broken hips or crushed vertebrae in elderly women. Proper nutritional care, particularly sufficient calcium intake, also plays an important role in preventing osteoporosis. As their life span increases, more men are developing osteoporosis. One in four men over the age of fifty will break a bone due to osteoporosis. One in two women over the age of fifty will. Exercise can help bone density increase during the young adult years and can help prevent bone loss in later years.

Although insufficient stress can cause bone weakening, too much stress can misshape, misalign, and even fracture a bone. The most common aerobic exercise injury in this category is the lower leg stress fracture, which can be very painful and is so thin that it is difficult to observe on an X-ray image. Set reasonable levels of intensity, duration, and frequency, and buy good shoes to help prevent such an injury.

Good posture is vital for maintaining proper bone alignment. If you walk around with your shoulders forward, eventually your spine and shoulder girdle bones will adjust to that posture and make it impossible to stand straight. Poor posture also leads to muscular problems, aches, and pains. Think of posture and alignment throughout your aerobics class as well as during the day.

THE MUSCULAR SYSTEM

The three kinds of muscle are skeletal (striated), cardiac, and smooth. Skeletal muscles, attached to the bones by tendons, make it possible for us to move around; the heart is composed of cardiac muscle; and smooth muscle is found in internal organs. Both cardiac and smooth muscle are involuntary, which means they contract without conscious thought. You don't have to think about making your stomach wall contract during digestion, nor do you command your heart to beat. Skeletal muscles are voluntary: You can make conscious decisions about how and when you want to move them. (Reflex movements and self-coordinating patterns of the skeletal muscles are the exception. During a reflex action, orders come from the spinal cord rather than the higher brain centers. The result is a very fast reaction that you don't consciously initiate.) Group fitness classes can develop both the cardiac and the skeletal muscles.

Muscles can only pull, not push; thus, they are paired together. One muscle pulls one way, the other muscle pulls the opposite way. When one is pulling, the other relaxes and stretches. The one doing the pulling is called the **agonist;** the one stretching is called the **antagonist.** When Popeye flexes his biceps, his lower arm is pulled closer to his upper arm. When he flexes his triceps (back of the upper arm), it pulls in the opposite direction, and his arm straightens out. When the biceps are working, the triceps are able to stretch and relax; when the triceps are working, the biceps are able to stretch and relax.

When you exercise muscles, it is important to work the muscle pairs equally. This way each stretches out the other, and strength balances are maintained. If you run on your toes throughout the aerobics section of a class, you have flexed (worked) your calf muscles the entire time. Stiffness will occur, and muscle imbalance may eventually lead to injury. Foot flexion exercises will work the muscles paired with the calf and allow the calf muscles to stretch. Because of this pairing, you can relieve a cramp in one muscle by flexing the opposite muscle: Relieve calf cramps by flexing the foot; relieve arch cramps by lifting up on the toes.

Don't confuse working a muscle with the pull of gravity or with the use of an eccentric (or negative) contraction. If you flex your arm using the biceps and then let it fall straight down, you are using gravity, not the triceps, to do the work. When you lower your arm slowly, the biceps are working in what is known as an eccentric contraction. An **eccentric contraction** is the controlled lengthening of a contracted muscle. You are using an eccentric contraction when you slowly lower a heavy box. Again, the triceps are not working. The opposite of an eccentric contraction is a concentric contraction. During a **concentric contraction,** the muscle is shortening. When you flex your arms, the biceps are doing a concentric contraction; they are shortening. Whether you are using concentric or eccentric contractions, you always want to move with control.

Muscles are composed of fibers. The power or strength of a contraction depends on how many muscle fibers are recruited by the nervous system. If you are doing something that takes all your strength, then most of the muscle fibers will contract at one time. If you are relaxing after class, only the fibers needed to maintain muscle tonus are used. During relaxation, only enough tension to maintain posture would be required.

Muscle spindles are specialized fibers that have stretch receptors. These spindles are responsible for the **stretch reflex.** When the muscle spindle's receptors are stretched suddenly, they send a signal to the spinal cord. The spinal cord sends back a message telling the surrounding muscle fibers to contract. The knee-jerk reflex is an example of this. When the doctor taps with a rubber hammer just below the knee, the patellar tendon, which attaches the thigh muscle to the bone, is suddenly stretched. The muscle spindles in the tendon react, the thigh muscle contracts, and the foot kicks.

Ballistic (bounce) **stretching** triggers the stretch reflex. Instead of relaxing and lengthening, the muscle gets the signal to contract. Proper **static stretching** does not excite the stretch receptors, so the muscle is able to relax and comfortably lengthen. Despite the stretch reflex, careful ballistic stretching can result in increased flexibility. However, it also carries a higher risk of tissue damage and muscle soreness than static stretching does.

Another kind of receptor, the Golgi tendon organ (GTO), sits among the muscle fibers. GTOs have high thresholds for tension, but if tension becomes too great during a muscle contraction, they alert the brain to send a back-off message to the muscles. The back-off or relax message actually stays in effect for a short while after the contraction is stopped. In **PNF** (proprioceptive neuromuscular facilitation) **stretching,** the response of the GTOs is purposefully elicited through an isometric contraction lasting 6 to 10 seconds. The muscle is stretched immediately after this contraction to take advantage of the relaxation phase induced by the GTO.

When the nervous system instructs a muscle to contract, it also alerts the antagonist (paired muscle) to relax. This is called reciprocal innervation. When you are trying to stretch a muscle, you can use reciprocal innervation by consciously contracting the opposing muscle. This is called **active** or **antagonist stretching.** For example, if you want to stretch your hamstring muscles, you can help them relax and lengthen by contracting your quadriceps muscles.

BENEFITS OF EXERCISING THE MUSCULAR SYSTEM

Muscles can improve in strength, endurance, and flexibility. The muscle-building exercises used in aerobic group fitness classes generally emphasize muscular endurance, but increases in strength can also occur, especially when exercise bands, weights, and stability balls are used. Flexibility is developed during the stretching segments of the class.

When muscles increase in strength, it may be the result of an increase in the size of the muscle fibers **(hypertrophy)** or improved neurological efficiency. For many years, it was believed that women's muscles did not hypertrophy like men's and that hormonal differences were the reason. Now, with better methods for measuring muscle tissue, we know that men's and women's muscles hypertrophy at the same rate.

So why don't women get big muscles? The increase in muscle size is not as apparent in women's muscles because their muscle fibers are smaller than men's and therefore the percentage gain is less noticeable. To picture this, imagine doubling the size of both a needle and a pencil. The percentage gain (100%) is the same for both, but the size difference would be much more apparent for the pencil. Another factor is the higher quantity of fat women have stored between muscle fibers. If some of this fat, which is less dense than muscle, is lost at the same time that muscle size is gained, little or no difference in muscle circumference will occur. It is even possible to lose circumference and gain strength.

Gender hormonal differences may explain why women have smaller muscle fibers. It may also be that with prolonged training, women's bodies will tend toward strength gains through neuromuscular efficiency rather than by continued hypertrophy. More research is needed to answer these questions. One thing is clear: The vast majority of women do not build bulky muscles. A very small percentage of women may experience more hypertrophy than they desire. A change in training methods can resolve this problem. Men generally gain muscle size with strength training, but the amount of gain varies considerably between individuals and even between muscle groups in an individual. For example, a man may hypertrophy more in his shoulders than in his chest or vice versa even though he has trained both equally and has made similar strength gains in each.

You may experience a temporary increase in muscle size while you are exercising due to the increased amount of blood being pumped to the working muscle. Some refer to this as being "pumped." The size of the muscle will begin to decrease when you stop exercising and will return to normal when increased blood flow is no longer needed. Because most women's muscles are relatively small, this increase in size is not very apparent. However, if you are going to take body measurements, be sure to do so before or well after exercising.

Anabolic steroids are drugs that can be taken to enhance strength gains, but they have dangerous side effects. They are most often associated with strength training and/or sports competitions. Today, many competitions, including the Olympics, consider anabolic steroid use illegal. Clearly these drugs do not belong in a health-related program.

Muscle endurance improves with exercise because the muscle cells become more effective at extracting oxygen and other nutrients from the blood and using them in the production of cellular energy. The oxygen goes into a structure inside the cell called the mitochondrion. The mitochondrion is often called the powerhouse of the cell, since it is inside these little factories that simple sugars (carbohydrates after digestion) are converted into cellular energy (ATP). The muscle adapts to endurance exercise by increasing the number and size of mitochondria. More mitochondria mean more available ATP, which means more fuel for contractions. With more fuel available, movement (or exercise) can be sustained for a longer period of time. Think of all the ATP mitochondria must produce for an hour of aerobics. Or for a marathon run!

Improving muscular strength, endurance, and flexibility results in greater work efficiency, an improved ability to meet emergencies, and a decreased chance of lower back pain and injury.

OTHER SYSTEMS

Other systems affected by exercise include the nervous and reproductive systems. The nervous system is a fantastic communications system. Electrical impulses speed along nerve pathways delivering messages from the brain and spinal column. Aerobic and neuromotor conditioning improves the coordination of these transmissions, which results in an ability to react with more speed, coordination, and strength. Skill and coordination improve as you learn which muscles to stimulate and which to inhibit. A clear example is the difference between a beginning and an advanced swimmer. Beginners use practically every muscle in their bodies to stay afloat. The advanced swimmer uses only the necessary muscles and uses them in a coordinated fluid movement. Beginning aerobics students experience a similar effect. They may start out feeling clumsy, but they quickly improve.

The effect of exercise on the reproductive system is difficult to study. Some researchers believe that exercise enhances sexual pleasure because of increased muscular strength and control. Two more serious issues regarding the effect of exercise on the reproductive system include the temporary loss of menstruation that sometimes occurs during high-level aerobic training and the effects of exercise on pregnancy. This loss of menstruation seems to be reversible, and a training regimen of lower intensity is recommended for women trying to conceive.

Guidelines for pregnancy and exercise have been published by the American College of Obstetricians and Gynecologists (ACOG). Exercise is healthy before, during, and after pregnancy for most women. A pregnant woman should consult her physician concerning the amount and type of exercise she can perform. There is some evidence that babies born to exercising mothers have fewer birth defects and that the mother's recovery time is faster. Women interested in exercising through pregnancy ideally should start exercising before they become pregnant, but most can begin during pregnancy and enjoy the benefits of being active. (For more information concerning exercise and pregnancy, see Chapter 2.)

OVERVIEW OF A WORKOUT

Exercise workouts are made up of several different components. This quick overview explains what you can expect as you begin your exercise class. Each of the components is discussed in much more detail in the chapters ahead. The workout begins with a 5- to 10-minute warm-up. During the warm-up, you will be doing easy, large-muscle activities to get your body warm and your heart beating a little faster. The warm-up also generally includes some dynamic stretches to ready your muscles to move through a good range of motion. The intensity of the warm-up should gradually increase until by the end you are just entering the intensity of exercise needed for the aerobic component.

The aerobic component consists of a variety of whole-body movements combined into a routine. Dance-style routines follow a 32–64 count pattern, which is taught in segments. Many styles and types of movements can be incorporated into these routines, making them a lot of fun to do. Some classes consist of fast-paced calisthenics, jump roping, etc. During the aerobic workout phase, you will be asked to monitor your intensity level using either heart rate, a talk test, ratings of perceived exertion, or the Omni Scale. You will receive instructions on how to do this early in the course, and worksheets are available online at www.pearsonhighered.com/bishopaerobics. You will also find copies of selected worksheets at the back of the book. The aerobic workout is followed by a standing cool-down. During this component, your exercise intensity is slowly brought down. If the class also includes separate resistance, or muscle-toning, exercises, they are generally performed after the standing cool-down, although they can also be done after the warm-up and before the aerobics. These exercises are followed by some stretching and, time permitting, some mind–body relaxation exercises. Music accompanies all of the class components. It is a great motivator for the workout portions and can be soothing and relaxing for the cool-down and stretch.

You only need a few things to be ready for class. Bring a positive attitude, some cool water to drink, a good pair of shoes, comfortable clothing that moves with you, and a towel if you sweat a lot or want one to put under you at times. Mats, ball, weights, steps, or other equipment is usually provided by the program unless otherwise specified.

SUMMARY

Wellness is both an attitude and a way of living. To be completely well, you must be in good physical, social, emotional, intellectual, and spiritual health. Individuals who practice healthy lifestyle habits will enjoy a higher quality of life and a reduced risk of disease and premature illness. Exercise, in addition to enhancing physical wellness, has a positive effect on the other four well-ness components. For this reason, it is one of the most powerful lifestyle changes you can make. At the same time, it is recognized that change is not always easy and that people in different stages of readiness to change require different strategies. Behavior changes are most successful when you have "bought in," when you feel that the change is important for you. We are living in the information age; knowing how and why something works enables you to decide if it is important and relevant to you. Knowing how the body works and how exercise works on the body enhances your ability to make informed decisions. You can choose the benefits that are important to you and make sure that the exercises that result in those benefits are included in your exercise program. Staying active is the key to physical wellness, and group fitness is a great way to do it.

COMMONLY ASKED QUESTIONS

What is the difference between fitness and wellness?

"Wellness" is a much broader term and is a way of life. Wellness involves lifestyle habits that support both a healthy body and a healthy mind. Fitness is a physical condition. Health-related fitness involves good levels of cardiorespiratory endurance, muscular strength and endurance, flexibility, and body composition. Skill-related fitness includes agility, balance, coordination, power, reaction time, and speed.

I look and feel fine, so why do I need to exercise?

Looks are about the outside of a person. On the inside, arteries may be filling with plaque, bones and muscles may be weak, etc. It is even possible for a person to look a healthy weight but still have a high percentage of body fat, because body fat can "hide" in the muscles and organs. People who don't exercise regularly are often unaware of how much better they can feel once they do start exercising. Plus, even if you feel fine now, years of not taking care of your body can cause problems to build up over time.

What is the difference between physical activity and exercise?

Physical activity is any movement produced by your skeletal muscles with an exertion level above resting. It includes exercise, recreational activities, sports, and daily activities. Exercise is a planned, structured activity that is repeated on a regular basis with a goal of achieving physical fitness.

Why are there so many exercise guidelines, and which should I follow?

Exercise scientists continue to study the effects of different levels of physical activity on health and fitness. As we learn more, guidelines change. Follow the most recent guidelines released by the American College of Sports Medicine or the United States Department of Health and Human Services. These guidelines are described in more detail in subsequent chapters of this text. Adjust guidelines to fit your personal levels of activity and fitness, health status, and goals.

KNOWLEDGE TIPS

1. Wellness is a way of life that involves taking responsibility for one's own well-being and practicing lifestyle habits that promote physical, social, emotional, mental, and spiritual health.

2. To lead a wellness lifestyle, you must be engaged in attitudes and behaviors that enhance quality of life and maximize personal potential.

3. Exercise is the remedy to inactivity, one of the heart disease risk factors. Exercise also helps to reduce the incidence of other risk factors, including obesity, hypertension, and high cholesterol.

4. Living a healthy lifestyle lowers your risk of premature death.

5. Exercise enhances all of the wellness components, albeit with a special emphasis on physical health.

6. Exercise causes short-term, or acute, responses, including an increased heart rate, increased systolic blood pressure, increased ventilation, and increased sweating.

7. Exercise causes long-term, or chronic, adaptations when it is done repeatedly over a period of time.

8. Aerobic exercises (continuous, rhythmic activities using large-muscle groups) use carbohydrate and fat for fuel.

9. Anaerobic exercises (intense activities of short duration) use carbohydrate for fuel.

10. The benefits of aerobically training the cardiovascular system include increased stroke volume, increased cardiac muscle strength, decreased resting heart rate, decreased blood pressure in individuals with hypertension, increased aerobic capacity, increased coronary circulation, decreased risk of heart disease, increased work capacity, increased level of HDL, increased oxygen delivery to the muscles, increased numbers of capillaries, and an increased number of mitochondria.

11. Two benefits of training the respiratory system are increased lung capacity and an increased ability to deliver oxygen to the blood.

12. The benefits of training the muscular system include increased strength, increased muscular endurance, increased flexibility, increased work capacity, decreased risk of lower back pain, and decreased risk of injury.

13. Some benefits of training the skeletal system are increased bone density, maintenance of good posture, and decreased risk of bone injury.

14. Other benefits of exercise include decreased mental tension, improved self-image, increased sense of well-being, regular digestion and excretion, improved sexual pleasure, and improved coordination and skill.

15. An aerobic group fitness class generally consists of the following components: warm-up, aerobic workout, standing cool-down, muscle strength and endurance exercises, stretching, and relaxation.

THINK ABOUT IT

1. What does living a wellness lifestyle mean?

2. What are the benefits of being physically active?

3. How much exercise or physical activity is enough?

4. What is the difference between aerobic and anaerobic metabolism?

5. What type of activities draw predominantly on the aerobic system? the anaerobic system?

6. Why are people more successful at making behavior changes when they use the transtheoretical model for behavior change?

7. What strategies help you stick with a program when you are in the action phase?

8. What are the components of an aerobic group fitness class?

REFERENCES

American Alliance for Health, Physical Education, Recreation, and Dance. *Health Related Physical Fitness: Test Manual.* Reston, VA: American Alliance for Health, Physical Education, Recreation, and Dance, 1980.

American College of Sports Medicine. *ACSM's Guidelines for Exercise Testing and Exercise Prescription.* 8th ed. Media, PA: Lippincott Williams & Wilkins, 2010.

American College of Sports Medicine. "The Recommended Quantity and Quality of Exercise for Developing and Maintaining Cardiorespiratory and Muscle Fitness in Healthy Adults." *Medicine and Science in Sports and Exercise* 30 (No. 6, 1998): 975–91.

American College of Sports Medicine. "Quantity and Quality of Exercise for Developing and Maintaining Cardiorespiratory, Musculoskeletal, and Neuromotor Fitness in Apparently Healthy Adults: Guidance for Prescribing Exercise." *Medicine and Science in Sports and Exercise* 43 (No. 7, 2011): 1334–59.

Blair, S. N. "Physical Activity, Physical Fitness, and Health." *Research Quarterly for Exercise and Sport* 64 (December 1993): 365–76.

Boyer, J. L. "Effects of Chronic Exercise on Cardiovascular Function." *Physical Fitness Research Digest* 2 (1972): 1.

Cooper, K. H. *Aerobics.* New York: Bantam Books, 1968.

Corbin, C. B., G. Welk, W. R. Corbin, and K. A. Welk. *Concepts of Physical Fitness: Active Lifestyles for Wellness.* 14th ed. New York: McGraw-Hill Higher Education, 2006.

Editors of the University of California at Berkeley Wellness Letter, *The New Wellness Encyclopedia,* New York: Houghton Mifflin, 1995.

Estivill, M. "Therapeutic Aspects of Aerobic Dance Participation." *Health Care for Women International* 16 (No. 4, 1995): 341–50.

Fahey, T. D., P. M. Insel, and W. T. Roth. *Fit and Well: Core Concepts and Labs in Physical Fitness and Wellness.* 8th ed. New York: The McGraw-Hill Companies, 2009.

Hoeger, W. W. K., and S. A. Hoeger. *Lifetime Physical Fitness and Wellness: A Personalized Program.* 9th ed. Belmont, CA: Thompson Wadsworth, 2007.

Housh, T. J., D. J. Housh, and H. A. deVries. *Applied Exercise and Sport Physiology.* 2nd ed. Scottsdale, AZ: Holcomb Hathaway Publishers, 2006.

Imm, P. S. "Perceived Benefits of Participants in an Employees' Aerobic Fitness Program." *Perceptual and Motor Skills* 71 (December 1990): 753–4.

Jordan, P. *Fitness Theory and Practice.* Sherman Oaks, CA: Aerobics and Fitness Association of America, 1993.

Kannel, W. B., and P. Sorlie. "Some Health Benefits of Physical Activity: The Framingham Study." *Archives of Internal Medicine* 139 (1979): 857–61.

Kraus, H., and W. Raab. *Hypokinetic Disease.* Springfield, IL: C. C. Thomas, 1961.

Mathews, D. K., and E. L. Fox. *The Physiological Basis of Physical Education and Athletics.* Philadelphia: W. B. Saunders, 1976.

National Osteoporosis Foundation. "Why Bone Health is Important," 2011. www.nof.org/aboutosteoporosis/bonebasics/whybonehealth.

Paffenbarger, R. S., and R. T. Hyde. "Exercise as Protection Against Heart Attack." *New England Journal of Medicine* 302 (1980): 1026.

Paffenbarger, R. S., R. T. Hyde, A. L. Wing, and C. Hsieh. "Physical Activity, All-Cause Mortality, and Longevity of College Alumni." *New England Journal of Medicine* 314 (1986): 605–13.

Pate, R. R., et al. "Physical Activity and Public Health, a Recommendation from the Centers for Disease Control and Prevention and the American College of Sports Medicine." *Journal of the American Medical Association* 273 (No. 5, 1995): 402–7.

Pollock, M. L. "How Much Exercise Is Enough?" *The Physician and Sportsmedicine* 6 (No. 6, 1978): 50–6; 58–60; 63–4.

___. *Exercise in Health and Disease.* Philadelphia: W. B. Saunders, 1984.

Pollock, M. L., and S. N. Blair. "Analysis into Action: Exercise Prescription." *Journal of Physical Education and Recreation* 52 (No. 1, 1981): 30–5, 81.

Pollock, M. L., J. H. Wilmore, and S. M. Fox. *Health and Fitness Through Physical Activity.* New York: John Wiley & Sons, 1978.

Prochaska, J. O., and C. diClemente. "Toward a Comprehensive Behavior Change." In *Treating Addictive Behaviors,* W. Miller and N. Heather, eds. New York: Plenum, 1986.

Smith, E. L. "Exercise for Prevention of Osteoporosis: A Review." *The Physician and Sportsmedicine* (No. 3, 1982): 72–83.

Thomsen, D., and D. L. Ballor. "Physiological Responses During Aerobic Dance of Individuals Grouped by Aerobic Capacity and Dance Experience." *Research Quarterly for Exercise and Sport* 62 (March 1991): 68–72.

U.S. Department of Health and Human Services. *Physical Activity and Health: A Report of the Surgeon General.* Centers for Disease Control and Prevention, National Center for Chronic Disease Prevention and Health Promotion. Atlanta: The President's Council on Physical Fitness and Sports, 1996.

___. *2008 Physical Activity Guidelines for Americans.* U.S. Department of Health and Human Services, 2008.

Watterson, V. V. "The Effects of Aerobic Dance on Cardiovascular Fitness." *The Physician and Sportsmedicine* 12 (No. 10, 1984): 138–45.

White, T. P., and Editors of the University of California at Berkeley Wellness Letter. *The Wellness Guide to Lifelong Fitness.* Rebus, NY: Random House, 1993.

Williford, H. N., M. Scharff-Olson, and D. L. Blessing. "The Physiological Effects of Aerobic Dance: A Review." *Sports Medicine* 8 (No. 6, December 1989): 335–45.

Wilmore, J. H. and Costill, D. L. *Physiology of Sport and Exercise.* 3rd ed. Champaign, IL: Human Kinetics, 2004.

2

Individual Differences:
Let's Talk About You

"I never looked at asthma, my condition, as being a handicap. My attitude was to beat asthma. I wasn't going to allow asthma to get the best of me."

JACKIE JOYNER-KERSEE

- Is there such a thing as a one-size-fits-all exercise program?
- Should I exercise if I have a health condition such as asthma or diabetes?
- What should I do if an exercise doesn't feel good or is hard for me?

EVEN though the information in this text is based on research and on strategies and techniques practiced by numerous professionals, exercise programs can and should be adjusted to accommodate each individual's needs. Research works with statistical measures such as the "mean" or "average" score, but people are not statistics; they can be average, above or below average, or above in one way and below in another. Sometimes, what is good for the "average" participant or for the "majority of" participants requires adjustments to meet individual needs. You, your instructor, and a health care professional (as needed) can work together to custom design the optimal program for you. Here is an example of this type of teamwork.

A student confided in her instructor that for years she had tried to do a proper curl-up but still couldn't get her back to round sufficiently. Partway through the curl-up, most of her back would lift off the floor as a unit. This put considerable stress on her lower back and resulted in back pain. The problem appeared to be more than weak abdominal muscles. A consultation with her physician revealed that two bones in her lower spine were fused. Armed with this information, her instructor modified the curl-up. When performing on a mat, the student was instructed to pull lightly with her

hands underneath her thighs at the point where she felt her lower back engage. The instructor also used a pilates approach to help the student gain as much rounding (mobility) of the spine as possible. Finally, the instructor suggested that the student perform curl-ups on a stability ball so that her back was supported on a comfortable surface throughout the movement. These adaptations allowed the student to reduce the stress on her lower back and to strengthen her abdominal muscles safely and effectively.

If you experience a problem with part of your exercise program, talk with your instructor or physician and as a team develop a safe and effective program.

Blindly following someone else's exercise program or technique is usually not a good idea. Group fitness participants often fall into the habit of imitating every movement the instructor makes. Instructors joke about how a whole class will follow their movements to wipe hair out of their eyes or scratch an itch. One day, as a test, I instructed my class in the hazards of exercises such as deep knee bends and then proceeded to put a series of these "bad" exercises into the routines. To my dismay, most of my class followed along.

Here is another story, with a twist, to illustrate the importance of paying attention to individual differences: A track coach once told me that for years the many high-jump coaches and athletes who carefully studied and copied the exact form of 1968 Olympic high-jump champion Dick Fosbury, the creator of the "Fosbury Flop," cheated themselves of jumping height by unwittingly imitating poor head positioning. He explained that Fosbury had hurt his neck high jumping into sawdust before the days of foam pits and, as a result, kept his neck in a protective rather than optimal position. I have had the opportunity to talk with Dick Fosbury, and guess what? Chuckling, he informed me that the story isn't true at all, but he quickly added that the point of the story is very true. According to Fosbury, he was not successful at imitating other great high jumpers of his day. He was able to achieve his gold medal height only by accommodating his body type and abilities and inventing (evolving) a new way to jump. Fosbury added that he believes strongly in studying and learning from other successful people; he does not believe that we can imitate perfectly what someone else does, nor should we try. Instead, real success comes when we take into account our individual differences and make the appropriate adjustments. On rare occasions, an individual's "adjustments," like Dick Fosbury's, revolutionize how something is done; in most cases, only slight variations or adjustments are needed.

In group fitness classes, there are a number of situations that require individuals to make adjustments in order to optimize their workouts. Here are just a few examples.

- A student's fitness level may differ from the level of workout being presented. In this case, intensity can be increased or decreased by techniques described in Chapters 8 to 11, such as increasing or decreasing arm work or amplitude (i.e., "largeness" of movements) during aerobics, or increasing or decreasing the amount of load (weight) used during resistance training.
- A student with an injury or physical disability may require modification of an exercise or exercise position. For instance, a person with a sore shoulder may need to eliminate overhead arm movements. A person with a hearing impairment may need louder music, preferential positioning near the instructor, and hand cues as well as verbal cues from the instructor.
- An overweight student may discover that the jumping in high-impact aerobics is too hard on his or her joints. In most cases, moderate- or low-impact movements can be easily substituted for high-impact movements. Additional options would be to switch to water aerobics or to use a cardiorespiratory endurance machine, such as an elliptical trainer or a rower.

- As a woman's pregnancy advances, she needs to make adjustments in her workout to ensure the safety of the developing baby and to provide personal comfort.
- A person on medications that affect heart rate will need to substitute ratings of perceived exertion (see Chapter 4) for pulse monitoring to estimate exercise intensity.

Good fitness instructors will demonstrate how to perform exercises at several levels of intensity to accommodate students who range from less fit beginners to highly fit advanced students. It is important for individuals to learn which of the demonstrated levels of intensity is appropriate for them and to be aware that the correct level of intensity will vary according to the type of exercise being performed. Although instructors present many modifications and levels, some individual modifications may not be demonstrated to the whole class. Instructors have to be careful of demonstrating advanced moves and positions in a class of mixed abilities because too often students, regardless of fitness level, follow every movement of the instructor. If you require modifications not presented by the instructor, be sure to ask for help. An instructor will happily share ways with you, one on one, to increase (or decrease) the intensity of your program.

Your experience with group fitness exercise and your age can both influence the type of program you want and need. Veterans are more apt to want variety and challenging step combinations, whereas beginners are happy when instructors stay with simple combinations and lots of repetition. People who have taken classes for a while with one instructor become accustomed to that person's patterns and sequences and may find it difficult, at least initially, to follow a new instructor. Age differences can involve everything from goals to music tastes. College students in their twenties want different things out of their exercise programs than do students in their forties or sixties. As your goals change, so too should your program.

Gender raises a number of exercise programming issues. Women need special considerations for exercising during pregnancy or the discomfort of menstruation. The average man has more strength than a woman, especially in the upper body, and may need different exercises or more resistance during exercises to improve strength. Different movements may make men and women feel uncomfortable exercising. Men, for example, may feel self-conscious handling dance steps, whereas women may be embarrassed when they can't perform a full set of a muscle endurance exercise. As with all gender issues, there is a certain amount of crossover— women who feel they have two left feet and men who can't do a push-up yet, for example.

Music preference also plays a role in how much an individual enjoys a group fitness workout. Some instructors use a wide variety of music; others concentrate on one type of music. Many use music sets that are specially produced, with a mix of songs set to a steady beat. The music and class style can range from salsa to funk to rock and roll to swing to country-western to boxing jabs and kicks. Most instructors are open to music suggestions, but don't expect an instructor to use your music immediately; it takes some time to put together an effective routine. When choice is available, look for an instructor who uses a style and type of music that makes *you* want to get up and move.

Injury or disabilities may limit you from performing certain exercises. Many times there are simple substitutions, alternative positions, or even alternative activities that you can perform while the class performs the original action. Some conditions, such as hearing loss, may require bringing in resources such as an interpreter, or having the instructor wear a microphone. Most college campuses are equipped to handle these situations; sometimes you just have to ask the question.

Some things in this text are necessarily based on the "average" person. For example, research tells us that the fastest our heart can beat can be estimated by plugging our age into a formula. The newest formula (see Chapter 4) estimates a 20-year-old's maximum heart rate to be 206 beats per minute. Some 20-year-olds, however, have maximum heart rates greater than 230 bpm, whereas others cannot exceed 170 bpm. This does not mean that the formula should be thrown out—it provides a good estimate for most people—but it does mean that for a few people some fine-tuning will be required.

The remainder of this chapter describes some of the special conditions for which modifications can and should be made.

EXERCISE AND BACK CARE

An alarmingly high number of people experience lower back pain at some time in their lives. Strong, flexible muscles, good posture, and good exercise techniques can all help prevent lower back pain. If you already suffer from chronic back pain, it is important to start with a medical examination to determine the underlying cause(s). When appropriate, the doctor or physical therapist will provide you with exercises to alleviate pain and correct muscular weakness and inflexibility. It is also important to know which exercises you should avoid. Inform your instructor, talk about

what to avoid, and establish a time during class when you can do your prescribed exercises.

When the hamstring (back of thigh) muscles are too tight, they pull the pelvis down, thus rounding your lower back. When the hip flexor (front of thigh) muscles are inflexible, they pull the pelvis forward, thus causing a swayback. Both of these positions cause lower back pain. A good stretching program can alleviate these problems. Weak abdominal muscles and poor posture are the other two biggest culprits in back pain—both of which can be corrected with proper exercise, attention and awareness, and correction of your posture during daily tasks. There are tips throughout the text on how to properly care for your back, including a set of guidelines for back care in Chapter 6, but here is a summary of some of the most important points.

1. When standing for any length of time, stand with your knees slightly bent.
2. When standing or sitting, keep your pelvis in a neutral position that allows normal (not exaggerated) curvatures of the spine.
3. Stabilize your back during exercises by contracting your abdominal muscles.
4. Take breaks from sitting or standing in one position.
5. Strengthen your abdominal and back muscles.
6. Develop good flexibility in both the hamstrings and hip flexors (quadriceps and iliopsoas).
7. Use your legs when lifting heavy objects.
8. Turn with your feet, not your waist, when picking up or putting down heavy objects.
9. Carry heavy objects close to your body.
10. And finally, here is one exercise you can—and should!—perform anywhere, anytime: Tuck your chin in and pull your shoulders back slightly. You will feel immediate relief in your upper back and neck.

EXERCISE AND ASTHMA

Asthma is a condition in which the muscles surrounding the airways constrict, thus causing shortness of breath, wheezing, and coughing. Allergies, infections, emotion, air temperature, and exercise can trigger an attack. When exercise is the trigger, it is called exercise-induced asthma (EIA). The labored breathing caused by bronchial constriction may discourage people with asthma from exercising. However, people with controlled asthma can—and should—exercise. Here are some of the benefits of exercising with controlled asthma.

- Tolerance to exercise increases. Research has shown that for most people with asthma, aerobic exercise improves their cardiorespiratory system, which, in turn, raises the exertion level at which symptoms begin to occur. This means that a person with asthma can be more physically active while experiencing fewer difficulties.
- Boosts self-esteem and self-confidence. Being able to do something good for your body and being able to perform as well (or better) than others boosts self-esteem. Individuals with asthma often get trapped into a downward cycle of reducing activity each time symptoms appear. This ultimately results in an inactive lifestyle. As individuals successfully work out, self-confidence grows. Amy Van Dyken, four-time Olympic gold medalist in swimming; Jackie Joyner-Kersee, triple Olympic track and field gold medalist; Bill Koch, America's Cup champion in cross-country skiing; Mary Jo Fernandez, two-time Olympic gold medalist and pro in tennis; and Jerome "The Bus" Bettis, all-pro running back for the Pittsburgh Steelers, all have asthma. These people are inspiring, and want other asthmatics to know they can enjoy and benefit from exercise.
- Allows the person to gain all the wellness benefits of regular exercise.

If you have asthma, consult with your physician before beginning an exercise program, then share pertinent information with your instructor. If you experience EIA, try to recognize early symptoms and then lower your intensity or take a break as needed. If you use bronchodilator medication, bring your inhaler to class, let your instructor know where it is prior to each session, and use it at the first sign of wheezing. Taking medications prior to vigorous exercise may help prevent EIA. Check with your physician concerning your medications.

Here are some additional tips for exercising with controlled asthma.

1. Use a long warm-up. Symptoms often occur in the first 15 minutes. A longer warm-up allows you to ease into the activity and to handle any symptoms that might occur. Try to schedule your exercise classes/activities so that you can arrive early and begin to warm up ahead of time as needed. A good warm-up, even if you have symptoms, often leads to a period of time when more intense exercise can be performed with fewer problems.
2. If the continuous nature of an aerobic activity doesn't work for you, as it doesn't for some people with asthma, try doing an interval approach. Do a series of 5 minutes of workout alternated with rest or walking in place. Discuss this with your instructor and physician.
3. Be particularly careful on days when environmental conditions are more likely to trigger an attack, such as days when it is hot or cold, or when there is a high pollen count or smog alert. Avoid exercising in an environment that triggers your asthma.
4. Drink plenty of fluids.
5. Increase the length of the cool-down as needed. EIA attacks can occur after exercise as well as during it. A good cool-down helps. Try to schedule your exercise classes/activities so that you have ample time to cool down.
6. Be prepared in the event of an asthmatic attack, and educate those around you so that they can get you assistance, if needed.
7. Do not exercise if you are experiencing symptoms such as wheezing prior to class.
8. Consider water aerobics. Most people with asthma have fewer symptoms in the moist, warm air of an indoor pool.
9. Set an appropriate exercise intensity and duration in consultation with your physician and instructor, and then work to gradually increase your symptom-free exercise time.

EXERCISE AND OBESITY

We know that one of the greatest health concerns in the United States is obesity, and we know that exercise along with good nutrition can help reduce it. Yet, many exercise programs do not make overweight individuals feel comfortable. Here are some guidelines that can help you if you are overweight and in a group fitness class. Also see the box, Do I Belong Here?

1. Feel no compulsion to keep up. It is critical that you work at an intensity that will allow you to keep going rather than start hurting and want to quit. Use low-intensity versions of movements. Walk in place if the movements are too hard. Take rests as needed. You may only be able to do a few minutes of activity in a row—that's okay. Endurance will come.
2. Enjoy the music, and use little movements to feel connected to the workout when you are resting. Keep time with your head and shoulders. Tap your toe.

3. Lower the workout intensity by eliminating or decreasing the size of arm movements as needed—especially those above shoulder height.

4. Avoid movements that create joint pain. Work toward smooth fluid movements rather than bouncy ones. Ask the instructor for alternative exercises if one is uncomfortable.

5. Consider using some of the cardio machines that are easy on the joints for cross-training on days you don't have aerobics class. The elliptical trainer, stationary bike, and recumbent stepper (performed in a sitting position) are all good choices.

6. Water activities are also excellent cross-training activities that reduce joint strain and prevent overheating. If you are self-conscious in a bathing suit, see if the facility will allow you to wear a t-shirt with your bathing suit.

7. Perform resistance training exercises to increase strength and stamina so that daily tasks such as climbing stairs become easier. Again, avoid exercises or weight loads that aggravate your joints.

8. Find a supportive exercise partner. It helps when you have someone to go to class with or meet there who is looking forward to seeing you.

9. Remind yourself that research shows that overweight and fit individuals have less health risk than the lean and unfit.

10. Know that you can look good exercising. Queen Latifah is a big woman, and her moves are smooth!

If you don't feel well exercising, check with your physician. Obese and overweight individuals are at risk for other health problems such as diabetes and arthritis. Exercise is still usually recommended, but additional

---

DO I BELONG HERE?

One overweight student confessed that when she went on vacation, she visited a club to take a step class. She had been enjoying an intermediate step class at home, but when she walked into this class, she felt as though everyone questioned whether she could handle the class. She assured them she could. At the end of the class, some well-meaning members congratulated her on doing so well but said it in such a way that it had the "you did a great job considering how heavy you are" feeling to it. She just wanted to enjoy an hour of exercise.

How about this student on his first day of class? He's concerned he'll be expected to wear form-fitting clothes, and he's not sure his form is something he's ready to share. He wonders whether others will question why he signed up. He can't do the basic steps without getting confused, and what if everyone is watching when he only completes 3 out of 10 push-ups? Maybe, he thinks … I'll drop this class.

Everyone belongs!! Here are a few ideas that might make you feel more comfortable.

- Sign up for class with a supportive friend.

- Look around at others, and smile. You'll find when you look up that "the whole class" isn't looking right at you and that the ones you smile at will either become new friends or stare less.

- Position yourself to one side so that you can see the instructor and most of your classmates well. This way you are watching them instead of the reverse.

- Proclaim improvements and make positive comments about getting through the class. Others will likely start to agree and cheer you on.

- Modify exercises so that you can complete them. Or do one move for every two or three that the instructor does. This will let you keep going and finish with the group.

- If you tire easily, walk in place, tap your toe, or move your arms to the music.

- Don't want to wear the form-fitting attire? How about a t-shirt that says something like, "I'm here for my health, what are you here for?" Or "Are you looking at me?" Or, "Wow, look at me!" or something even better you think up.

- Socialize. You'll find others will enjoy a word of encouragement, too.

adjustments may be needed. (Obesity, weight management, and nutrition are further discussed and defined in Chapter 13.)

EXERCISE AND DIABETES

Diabetes mellitus is a group of metabolic diseases in which the pancreas fails to produce sufficient insulin (Type I) or the body is unable to effectively use the insulin it does produce (Type II). Insulin's role is to regulate the amount of sugar **(glucose)** in the blood and move the sugar into cells when it is needed. Muscle cells, for example, use the glucose to produce energy for movement.

If diabetes is untreated, the blood sugar can reach dangerously low, or high, concentrations. If blood sugar drops too low, a person becomes hypoglycemic. This can be caused by taking too much diabetic medicine, delaying or missing a meal, exercising more than normal, or drinking alcoholic beverages. When hypoglycemic, a person should eat an easily digested carbohydrate or glucose tablets and get the blood sugar up before exercising.

If blood sugar is too high, the person becomes hyperglycemic and needs insulin. Hyperglycemia can happen if a person with diabetes misses a dose of diabetes medicine, eats too much, or doesn't get enough medicine. Infection, illness, and stress can also raise blood sugar. When blood sugar is not controlled, a person has a higher risk of serious diseases such as kidney failure, nerve disorders, eye problems, and heart disease.

People with Type I (insulin-dependent) diabetes control their glucose levels through diet, exercise, and insulin injections or an insulin pump. The vast majority of people with diabetes have Type II (non–insulin-dependent) diabetes. Some people with Type II diabetes can control their blood sugar using a good exercise and diet regimen. These individuals seldom have a low blood glucose problem. Other people with Type II diabetes need to augment their body's production of insulin with either oral medication or injections.

People with diabetes should exercise for several important reasons.

- Aerobic and strength exercises help make muscle cells more permeable to glucose. This means that glucose can more easily leave the bloodstream and enter the muscle cell where it can be used for energy.
- Aerobic exercise seems to allow the body to be more effective at using available insulin.

- Exercise helps control body weight and composition. This is important because obesity is a risk factor for Type 2 diabetes. For Type 2 diabetics who are overweight, losing weight may bring blood sugar levels back into a normal range.
- Exercise helps reduce the amount of cholesterol and other fats circulating in the blood, thus effectively lowering an otherwise elevated risk for heart disease.
- Regular, moderate exercise helps a person with diabetes maintain normal blood glucose levels and, in some cases, may reduce the amount of insulin a person needs to take. Any changes should, of course, be made under the guidance of a physician.

If you have diabetes and are starting an exercise program, get a thorough medical examination and discuss your exercise plan with your health care team. You will probably be able to take part in both aerobic and resistance training (weight training) exercise. When you are cleared for exercise, you will need to make ongoing adjustments to your exercise, meals, and medicines as you get in shape. You will want to follow all of the normal exercise procedures of warming up and working at an appropriate intensity, but you will also need to add some additional safety steps that take your diabetes into account. You should stay well hydrated and take extra good care of your feet. Wear good aerobic or cross-trainer shoes, wear good smooth socks that wick away moisture, keep your feet dry and free of athlete's foot, and inspect them frequently. See the Workout Tips for People with Diabetes box for some safety tips concerning blood sugar monitoring. Report any problems to a doctor immediately. And finally, keep your instructor informed so that you can work together to provide you with the best exercise experience.

EXERCISE AND PREGNANCY

Exercise is a positive health habit that, in most cases, can be continued through pregnancy. It is important, however, to recognize the demands pregnancy places on a woman's body and to make adjustments accordingly. (See the "Exercise During Pregnancy" box). It is better to start an exercise program before pregnancy, but it is certainly possible to begin with light exercising during pregnancy. Women who have been exercising regularly prior to conception may be able to continue in a regular group fitness class, as long as they make appropriate adjustments to their intensity and avoid contraindicated exercises. As pregnancy advances, many women prefer to take a class specifically designed for pregnant women or continue with a non-weight-bearing activity such as cycling or swimming.

WORKOUT TIPS FOR PEOPLE WITH DIABETES

If you have diabetes, make sure to do the following when you exercise.

- Get a thorough medical exam before you start a new exercise plan.

- Watch for low blood glucose levels. If you take insulin or oral diabetes medicine, you may have low blood sugar during or immediately after exercise, or up to a day later. Medications can be adjusted to prevent this. Careful monitoring of blood glucose may be required before, during, and after exercise.

 Update your exercise plan regularly with your doctor. Regular exercise may result in a need for less insulin or lower doses of diabetes pills. Your doctor can also teach you how to adjust your medicine for the days when you perform a different exercise plan.

BEFORE EXERCISE

- Ask your health care team whether you should check your blood glucose level before exercising.

- If you take diabetes medicines that can cause low blood glucose, ask your health care team whether you should

    change the amount you take before you exercise

    have a snack if your blood glucose level is below 100

DURING EXERCISE

- Wear your medical identification (ID) bracelet or necklace or carry your ID in your pocket.

- Always carry food or glucose tablets so you'll be ready to treat low blood glucose.

- If you'll be exercising for more than an hour, check your blood glucose at regular intervals. You may need snacks before you finish.

AFTER EXERCISE

- Check to see how exercise affected your blood glucose level.

Source: http://www.diabetes.niddk.nih.gov/dm/pubs/physical_ez/index.htm.

If you are pregnant or considering pregnancy, discuss an exercise plan with your physician.

 If your doctor agrees that exercise is healthy for you, discuss frequency, intensity, duration, and additional nutritional requirements. During flexibility work, be careful not to overstretch, because your ligaments will tend to be looser and more relaxed. If you feel clumsy or uncoordinated, try not to let it frustrate you. Instead, simplify the steps or walk in place and enjoy the music. Finally, make sure your instructor is aware of your pregnancy (or recent childbirth), and provide him or her with the names and phone numbers of your physician, the hospital, and the relative you want contacted in case of an emergency. If you will enter into your second or third trimester during a semester-long course, talk with the instructor ahead of time concerning alternatives in the event that a weight-bearing aerobic class (i.e., aerobic dance) becomes uncomfortable for you. You might, for example, be able to leave the floor after the warm-up, cycle during the aerobic portion of class, and then return to class for muscle toning and stretching. This kind of solution is preferable to dropping the course.

 Some women are able to begin exercising within days of giving birth, but most need 4 to 6 weeks to recover and manage the new responsibilities of taking care of a newborn. When cleared to exercise by their physicians, women find that exercise helps them regain their shape, rebuild their fitness, and enjoy a greater sense of well-being.

EXERCISE AND JOINT PAIN

Joint pain can be the result of disease or injury. Because there are many causes, some of which can be serious, a person with joint pain should consult a physician prior to beginning an exercise program. There are some things that you can do to prevent joint pain and/or to keep from aggravating pain with which you are allowed to exercise.

1. Do not perform an exercise that hurts. Ask for a modification or second exercise that may attain the same benefit. For example, a stretch

EXERCISE DURING PREGNANCY

WHAT ARE SOME OF THE BENEFITS OF EXERCISE DURING PREGNANCY?

Exercising at least 30 minutes on most, if not all, days of the week can help to reduce backaches, constipation, bloating, and swelling; prevent or treat gestational diabetes; increase your energy; improve your mood; improve your posture; promote muscle tone, strength, and endurance; and help you sleep better. It may also improve your ability to copy with labor, making it easier to get back in shape after the baby is born.

WHAT CHANGES OCCUR IN MY BODY THAT MAY AFFECT MY EXERCISE ROUTINE?

The hormones produced during pregnancy cause the ligaments that support your joints to relax, making the joints more mobile and more at risk of injury. The extra weight in the front of your body shifts your center of gravity and places stress on joints and muscles, especially those in the pelvis and lower back. This can make you less stable, cause back pain, and make you more likely to lose your balance and fall, especially in later pregnancy.

WHAT SHOULD I BE AWARE OF WHEN EXERCISING DURING PREGNANCY?

Certain positions and activities can be risky for you and your baby. While exercising, try to avoid jumping, jarring motions, or quick changes in direction that may strain your joints and cause injury. Becoming overheated during pregnancy may cause loss of fluids, leading to dehydration and other problems.

Follow these guidelines:

- After the first trimester, avoid doing any exercises on your back.
- If it has been some time since you have exercised, start slowly. Begin with as little as 5 minutes of exercise a day, and add 5 minutes each week until you can stay active for 30 minutes a day.
- Avoid brisk exercise in hot, humid weather or when you have a fever.
- Wear comfortable clothing that will help you to remain cool.
- Wear a bra that fits well and gives lots of support to protect your breasts.
- Drink plenty of water to help keep you from overheating and dehydrating.
- Make sure you consume the extra calories you need during pregnancy.

WHAT ARE WARNING SIGNS THAT I SHOULD STOP EXERCISING?

Stop exercising and call your health provider if you have any of these symptoms: vaginal bleeding; dizziness or feeling faint; increased shortness of breath; chest pain; headache; muscle weakness; calf pain or swelling; uterine contractions; decreased fetal movement; or fluid leaking from the vagina.

Source: Adapted from American College of Obstetricians and Gynecologists, "FAQ: Exercise during Pregnancy," 2011, www.acog.org/~/media /For%20Patients/faq119.pdf?dmc=1&ts=20120710T1945049211.

that requires a kneeling position is contraindicated for someone with knee pain. A similar exercise in a lying down position can usually be substituted.

2. Wear good shoes. Most of the complaints about group fitness classes have to do with the feet, shins, and knees. Supportive, well-cushioned shoes can help prevent many of these problems. See Appendix 2 for more details.

3. Exercise using good alignment and technique. If you start to tire and break form, take a break and begin again when you can do the exercise correctly. You want joints to move in their proper direction (planes) and not experience unnecessary torque or shearing forces. Information on exercise technique is provided throughout this book. You can also ask your instructor to check your technique.

4. When adding resistance such as weights, do it gradually, and never add resistance when joint soreness exists. If a joint does become painful, rest, ice it, and seek a physician's advice.

5. Develop flexibility to allow a healthy range of motion around the joint, and develop strength in the muscles to help support joints.

EXERCISE AND HYPERTENSION

Blood pressure that is higher than normal results in a condition called **hypertension**. Hypertension affects more than 30% of people in the United States; as many as half of these people are unaware that they have high blood pressure. For this reason, it is often referred to as the silent killer. People with hypertension have a higher risk of developing heart disease or suffering a stroke. Hypertension places an increased strain on the heart, so the additional strain of exercise must be carefully applied and monitored. Exercise can, however, be therapeutic because it helps improve the efficiency of the cardiovascular system. Before exercising, individuals with high blood pressure need to obtain both medical clearance and guidelines about how much and how intense the exercise should be.

If you have hypertension, be sure to tell your instructor and make sure that he or she is prepared in the event of an emergency. Your instructor should also be informed of any medications you are taking and any changes in medication that occur during the course. Some medications influence heart rate; in this event, your instructor will teach you how to use ratings of perceived exertion (RPE; see Chapter 4) to monitor your exercise intensity. Also be sure to let the instructor know of any symptoms you experience.

Certain exercises tend to raise blood pressure more sharply than others. These should be avoided unless otherwise approved by your physician. Isometric exercises (in which you push against an immovable object) may spike blood pressure and should be avoided. Resistance training (such as lifting weights) can be a healthy part of an overall fitness program for some people with hypertension, but it should not be considered the best kind of stand-alone program because it does not help reduce blood pressure the way aerobic exercise does. If you have hypertension, or are at risk for hypertension, check with your physician to see whether you should use resistance exercises and, if so, at what intensity.

Individuals with hypertension should begin exercising with an extra-long warm-up. As with all exercisers, they should start at a low intensity and gradually build up to a moderate intensity. Low-impact aerobics may be a better choice than high-impact or step aerobics. A longer cool-down is also recommended. Individuals with hypertension may also experience more orthostatic hypotension—the dizziness and light-headedness that accompany standing up too quickly. Therefore, they should be careful as they move from floor exercises to standing exercises and avoid exercises that involve dropping the head below the knees.

EXERCISE AND LOW-RISK CORONARY ARTERY DISEASE

Building fitness, especially cardiorespiratory fitness, is very important in both the prevention and rehabilitation of **coronary artery disease (CAD)**. It is one of the keys to maintaining a good quality of life. Individuals with moderate- to high-risk CAD should begin exercising in a rehabilitation program under a physician's care. After being thoroughly evaluated by a physician, people with low-risk CAD may be recommended to a regular exercise program. If you have low-risk CAD, be sure to obtain an exercise prescription from your physician, and then share this with your instructor. The instructor may want to talk directly to your physician. Start with low-intensity exercise; gradually work on duration first, and then intensity. Monitor your intensity frequently using heart rate (if you are not on heart-rate-altering medications) or ratings of perceived exertion. If resistance equipment such as weights or exercise bands are used in class, clear this with your physician. When performing resistance exercises with or without weights, be sure to breathe. Holding your breath, overzealously gripping weights, and performing isometric exercises may unnecessarily drive up your blood pressure. Be sure to tell the instructor of any abnormal symptoms you experience before, during, or after exercise. Finally, check to make sure an emergency protocol is in place in case you need help.

EXERCISE AND AGING

There is no age limit on who can enjoy the benefits of exercise. Through exercise, older adults can:

- improve their muscular strength and endurance, flexibility, and aerobic capacity
- take off or prevent unwanted fat and increase muscle mass
- help control the swelling and pain of arthritic joints
- enjoy the company of others during group exercise (such as low-impact or aquatic aerobics classes), including other active seniors

- boost metabolism (metabolism slows as you age), which helps combat weight gains that are common among the sedentary elderly

The Surgeon General states that muscle-strengthening exercises can reduce the risk of falls and fractures in older adults and can improve their ability to live independently.

If you are an older adult in a college group fitness class, you may need to make some modifications. Most high-impact aerobic steps can be modified into low-impact steps. Ask your instructor to demonstrate this. At times you may want to simply walk in place. If having your arms overhead is tiring or makes you light-headed, use lower arm positions or leave them by your sides. If you are on any medications that alter heart rate (ask your physician), you may want to use other ways (see Chapter 4) to monitor your exercise intensity. If you don't have any joint problems and are adding weights for the first time, start with small amounts of weight and gradually work up. If you have arthritis, high blood pressure, or heart disease, ask your physician about using weights or exercise bands. If you are on any medications, also check with your physician for any exercise implications. For example, nitroglycerine taken right before exercise can cause hypoglycemia (low blood sugar). Wear layers of clothing so that you don't become too hot or overcooled in class, or en route to or from class. A longer cool-down may be needed. If you find this to be true, lower your intensity sooner in the aerobics portion of class, or spend additional time walking after class. Finally, if you have difficulty with some exercise positions, speak to your instructor about alternatives or using equipment such as a mat that will make you more comfortable. Older individuals in college courses are often inspirations to their younger counterparts—real "wellness" role models!

SUMMARY

You are an individual—unique. An exercise program can be adjusted to meet your special needs. Programs are designed around the "average person" but are not intended to be limited to this. Good instructors try to provide and demonstrate alternative exercises, positions, and intensity levels. Being able to take advantage of this information and working with the instructor concerning individual needs will provide you with the very best program. Individual differences may be due to age, gender, ethnicity, pregnancy, aging, disability, injury, disease, or personal preferences.

COMMONLY ASKED QUESTIONS

It seems like everyone does the same thing at the same level during group instruction. Is there any room for individual differences in a group exercise class?

Absolutely. A good instructor will work with you to make sure you know how to adjust the class to meet your specific needs. Your instructor can guide you in scaling back or ramping up the workout to meet your needs and goals. If you have any special medical conditions, be sure to give your instructor the necessary information and permission from your health care provider so that the instructor can modify your workout appropriately.

Is it okay to exercise if I have asthma or diabetes?

Yes, as long as the asthma or diabetes is well controlled. In both cases, you should check with a physician first to monitor medication needs or other potential issues. Also be sure that there is a good channel of communication between you, your instructor, and your physician.

Is it okay to exercise while pregnant?

Almost always, but there are exceptions. You, your physician, and your instructor will need to make sure the workout is appropriate. Changes may be needed as you progress in the pregnancy.

I know that exercise can help lower risk of heart disease and high blood pressure, but is it safe to exercise when I already have some of these issues?

Exercise not only can help prevent these conditions, but also can help you regain health. The key is to make sure you are medically cleared for regular group exercise. Depending on the severity of your condition, you may need to start in a more supervised setting. Check with your physician.

Group fitness classes seem to cater to slender and fit people. Is there a place for the overweight beginner?

Definitely. Meet with your instructor to find out how to tailor the workout to match your fitness level. For tips on feeling comfortable in a group fitness class, see the box, Do I Belong Here? on page 22.

KNOWLEDGE TIPS

1. Group exercise programs can be adjusted to accommodate people's individual differences.

2. Individual differences arise for numerous reasons, including experience, age, gender, ethnicity, pregnancy, aging, disability, injury, disease, and personal preferences.

3. Any exercise modifications due to pregnancy, illness, disease, disability, or injury should be made in conjunction with a physician.

4. Flexibility and strength work can prevent and in some cases relieve back pain.

5. People with asthma who exercise aerobically can raise the exertion level at which symptoms occur. This allows them to enjoy more symptom-free activity.

6. Aerobic exercise can be modified to accommodate the comfort and abilities of obese individuals.

7. Exercise can help people with diabetes control blood sugar, lose weight, and improve the body's use of insulin.

8. Aerobic exercise can help lower blood pressure.

9. Aerobic exercise can reduce the risk of cardiovascular disease and is therapeutic for those who already have it.

10. People of all ages can enjoy exercise. For older adults, exercise helps improve coordination, strengthen muscles, sustain bones, decrease falls, and increase the ability to live independently.

THINK ABOUT IT

1. Why is it important to adjust an exercise or exercise plan to meet the needs of an individual?

2. Think about a friend in the class and identify ways that you are the same and different and how these characteristics might influence your individual exercise plans.

3. Is it possible to exercise safely if you are asthmatic? diabetic? overweight? hypertensive?

4. What are some things you can do to prevent low back pain?

5. Who should make the decisions about exercising while pregnant?

6. Can you think of one way you would individualize your aerobic exercise to better meet your needs?

REFERENCES

American College of Obstetricians and Gynecologists. *Getting in Shape After Your Baby Is Born.* (AP131). Washington, DC: American College of Obstetricians and Gynecologists, 2000.

___. *Exercise During Pregnancy.* (AP119). Washington, DC: American College of Obstetricians and Gynecologists, 2003.

___. *Easing Back Pain During Pregnancy.* (AP115) Washington, DC: American College of Obstetricians and Gynecologists, 1997.

American Council on Exercise. *Aerobics Instructor Manual: ACE's Guide for Fitness Professionals.* San Diego, CA: American Council on Exercise, 2000.

Estivill, M. "Therapeutic Aspects of Aerobic Dance Participation." *Health Care for Women International* 16 (No. 4, 1995): 341–50.

Kenney, W. L., J. H. Wilmore, and D. L. Costill. *Physiology of Sport and Exercise.* Champaign, IL: Human Kinetics, 2012.

Lokey, E. A., Z. V. Tran, C. L. Wells, B. C. Myers, and A. C. Tran. "Effects of Physical Exercise on Pregnancy Outcomes: A Meta-analytic Review." *Medicine and Science in Sports & Exercise* 23 (No. 11, 1991): 1234–9.

Wells, C. L. *Women, Sport, and Performance.* Champaign, IL: Human Kinetics, 1985.

Fitness Components and Exercise Principles

3

*"Failure comes only when we forget
our ideals and objectives and principles."*

JAWAHARLAL NEHRU

- Do I have to play sports to get fit?
- What types of exercises do I need to do to be healthy?
- Are there some basic rules or guidelines to follow for exercise?

COMPONENTS OF FITNESS

Exercising for health is different from training for competition. To fine-tune your performance for competition, you have to train long hours at high intensities. You may also have to place your body in mechanically difficult positions. For example, volleyball players and weight lifters drop into deep knee positions that place stress on their knee ligaments. Gymnasts constantly hyperextend their backs, thus placing pressure on their vertebral discs, and pitchers risk injuring their elbows when they throw curve balls. The motivation for such intense practice and performance comes from a deep-seated drive to excel and a desire to win recognition and awards.

Many positive outcomes are associated with competition—health can be one of them. However, a higher risk of injury is associated with high-intensity training. It may also surprise you to learn that not all highly skilled competitors are physically fit. For example, some excellent golfers and baseball players carry extra pounds of fat and lack good cardiorespiratory conditioning.

To exercise for health, you can train at a moderate intensity, enjoy the physiological and psychological benefits of exercise, and at the same time limit the risk of injury. It's time to discard the myth that it is good to exercise until you drop. Lifetime fitness is built on activities that are enjoyable and, when done correctly, free from pain. There are five health-related components of physical fitness:

1. cardiorespiratory endurance
2. body composition
3. flexibility
4. muscular strength
5. muscular endurance

Sometimes muscular strength and endurance are considered one component (muscular fitness), thus making the total number of health-related components four. Any improvement in these five areas will improve your health (see the box, Can You..., on page 30). There are also skill-related components of fitness:

1. agility
2. balance
3. coordination
4. power
5. reaction time
6. speed

Strength is often included as a seventh component because it plays an important role in skilled performance. Kinesthetic awareness (awareness of where your body is in space) may also be included as a skill-related component. Because group fitness classes are primarily concerned with developing and maintaining physical health, they emphasize exercises that concentrate on the five health-related components. This emphasis does not exclude the possibility of improving some of the skill-related components, especially coordination, agility, and balance.

CAN YOU ...

... identify exercises or activities that will result in positive changes in each of the following health-related fitness components?

- cardiorespiratory endurance
- body composition
- flexibility
- muscular strength
- muscular endurance

Skill-related components can play a role in staying healthy because when you are good at something (skilled), you tend to do it more often. And being physically active is the key ingredient to health-related fitness. Group fitness classes tend to keep skill requirements low so that they have a broad appeal. One reason why Zumba has been successful is that it emphasizes moving to the beat, not doing the right number of steps exactly the right way. Repetition is also important in group fitness because it helps everyone get the movements down. Skilled movement plays a somewhat bigger role in advanced dance and step classes, because these classes often use more intricate movement patterns and power steps. Functional fitness classes incorporate agility and balance moves as well as aerobic and strength moves. Classes that focus on muscular fitness emphasize good technique and alignment, but you are not developing skills in the same sense as learning a sport. However, the technique and alignment you learn in fitness classes, including yoga and Pilates, are foundational to movement and translate well into many recreational and sport activities. When you first start a group fitness class, you may feel a little clumsy or uncoordinated, but after only a few classes these feelings will start to diminish—and before you know it, you will be comfortable with the routines.

CARDIORESPIRATORY ENDURANCE

Cardiorespiratory endurance is the ability to perform large-muscle movements over a sustained period of time. Defined another way, it is the ability of the circulatory (heart, blood, blood vessels) and respiratory (lungs) systems to deliver fuel, especially oxygen, to the muscles during continuous exercise. Fit individuals have a heart–lung capacity that allows them to persist in physical activity for relatively long periods of time without undue fatigue. (The terms "cardiovascular endurance" and "cardiorespiratory endurance" are often

used interchangeably. The latter will be used in this text because it reflects the important relationship between the respiratory and circulatory systems.)

Cardiorespiratory endurance is improved during the aerobic portion of the exercise class. Some of the health benefits associated with cardiorespiratory endurance include a stronger heart, improved circulation to the heart, increased oxygen transportation by the blood, an increased level of high-density lipoproteins (HDL), a lower risk of coronary heart disease, a better chance of surviving a heart attack, a decreased level of blood fat (cholesterol), a lowered resting heart rate, lower blood pressure, improved body composition, and a better chance of living a longer, healthier life.

BODY COMPOSITION

Body composition refers to the relative amounts of lean body mass and fat in your body. **Lean body mass (LBM)** includes bones, muscles, and connective tissue. **Fat** includes subcutaneous fat (the fat deposits stored *between* the muscles and the skin) and intramuscular fat (the fat stored *within* the muscles). The percentage of fat you have can be measured several ways, including the skin-fold technique, underwater weighing, and electrical impedance (see Chapter 13). A certain amount of fat is essential for health. Too high or too low of a percentage of fat is unhealthy.

Body composition can be changed by decreasing the body's amount of fat, increasing the body's amount of lean body mass, or both. You can change your body composition through a sound diet and exercise program. Fat (along with carbohydrate) is metabolized during aerobic exercise, whereas muscle (lean body mass) can be added through strength training exercises. Increasing muscle mass has the added benefit of increasing your resting metabolic rate, which means your body is burning more calories while at rest. This can help you maintain a healthy weight after a weight-loss diet.

Maintaining a healthy body composition reduces the risk of heart disease, stroke, some cancers, diabetes, hypertension, high blood cholesterol, and arthritis. In addition, it makes you look and feel better, and it increases your body's work capacity.

FLEXIBILITY

Flexibility is the ability to move a joint or a combination of joints through a full range of motion. Muscles, tendons, ligaments, and bone structures all determine a joint's range of motion. When bones articulate well and muscles and tendons are properly elastic, movement is full and comfortable. When muscles and tendons tighten and shorten, the range of motion in the joint is restricted. Simple tasks such as turning in a car seat to check traffic or picking something up off the floor can become difficult. When ligaments and tendons are overstretched or damaged, the joint becomes loose and dislocates easily. Strengthening the muscles around a joint may help stabilize a loose joint, or surgery may be required. (Consult your physician for advice on which exercises are appropriate for rehabilitating a loose or injured joint.)

Working on flexibility by stretching during the warm-up and cool-down periods of an aerobics class helps maintain and improve range of motion. The warm-up involves a type of stretching called dynamic stretching. This is an active stretch of the muscles achieved through easy rhythmic movements. Following this, or intermixed with it, may be some static or held stretching. This stretching regimen prepares the body for more vigorous movement. The best way to develop or improve flexibility is to perform static stretches after a good workout, when the muscles are really warm and pliable. Health benefits associated with good flexibility include freedom of movement (which represents independence for older individuals), improved postural alignment and physical appearance, greater work efficiency, less risk of muscle or joint injury, and decreased chance of developing lower back pain. Flexibility can also enhance sport skill performance, decrease muscle tension, and promote relaxation.

MUSCULAR ENDURANCE

Muscular endurance is the ability of a muscle, or group of muscles, to apply a submaximal force repeatedly or to sustain a muscular contraction for a period of time. Leg lifts are an example of repeatedly applied force. Holding the leg in a raised position for 10 seconds is an example of a sustained contraction. During leg lifts, the muscles go through a range of motion while applying force. This is an example of a **dynamic contraction**. During a dynamic contraction, muscle fibers contract and shorten. When the leg is held in one position, the muscles are in a **static** or **isometric contraction.** During a sustained isometric contraction, muscle fibers contract but don't shorten.

Most muscle-toning exercises are done using dynamic contractions, because they strengthen the muscle through its entire range of motion. Muscular endurance is usually developed by performing a high number of repetitions (approximately 8 to 15) with light to medium resistance. Higher numbers of repetitions may be used depending on the objective. Isometric contractions strengthen a muscle in a particular position, which can be particularly useful for therapeutic purposes and improving posture. The wall sit is a good example. People with high blood pressure should check with their physician before doing isometric contractions, which can cause a rapid rise in peripheral resistance (blood pressure). The benefits of improving muscular endurance include less fatigue during regular activity, an increased ability to do work, and a reduced risk of injury.

MUSCULAR STRENGTH

Muscular strength is the ability of a muscle, or group of muscles, to exert force against a resistance. The number of pounds you can lift one time with your arms is a measure of maximal muscular strength. You can improve your muscular strength by lifting relatively heavy weights in a small number of repetitions. Aerobic exercise classes have traditionally placed more emphasis on endurance than on strength, but the use of exercise bands, weights, weighted balls, bars, and stability balls have enabled participants to improve both muscular endurance and strength. Strength training, like endurance training, usually emphasizes dynamic contractions. The health benefits related to muscular strength include an increased ability to do physical work, a decreased risk of injury, and a decreased risk of back pain.

PRINCIPLES OF EXERCISE

As you work to improve or maintain your fitness level in each of the five health-related components of fitness, use the following principles of exercise to guide you.

THE PRINCIPLE OF OVERLOAD

When the human body is stressed repeatedly over a period of time, it responds by adapting to the stress.

OVERLOAD: FOR ONCE IT'S A GOOD THING!

Remember, overloading in exercise is a good thing as long as you do it gradually. Here are some examples of how you can create progressive overloads. Can you apply these ideas to specific exercises?

- **Flexibility:** Stretch the muscle just longer than its normal length.

- **Strength:** Increase the amount of resistance against which the muscle normally moves, OR increase the number of repetitions and/or sets of an exercise you perform.

- **Muscular endurance:** Increase the number of repetitions (or sets of repetitions) you normally perform, OR increase the resistance against which the muscle is moving while maintaining a moderate to high number of repetitions, OR hold an isometric contraction for a longer time than normal.

- **Cardiorespiratory endurance:** Place a demand that is greater than normal on the heart and lungs by sustaining a longer bout of aerobic exercise, OR increase the intensity of the exercise by working at a higher level (higher heart rate), OR perform aerobic exercise on more days of the week.

Regular exercise stresses the body, which adapts by becoming stronger and more efficient. Another word for "stress" is "overload." When the muscles, including the heart muscle, are overloaded or stressed more than normal amounts, fitness gains occur. This is the **principle of overload.** When you overload, you are temporarily increasing the amount or intensity of an exercise. As your body adapts, you experience a training effect and the exercise becomes easier. To continue to improve your physical fitness, you have to continue to overload. For example, if you can normally do 10 push-ups, create an overload to the arm and chest muscles by doing 11 or 12. When 12 becomes easy, overload again by doing 13 or 14, and so on. Overload can also be achieved by doing a harder version of the push-up rather than more push-ups. See the Overload box above to begin applying the principle of overload. When you reach your desired level of fitness, you can stop overloading. To maintain your fitness level, continue to perform your new "normal" amount. Doing less than normal will result in deconditioning.

A minimum amount and intensity of exercise must be performed before fitness improvement begins. This minimum level of exercise is called the **threshold of training.** To improve your physical fitness, you must engage in activities at an intensity above your threshold of training. The threshold of training for a beginner is relatively low. As you become more fit, your threshold of training will increase.

THE PRINCIPLE OF PROGRESSION

The **principle of progression** is an extension of the principle of overload. Basically, this principle means that you should gradually increase your overload over a period of time. Too rapid an overload can make you really stiff and sore or even result in injury. Overload and progression are so interrelated that fitness professionals usually speak in terms of doing appropriate progressive overloads. Beginners will want to progressively overload by increasing the duration and frequency with which they perform activities before adding intensity. For example, a beginning aerobics student who can do only 10 minutes of continuous low-intensity aerobics will want to slowly extend that to about 20 minutes of aerobic activity for 3 to 5 days before thinking about increasing to a moderate intensity workout. Similarly, with push-ups, beginners would want to improve from five modified (on knees) push-ups to 10 to 15 before attempting push-ups performed on the toes. More advanced participants can gradually add intensity. People who fail to progress may be exercising too infrequently or not overloading enough to stimulate change.

THE FITT PRINCIPLE

The FITT principle describes exercise and provides guidance about the appropriate amounts and intensity of exercise needed to attain health and performance benefits. The optimal range of exercise for health-related physical fitness is called the **fitness target zone.** The lower limit of the zone is the threshold of training; the upper limit is the ceiling, or maximum amount and intensity of exercise recommended for health. The best-known target zone is the one for cardiorespiratory endurance. However, target zones exist for each of the health-related components of fitness.

Three variables are involved in locating and exercising within your target zones: the frequency with which you train (number of times per week), the intensity at which you train, and the amount of time you train per session. These three variables are often remembered by the acronym **FITT**—the *F* stands for **frequency,** the *I* for **intensity,** and the first *T* for **time** (or **duration**). Each of the health-related fitness components has optimal ranges (fitness target zones) for these three variables. The last *T* stands for **"type of exercise."** Therefore, to describe your exercise using the FITT principle, you would specify the Frequency, Intensity, and Time you perform a certain Type of activity.

The target zone for aerobic endurance is described in more detail in Chapter 4. The target zones for flexibility and muscular strength and endurance are described in Chapters 7 and 8. Each of these chapters will discuss how to adjust the frequency, intensity, and duration of your exercise so that you get the most out of your workout.

THE PRINCIPLE OF INDIVIDUALITY

Everyone is unique, and this includes people's responses to exercise. The **principle of individuality** holds that no two people react exactly the same way to exercise. Two men with the ability to lift the same amount of weight can have significantly different muscle circumferences. Two women eating the same diet, attending the same exercise class, and working out at the same intensity may lose inches or pounds in different places at different rates. This means that the only person you can really compare yourself to is you. Your rate of progress and the way you progress are unique to you.

Many fitness tests provide norms, averages, or percentiles for you to compare your scores against. These are helpful guidelines, but they should not be considered the gold standard. Norms simply state what a tested group of people were able to do. The norms for a push-up test performed by athletes would be considerably higher than the norms for a push-up test performed by senior citizens. The best fitness test norms are age adjusted and based on scores from large populations. The fitness tests in the worksheets available online at www.pearsonhighered.com/bishopaerobics

and at the back of this book were selected with these criteria in mind. Compare yourself to these norms, but most importantly, compare yourself to yourself.

THE PRINCIPLE OF SPECIFICITY

Would you ever practice stretching your shoulders so that you could touch your toes or do a set of abdominal curls to tone your legs? Of course not. You would select exercises that would accomplish your goal. When you make these selections, you are using the **principle of specificity,** which states that placing a specific demand on the body results in a specific adaptation.

If you create a demand on the body by doing strength exercises, the body adapts by building stronger muscles. If you create a demand by doing aerobic exercises, the body adapts by improving the cardiorespiratory system. Note that the adaptation is specific to the demand—strength exercises result in strength, not in cardiorespiratory endurance.

Different occupations place different demands on the body. As a result, pianists have strong fingers, construction workers have well-developed shoulder and arm muscles, ice cream scoopers have one strong arm, and fitness instructors have toned muscles and healthy hearts. (If an occupation does create muscle imbalances, as in the ice cream scooper with only one strong arm, an exercise program can often correct the imbalance.)

THE PRINCIPLE OF REGULARITY

Sometimes referred to as the **principle of reversibility** or the **use/disuse principle,** the **principle of regularity** is succinctly defined by the well-known phrase "use it or lose it." Within two weeks of the time you stop exercising, your body begins to adapt to the lack of activity. The loss of competitive edge can be even faster. Cardiorespiratory and flexibility losses occur more rapidly than strength and endurance losses. Nobody is protected from these negative adaptations. The only way to be fit is to be active on a regular basis. (Worksheet 3.1, available online at www.pearsonhighered .com/bishopaerobics will help you track your progress and stay motivated.) Varsity college athletes who stop exercising when they graduate are ultimately no better off than people who never exercised. So—keep moving!

THE PRINCIPLE OF OVERUSE

Overuse results from violating the principle of overload. When you overdo (which is the essence of the

principle of overuse), you create problems. Injuries, especially chronic injuries such as shinsplints and tendinitis, start to appear. Some people actually become addicted to exercise, a sign of which is the refusal to exercise fewer than seven days a week. Addiction leads to overtraining. Signs of overtraining are the previously mentioned chronic injuries and an elevated resting heart rate. Overuse may also be the result of a violation of the principle of individuality. A person trying to keep up with another person may overload too quickly. Three sets of 10 push-ups may be an appropriate load for one individual but may be overuse for another.

WORKOUT COMPONENTS

There are several parts, or components, to a workout. It begins with a warm-up, is followed by either a cardio workout or muscular fitness workout or both, and ends with a cool-down. The warm-up consists of 3 to 5 minutes of general body-warming exercises, such as light jogging, jump roping, or jumping jacks and then usually a series of dynamic stretches such as walking lunges, the inchworm, arm swings, or power skips. The cardio section of the workout can take many forms but is usually either a continuous aerobic workout or a series of aerobic intervals (changes in intensity). The muscular fitness portion may involve body weight exercises or use of equipment such as bands, balls, or barbells. The cool-down consists of two parts. The first follows the cardio portion of the workout, gradually bringing the body back down to normal levels and the second is a series of static stretches that can follow the cardio cool-down or a muscle workout. The cool-down generally lasts 5 to 10 minutes. (The warm-up and cool-down are discussed in more detail in Chapter 7, and the cardio and muscular fitness workout components are discussed in Chapters 9 and 10, respectively.)

SUMMARY

Even though you may not know it, you are probably an expert at using the principles of exercise. For example, have you ever increased the frequency, intensity, or duration of your workout to make it more challenging (overload)? Have you ever asked someone for a better exercise to achieve a goal like a flatter abdomen or thinner thighs (specificity)? Have you ever wondered why your friend is adapting more quickly or more slowly than you are to certain parts of the class (individuality)? Have you ever noticed how you have more energy when you are on an exercise program

than when you stop your program (regularity)? Now you can consciously put these principles to work for you. Think through the group fitness class you are in now and see if you can identify the principles of exercise at work and identify which of the health-related components of fitness are being targeted.

COMMONLY ASKED QUESTIONS

How often do I need to work out?

The answer to this depends on your goals. For general health, you need to accumulate 150 minutes of moderately vigorous physical activity or 75 minutes of vigorous activity each week or a combination of the two. You can break these times down over fewer or more days. For example, you can obtain the 150 minutes by being active 30 minutes 5 times a week or being active 50 minutes 3 times a week. You need to engage in some form of muscle fitness 2 to 3 days a week, and activities that increase flexibility 3 to 7 days a week. Much more information is available in later chapters.

Why do I get so sore when I start an exercise program?

Whenever you use muscles in a new way, ask them to handle more resistance, or stretch them more than normal, you will get sore. A little soreness is okay, but if you are really sore you should lower the intensity of your workout and then gradually build up to a higher intensity. Delayed muscle soreness is due to injury or damage to the muscle. Although that sounds bad, the breaking down and building back up of the muscle fibers is actually what makes your muscles stronger. But be careful. Too much muscle damage or not enough recovery time can result in declining strength or injury. Interestingly, you can become sore as much as 24 to 48 hours after a workout. So the soreness you are feeling may actually be related to something you did two days ago!

Do I have to keep overloading my program if I am happy with my fitness level?

No, you can simply stay on a maintenance program. You might consider mixing things up a bit to prevent boredom and to target your muscles a little differently.

What should I increase first, frequency, intensity, or time?

There is no one completely correct answer to this question. That said, frequency and time (duration) are usually increased before intensity. If you are a beginner, you will want to work toward 150 minutes/week of moderately intense physical activity, as recommended in the *2008 Physical Activity Guideline for Americans*. More advanced individuals can work toward the guideline of 75 minutes of vigorous activity. If, for example, you are active 15 minutes twice a week, you can increase the minutes by being active on more days or by being active longer on the two days. Once you meet the number of minutes per week, you can increase intensity as desired.

Why do I feel exhausted instead of energized after I work out?

It could be that you are trying to work out at too high an intensity level. You need to gradually overload. The reason may also be overuse—muscles, for example, need time to rest and rebuild. Or your problem may be related to other factors, such as poor eating habits, not getting enough sleep, or dealing with an emotionally stressful situation.

What is the difference between muscular strength, endurance, and power?

Muscular strength is used for all-out efforts or nearly all-out efforts—for example, when you pick up a heavy box and load it in the trunk, or pull back on a dog trying to bolt after a cat. Muscular endurance comes into play when you do something over and over, or hold a position for an extended period of time—for example, if you want to bring numerous bags of groceries up the stairs into an apartment or maintain a good position while water skiing. Power is a combination of strength and speed. It is useful in many sports. A daily activity that involves power is being able to jump quickly out of the way.

KNOWLEDGE TIPS

1. The five health-related fitness components are cardiorespiratory endurance, body composition, flexibility, muscular strength, and muscular endurance.

2. The six skill-related components of fitness are agility, balance, coordination, power, reaction time, and speed; strength is often included as a skill-related component as well.

3. Group fitness workouts designed to improve all of the health-related components of fitness and some of the skill-related components of fitness.

4. To overload, you must go just beyond the point of comfort by increasing frequency, intensity, or time.

5. A progressive overload is one that occurs gradually over time.

6. The FITT principle uses the variables of frequency, intensity, time, and type of exercise to describe beneficial fitness target zones for the health-related components of physical fitness.

7. Individuals respond to exercise differently.

8. The body makes specific adaptations in accord with the demands placed on it.

9. Deconditioning occurs with disuse.

10. Overuse results in undue fatigue, chronic injury, and other problems.

THINK ABOUT IT

1. What is the difference between health-related and skill-related fitness? Can you name the components for each?

2. How is exercising for health different from exercising for sport and competition?

3. Which components of physical fitness are targeted in a group fitness workout?

4. Identify one or more health benefits for each health-related component of fitness.

5. Describe a progressive overload for both cardiorespiratory endurance and muscular fitness.

6. Explain why varsity athletes are no better off than anyone else if they stop being physically active. Which principle of exercise speaks to this?

7. Is it healthy to perform both aerobic and muscular resistance training in the same day? Explain why or why not.

8. Does an individual have to be skilled in order to be fit? Explain your answer.

9. Explain the FITT principle.

10. What are some signs that a person is overdoing his or her fitness program?

REFERENCES

American College of Sports Medicine. *ACSM's Guidelines for Exercise Testing and Exercise Prescription.* 8th ed. Media, PA: Lip-pincott Williams & Wilkins, 2010.

Corbin, C. B., G. Welk, W. R. Corbin, and K. A. Welk. *Concepts of Physical Fitness: Active Lifestyles for Wellness.* 14th ed. New York: McGraw-Hill Higher Education, 2006.

Physical Best and NASPE. *Physical Education for Lifelong Fitness: The Physical Best Teacher's Guide.* 2nd ed. Champaign, IL: Human Kinetics, 2005.

4

The Aerobic Target Zone

"Life begets life. Energy creates energy. It is by spending oneself that one becomes rich."

SARAH BERNHARDT

- How much aerobic exercise do I need to do?
- How will I know if I'm exercising hard enough?
- Why do I see people taking their pulse or looking at their heart-rate monitors during aerobic exercise?

EROBIC exercise has a lot of benefits; the amount and type of benefits you will experience depend on the intensity with which you perform. In Chapter 1, you learned that you can get substantial health benefits by doing a minimum of 150 minutes per week of moderate-intensity aerobic physical activity *or* 75 minutes per week of vigorous-intensity aerobic activity *or* an equivalent combination of moderate and vigorous activity. Research tells us that moderate-level activity (brisk walk) is the minimum level most people must reach in order to gain benefits. But greater gains in health and fitness occur when a person performs exercise at a higher level, one which substantially increases heart rate and breathing. The aerobic target zone described in this chapter ranges between moderately vigorous to vigorous intensity to promote optimal benefits but with the allowance that levels below the zone can benefit those in class who are just getting started and need to build endurance. If you perform the aerobic portion of class at a level similar to a brisk walk, you may need to supplement class with additional exercise to achieve your 150 minutes. If you jog and jump your way through class, you will probably achieve or come close to your 75-minute minimum of vigorous activity for the week.

Like all target zones, the **aerobic target zone** is composed of three variables: frequency, intensity, and time (duration). In this chapter, you will learn how often, how hard, and how long to perform aerobic exercise to improve your cardiorespiratory endurance and to enjoy the associated health benefits.

Please note that this chapter is only about the target zone for aerobic exercise. (The target zones for flexibility, muscular strength, and muscular endurance are described in Chapters 7 and 10.)

FREQUENCY

How often should you be physically active? According to the *2008 Physical Activity Guidelines for Americans*, it is preferable to use a frequency pattern that spreads the required accumulation of aerobic minutes over the week. The American College of Sports Medicine (ACSM) 2012 guidelines are similar but make more specific recommendations with respect to the number of days per week. The ACSM recommends that moderate-intensity exercise (150 minutes) be performed over 5 or more days of the week, vigorous-intensity exercise (75 minutes) over 3 or more days a week, or a combination of moderate- and vigorous-intensity exercise 3 to 5 days or more a week. As an example, you can walk briskly 5 times a week, or jog 3 times a week, or do a combination run/walk 3 to 5 times a week, depending on how much you walk and how much you jog.

A frequency of 5 times a week is enough to help you attain most of the benefits of health-related fitness. Exercising more than this may result in more benefits, but the gains are smaller in comparison with the time commitment. Competitions are won with narrow margins, so the small additional fitness benefits can be important for competitive athletes—provided that overuse or other injuries do not limit gains. The other group of individuals who may benefit from exercising more days are those trying to achieve weight loss. People who exercise at low-end intensities (see the next section) may need to exercise more than 3 days a week to burn enough calories to meet weight-loss goals. When weight loss is the primary goal, frequency can range from 3 to 7 days a week, depending on the intensity, duration, and type of exercise. (For more information on weight loss and exercise, see Chapter 13.) According to the *2008 Physical Activity Guidelines for Americans*, people can gain additional health benefits by increasing to 5 hours (300 minutes) a week of moderate-intensity aerobic physical activity, or 2 hours and 30 minutes a week (150 minutes) of vigorous-intensity physical activity, or an equivalent combination of both.

High-frequency exercisers (e.g., those working toward weight loss, instructors, and individuals training for competition) can minimize impact stress by using low-impact, nonimpact, or non-weight-bearing activities in combination with, or in place of, high-impact aerobics. Low-impact exercises include step, low-impact, and aqua (water) aerobics as well as brisk walking; nonimpact exercises include slide aerobics, some special forms of aerobic dance, and non-weight-bearing exercises such as swimming, rowing, cycling, and deep-water running. (Activities and their impact stress will be discussed in more detail later in Chapter 8.)

Exercise addicts are people who feel compelled to work out every single day. Addicts are more prone to overuse injuries such as shin splints and tendinitis and may develop such an obsession for exercise that they begin to value it above everything else. Like any addiction, this leads to an unhealthy lifestyle. Physical fitness must always be balanced with the other wellness components: social, emotional, intellectual, and spiritual health.

INTENSITY

This section contains a number of abbreviated terms. To make your reading of the text easier, here is a quick reference list of abbreviations.

HR	= heart rate
EHR	= exercise heart rate
RHR	= resting heart rate
THR	= training heart rate range (target zone)
MHR	= maximum heart rate
PreHR	= pre-exercise heart rate
RecHR	= recovery heart rate
HRR	= heart rate reserve (MHR−RHR)
VO_2max	= maximum volume of oxygen consumed

How hard should you exercise? And how do you know whether you are exercising that hard? The "how hard" is what is referred to as the *intensity* of the exercise. The physical activity guidelines talk about moderate and vigorous intensity for aerobic activity—but again, how hard is moderate intensity? Vigorous intensity? One way to know is to look at a list of activities that fall into these categories (see Table 4.1). That helps somewhat, but it doesn't really give you an idea of how hard you are working during an aerobic dance or spinning class or whether you stay at the same intensity during the class. Fortunately, there are several ways to measure intensity during an activity. These include monitoring your heart rate, ratings of perceived exertion, and the talk test. Using one (or more) of these methods will allow you to adjust your intensity as needed and thereby get the most out of your workout.

To fully understand how to measure intensity, and to find the correct level of intensity for you, it is important to understand the role of oxygen in aerobic activity. Remember from Chapter 1 that the word "aerobic" means "with oxygen." It is only when a steady supply of oxygen is available to the muscles that aerobic exercise can be performed. The oxygen you breathe into your lungs is picked up by red blood cells and delivered to your muscles. Inside the muscle cells, oxygen is used in the chemical processes that convert

Table 4.1 Classification of Activity Intensity by Type of Activity

MODERATE-LEVEL ACTIVITIES	VIGOROUS ACTIVITIES
• Biking slowly	• Aerobic dance
• Canoeing	• Basketball
• Dancing	• Fast dancing
• General gardening (raking, trimming shrubs)	• Jumping rope
• Tennis (doubles)	• Martial arts (such as karate)
• Using a manual wheelchair	• Race walking, jogging, or running
• Using hand cyclers (also called arm ergometers)	• Riding a bike on hills or riding faster
• Walking briskly	• Soccer
• Water aerobics	• Swimming fast or swimming laps
	• Tennis (singles)

Source: U.S. Department of Health and Human Services, *2008 Physical Activity Guidelines for Americans* (modified).

food (carbohydrates, fats, and proteins) into energy for muscular contraction. The more intensely you exercise, the more oxygen your muscles need. The more oxygen you are able to supply, the more exercise you will be able to do. As you increase your exercise intensity, your breathing becomes faster and deeper to bring in more oxygen, your heart beats faster to speed up the delivery of the oxygen, and your muscles use more food and oxygen to produce movement. As exercise becomes more and more intense, the rate and volume of oxygen entering the body continues to increase until finally the body is consuming oxygen as rapidly as it can. This maximum volume of **oxygen consumption** (measured in liters per minute or milliliters per minute per kilogram of body weight) is called **VO$_2$ max;** you may also see it referred to as "maximum oxygen uptake (MOU)." If exercise intensity is increased any further, the muscles' demand for oxygen cannot be met. You can exercise at these very high intensities for only a short time before total exhaustion makes you stop.

Exercising near or at VO$_2$ max is not fun. In fact, it's agonizingly difficult. The good news is that you can improve your aerobic fitness and health by exercising at an intensity well below maximum. The question then becomes, What percentage of maximal effort does one need to exercise at in order to get a training effect? The answer turns out to be more complicated than once thought. Rather than being able to say that you need to get above one minimum (threshold) amount, newer research is finding that the threshold level depends, at least in part, on a person's fitness level. In addition, the threshold required to attain health benefits may vary depending on the health benefit (for example, decrease in blood pressure or increase in insulin sensitivity). Until research becomes more specific, a good take-away message is that to improve aerobic fitness, more-fit individuals need to exercise at a higher percentage of maximal effort than low-fit individuals. So whereas a beginner can benefit from working out at 50% of VO$_2$max, a more conditioned individual may need to bump that up to 70%, and a highly trained individual up to 85%. Table 4.2 shows the ACSM's percentage ranges for VO$_2$max that match light, moderate, and vigorous workout levels. The bottom of the range represents the threshold.

This is all fine and good if you have a way to measure how much oxygen you are using, but who can count oxygen molecules while exercising? Clearly, the average person can't, but exercise scientists can, using a supervised laboratory test during which a person exercises on a stationary bicycle or treadmill while hooked up to machines that monitor oxygen consumption and heart rate. These kinds of tests are the most accurate and are wonderful research tools, but they are too elaborate and individualized to be of any practical benefit to group fitness participants. Fortunately, there are several other ways, one of which is based on the link between oxygen consumption and heart rate. Another approach is to teach people to determine appropriate intensity levels by gauging their sense of how hard they are exercising. The simple talk test is yet another option. These will all be described in the following sections.

Table 4.2   Classifications of Exercise Intensities for Cardiorespiratory Endurance

ACTIVITY INTENSITY	TALK TEST	BORG RPE (6–20 SCALE)	OMNI	%HRmax	%HRR	%VO$_2$max
very light	sing	< 9 (< very light)	0 to 1 (extremely easy)	< 57	< 30	< 37
light	sing/easy conversation	9–11 (very light to fairly light)	2 to 4 (easy to somewhat easy)	57–63	30–39	37–45
moderate	brief sentences and words	12–13 (fairly light to somewhat hard)	5 to 6 (somewhat easy to somewhat hard)	64–76	40–59	46–63
vigorous	a few words	14–17 (somewhat hard to very hard)	7 to 8 (somewhat hard to hard)	77–95	60–89	64–90
near-maximal to maximal	barely able or not able to talk	≥ 18 (≥ very hard)	9 to 10 (hard to extremely hard)	≥ 96	≥ 90	≥ 91

Data are from: American College of Sports Medicine, *ACSM's Guidelines for Exercise Testing and Prescription*, 8th Edition (Baltimore, MD: Lippincott Williams & Wilkins, 2010); Office of Disease Prevention and Health Promotion, U.S. Department of Health and Human Services, *2008 Physical Activity Guidelines for Americans: Be Active, Healthy, and Happy!* ODPHP Publication no. U0036 (Washington, DC: U.S. Department of Health and Human Services, 2008). Available at: www.health.gov.paguidelines; R.J. Robertson and others, "Validation of the Adult OMNI Scale of Perceived Exertion for Cycle Ergometer Exercise," *Medicine & Science in Sports & Exercise* 36, no. 1 (2004): 102-108; A.C. Utter and others, "Validation of the Adult OMNI Scale of Perceived Exertion for Walking/Running Exercise," *Medicine & Science in Sports & Exercise* 36, no. 10 (2004): 1776-1780, G. Borg, *Borg's Perceived Exertion and Pain Scales* (Champaign, IL: Human Kinetics, 1998): 27-38; American College of Sports Medicine, "The Recommended Quantity and Quality of Exercise for Developing and Maintaining Cardiorespiratory, Musculoskeletal, and Neuromotor Fitness in Apparently Healthy Adults: Guidance for Prescribing Exercise," *Medicine & Science in Sports & Exercise* 43, no. 7 (2011):1334–1359.

MONTIORING INTENSITY BY HEART RATE

While doing some research in the 1960s, Dr. Martii Karvonen discovered a nearly linear relationship between oxygen consumption and heart rate during aerobic exercise. In other words, when one goes up, the other goes up at about the same rate. This means that measures of heart rate can be substituted for oxygen measures. Because heart rate is easy to monitor by feeling your **pulse** (the wave of pressure felt in the arteries when the heart beats), it is a very practical way to monitor exercise intensity.

Even if it were possible to pick the one heart rate that is most beneficial to work at, it would be very difficult to stay right at that number. Instead, it is common practice to determine a range of heart rates to stay within; this is referred to as the **training heart-rate range** (or **target heart-rate zone**), usually abbreviated **THR** (or **THZ**) and often simply referred to as the "aerobic target zone."

Two formulas have been developed to calculate this target zone. The **maximum heart rate formula** determines the zone by taking percentages of your **maximum heart rate (HRmax)**—the fastest your heart can beat in a minute. It is pretty easy to calculate because all you need to know is your HRmax and the intensity range (moderate, vigorous, etc.) in which you want to exercise. The second formula, aptly named after the man who discovered the link between oxygen and heart rate, is called the **Karvonen formula**. This produces a more individualized range because it uses a percentage of **heart-rate reserve (HRR)**; to get your HRR, you subtract your resting heart rate from your maximum heart rate. The resting heart rate is the rate at which your heart beats when you are at complete rest and is often lower in well-trained individuals. One advantage of the Karvonen formula is that you can refigure your zone if your resting heart rate goes down.

Determining your true resting heart rate takes several days, so many people start off using the maximum heart-rate formula and then, when they are ready, use the Karvonen formula. Look again at Table 4.2, and you will see heart rate ranges that coincide with light, moderate, and vigorous workouts based on percentages of both HRmax and HRR. How to use these ranges will be discussed shortly.

First, to calculate your target zone using either formula, you need to know your maximum heart rate. The most accurate way to determine your MHR is to exercise to absolute exhaustion while your heart rate is monitored by an EKG (electrocardiograph) machine. Fortunately for you, there is a faster and easier way to estimate your MHR. Researchers discovered that the MHR drops an average of one beat each year of an individual's life. Through statistical extrapolation, researchers determined that a newborn's MHR is about 220 beats per minute (bpm). A one-year-old would have an MHR of 219 bpm, a two-year-old 218 bpm, and so on. So, until recently, to calculate your MHR all you had to do was subtract your age from 220. For a 20-year-old, this would mean a MHR of 200 bpm. More recent research has found that this formula generally overpredicted maximum heart rates in people aged 20–40 and under-predicted them for individuals over 40. A new formula has been developed, and it is this newer version that will be used in the examples in this book. (Please note, however, that at this time, both formulas are still being used by professionals in the exercise field.) The new formula is as follows:

$$207 - (0.7 \times age) = MHR$$

By this formula, a 20-year-old will have a MHR of 193 bpm.

$$207 - (0.7 \times 20) = 207 - 14 = 193 \text{ bpm}$$

MAXIMUM HEART-RATE FORMULA (ZERO TO PEAK FORMULA)

Now that you know how to calculate your maximum heart rate, you can use the maximum heart-rate formula to develop a training range. You will want to pick a percentage range that matches the intensity level at which you wish to exercise. For example, for moderate intensity, the percentage range is 64% to 76% of HRmax. You can calculate using these numbers or round them off a bit. If you feel the right intensity for you is between light and moderate (see Table 4.2), you can calculate a range of 60% to 70%. Or perhaps you are ready for a vigorous workout, in which case the range is 77% to 95%. You might choose 75% to 85% to start and then work up to the higher end of the range. The key is to individualize it to your present fitness level and then challenge yourself a little (overload) if you want to improve your aerobic fitness.

The THR for a 20-year-old person is calculated below using a vigorous intensity range of 75% to 85%. A space for figuring your THR is provided online at www.pearsonhighered.com/bishopaerobics and at the back of this book on Worksheet 4.1. The HRmax is figured first, then the low end of the range, followed by the high end of the range.

STEP ONE	STEP TWO	STEP THREE
207	193	193
− (0.7 × 20)	× .75	× .85
193	144.75	164.05
(HRmax)	(lower limit of THR)	(upper limit of THR)

Rounding off, the THR for this individual is 145 to 164 beats per minute.

In most fitness classes, the heart rate is taken for 10 seconds (as described in the How Long Should You Count Your Pulse during Exercise? box later in this chapter). You can translate your beats per minute to beats per 10 seconds by dividing the top and bottom of the range by 6.

STEP FOUR

$$\frac{145}{6} = 24.2$$

STEP FIVE

$$\frac{164}{6} = 27.3$$

The THR = 24 to 27 beats/10 seconds.

If this were your range, and if you took your pulse during class and found it to be below 24, you would want to increase the intensity of your movements; but if your pulse were above 27, you would want to bring it down a little. And if the pulse were between those numbers? Perfect; keep going.

KARVONEN FORMULA

In the Karvonen formula, percentages of the heart-rate reserve (HRR) are calculated. The HRR is the HRmax minus the RHR in beats per minute. The RHR is added back in after a percentage of the HRR has been calculated. As described with the previous formula, you should select a range that fits your fitness level and goal. See Table 4.1. For example, someone wishing to do a vigorous workout but not at the high end of the range might choose 60% to 80% instead of the full 60% to 89%. This is, in fact, one of the most common ranges used for healthy adults who are ready for vigorous activity and is the range used in the example that follows. But, before you can use the Karvonen formula, you need to know your true RHR. To do this, you have to be lying down for 30 minutes or more. One of the best times to count your RHR is first thing in the morning before you get up. If you have been jarred awake by your alarm clock, relax for a few minutes. Then count your heartbeats by taking your pulse for a full minute. Do this on two or three different days, and then average your results. For example, if you count 70, 73, and 68 over three days, your average RHR would be $(70 + 73 + 68)/3 = 70.3$.

The example of the Karvonen formula that follows is for a 20-year-old with a resting heart rate of 75 beats per minute (bpm). (Notice that the HRmax calculation is the same as that used in the previous formula.) The range is calculated first in beats per minute and then converted to beats per 10 seconds. A space for figuring your THR is provided online at www.pearsonhighered.com/bishopaerobics and at the back of this book on Worksheet 4.2. The HRmax is figured first, then the

low end of the range, followed by the high end of the range.

STEP ONE	**STEP TWO**
207	193
− (0.7 × 20)	− 75
193 (MHR)	118 (HRR)

STEP THREE	**STEP FOUR**
118	70.8
× .60	+ 75
70.8	145.8 (lower limit THR in bpm)

STEP FIVE	**STEP SIX**
118	94.4
× .80	+ 75
94.4	169.4 (upper limit THR in bpm)

Figure 4.1 illustrates how both formulas have yielded similar ranges, even though the calculations were done using different percentages, 75% to 85% and 60% to 80%. This is because the two formulas are taking percentages of two different things: HRmax and HRR.

TAKING YOUR PULSE

When you press gently on an **artery**, you can feel the pulsing of the blood as it is pushed through the arteries by the heart. The arteries most commonly used for

Figure 4.1 (a) THR calculated using the Karvonen formula for a 20-year-old with 75 bpm for RHR. (b) THR calculated using the maximum heart-rate formula for a 20-year-old.

Scan to view video ▲

Figure 4.2 Radial artery.

Scan to view video ▲

Figure 4.3 Carotid artery.

taking the pulse during exercise are the radial and carotid arteries.

The **radial artery** is located on the inside of your wrist. You can feel it beside your forearm tendons on the thumb side (Figure 4.2). The **carotid artery** is just to the side (either side) of your voice box (larynx). You can feel it in the valley between your Adam's apple and your neck muscles (Figure 4.3).

To feel your pulse, use two fingers to press gently but firmly on the artery. Do not use your thumb; it also has a pulse and will cause you to miscount. If you can't feel your pulse, you may be pressing too lightly or too hard. Pressing too hard on an artery squeezes it shut so that you can no longer feel any pulsing. Try different pressures while sitting quietly until you can feel and count your pulse easily. Then practice taking it while you move around the room. If you have a lot of trouble counting your pulse, place your hand over your heart and count beats.

Although most people can use the carotid site without experiencing any problems, a word of caution is in order. Special receptors located in the walls of the carotid artery are responsible for detecting changes in pressure. If you put pressure on these baroreceptors while taking your pulse (or massage them while looking for your pulse), they send a message to the heart to slow down. This slowing heart rate can cause dizziness or faintness in some people. If your heart rate does slow down, your pulse count will not be accurate. Try taking your pulse at both your carotid and radial sites. If you find the carotid gives you a slower count, use the radial site.

When taking your pulse, count complete cardiac cycles. A pulse throb constitutes the end of a cardiac cycle. If the instructor says "go" and you immediately feel a throb, don't count it (or, call it zero). If the instructor says "go" and there is a pause and then a beat, go ahead and count it as number 1. Continue to count until the instructor stops you.

OTHER HEART RATES

Other heart rates in addition to the EHR are useful to monitor and compare. For example, the RHR is a useful indicator of cardiorespiratory fitness. As your fitness improves, your heart becomes stronger and your circulatory system more efficient. This means that your heart can beat fewer times per minute and still accomplish the same amount of work. Think of how many times you have to work the handle on an inefficient pump to get a gallon of water compared to the number of times you have to work the handle on an efficient pump. Your heart acts like a pump. As your heart and circulatory system improve, you will be able to see a decline in your RHR. Remember the principle of individuality; some people's RHRs will decline quickly and dramatically, while those of others will hardly decline at all. You can take your RHR periodically to see whether it is declining.

Besides heredity and exercise, a number of other factors influence the RHR. Medication, illness, stress,

HOW LONG SHOULD YOU COUNT YOUR PULSE DURING EXERCISE?

This is a great question that deserves more than a simple answer. If you have been exercising and stop to count your pulse, your heart rate will stay at the exercise rate for about 15 seconds, after which it starts to drop off fairly quickly. Therefore, it is important to complete your count within 15 seconds. It takes most people about 5 seconds to find their pulse, leaving about 10 seconds available for a pulse count.

Some people like to take a 6-second count because this can be converted to beats per minute simply by multiplying by 10. For example, if in 6 seconds I count 15 beats, my heart rate is 150 bpm. The only problem with this is that it is easy to miscount by 1 or 2 beats. If you are multiplying by 10, your possible error is 10 to 20 beats. If instead you use a 10-second count and multiply by 6, you drop your possible error to 6 to 12 beats. **Most professionals recommend the 10-second count.** This, however, means that you would need to multiply your result by 6 if you want to know your heart rate in beats per minute. Most of us are not as comfortable doing that while exercising. The solution: Simply divide your training range by 6; that way, you know how many beats to look for in the 10-second count.

overtraining, temperature, caffeine, and smoking are a few of the major influences. Because many of these influences are transient, you probably won't pick them up in a morning RHR reading. They will, however, often show up in a heart rate taken right before class. For example, your **pre-exercise heart rate (PreHR)** can be elevated if you are still digesting a meal, just drank a cup of caffeinated coffee or a can of soda, ran to class, or are anxious about a test in the next class. Take your PreHR before you begin exercising, plot it on the chart provided in Worksheet 4.3, available online at www.pearsonhighered.com/bishopaerobics, and see whether you can identify reasons for any fluctuations you discover.

Another useful heart rate to monitor is your **recovery heart rate (RecHR),** which reflects the speed with which your cardiorespiratory system can return to its pre-exercise state after you stop exercising. It is often used as an indicator of fitness because a physically fit person with an efficient cardiorespiratory system recovers from exercise more quickly than an unfit person exercising at the same intensity. The heart rate drops rapidly during the first minute of recovery, then more slowly, and gradually drops to normal. A good guideline is to be able to return to a heart rate below 120 bpm within 2 minutes. If you are not below 120 bpm in 5 minutes, your THR is probably too high for your fitness level. (You may also have performed too active a cool-down.) Continue to cool down until your pulse is below 120 bpm.

To monitor your RecHR, take your pulse immediately after the aerobic portion of class and again 1 minute later. Record your RecHR on the chart provided in Worksheet 4.3. Your instructor may want to use a 2-, 3-, or 5-minute recovery time instead of a 1-minute time. Any recovery time will work as long as you are consistent, although more fit people may want to use the shorter times because most of their recovery will occur in the first 2 minutes. You should see an improved recovery rate after about 6 to 12 weeks of aerobic conditioning.

Keeping track of these heart rates can make you more aware of the kinds of things (exercise, stress, caffeine, and others) that affect your body. Figure 4.4 is an example of a heart rate chart in progress for a 20-year-old individual. The THR is drawn in bold lines. The PreHR, EHR, and RecHR have been recorded for each exercise session. Lines connecting the same types of heart rates have been drawn to make it easier to see the trends. Some trends to look for include a more consistent EHR with practice, a lower RecHR over time, and an increased ability to work in the upper portion of the THR.

ALTERNATIVE METHODS OF MONITORING INTENSITY

A Swedish physiologist named Gunnar Borg discovered a relationship between the perception of exercise intensity and heart rate. He developed the **ratings of perceived exertion (RPE)** scales referenced in Table 4.2 on page 38. To use these scales, you look at the numbers and word descriptions and select the number that best represents how hard you feel (perceive) you are exercising. An aerobic training effect is associated with perceived exertion ratings of "somewhat hard" to "hard," approximately 12 to 16 on the original category scale and ratings of 4 to 5 on the category-ratio

Figure 4.4 Heart rate chart in progress.

SELECTING A HEART-RATE MONITOR

Heart-rate monitors have improved significantly and the cost of good ones has dropped, thus making them a more affordable tool for individuals embarking on an aerobics program. They generally consist of a lightweight wireless transmitter that is worn comfortably and securely around the chest (below the bustline) that picks up the heartbeat and sends a signal to a watchlike receiver worn on the wrist where it displays heart rate in beats per minute. Other versions make use of technology that measures heart rate by finger touch on the wrist receiver, but these are generally less accurate. A good monitor will track total exercise time, time in your training zone, and average heart rate. It will also have an alarm that lets you know when you drop below or exceed your training zone. More expensive models include more options, such as a calorie counter, data storage, and an improved ability to screen out heart-rate signals from other nearby monitors.

A heart-rate monitor is only as good as the formulas and information in its memory. A monitor that allows you to input information such as your resting heart rate, height, weight, gender, and age will be more accurate than one that does not. Although these devices are great training tools that offer immediate feedback and reinforcement, they are by no means necessary equipment for an aerobic workout. Heart rate can be monitored accurately and easily just by counting your pulse. Finger and earlobe monitors that you may encounter on older fitness equipment are not reliable.

---

scale. Research evidence indicates that the RPE scale is an effective way for adults to monitor aerobic intensity as long as standardized instructions are used to introduce it.

One big advantage of ratings of perceived exertion is that they can be used to monitor exercise intensity when heart rate is not reliable. If, for example, you are on a medication that affects heart rate, or if you aren't good at taking a pulse count, RPE can be a good method for estimating workout intensity. If your heart rate is a valid way to estimate intensity, you may want to compare heart rates with ratings of perceived exertion to see where your training range falls on the RPE scales.

The OMNI scale (Figure 4.5) also uses ratings of perceived exertion, but in contrast to the Borg scales, it has pictures of exertion and slightly different anchor words. (There are also OMNI scales for resistance exercise and scales for children as well as adults.) On the adult cardiovascular OMNI scale, low-fit beginners will want to aim for about 5, which falls between "somewhat easy" and "hard." For moderately fit individuals, 5 to 6 is a good goal, and for those with good fitness, 6 to 7 is appropriate. Highly fit and competitive individuals may choose to work at hard to very hard levels (8 to 10). You can use the scale to rate your overall perceptions of effort, or you can use the scale to focus on body parts. The latter might be useful for activities such as spinning, for which you could rate the legs as well as overall sensation.

Figure 4.5 OMNI Scale.

Another quick, easy (and less scientific) method for estimating intensity is the talk test. You should be able to talk comfortably while working out. If you can't, your workout intensity is too high. If you can sing comfortably, your intensity is probably too low.

WHEN TO MONITOR INTENSITY

Using the pulse check, the RPE or OMNI scale, or the talk test, you can monitor your level of exertion periodically during your workout. It is a good idea to check your intensity level 5 to 10 minutes into the aerobic workout to make sure you have reached your training intensity. Check again at the peak of the aerobic section to make sure you aren't too high. Check once again toward the end of the aerobic section to see whether you were able to maintain the training intensity to the end. If you check your intensity only at the end of class and find that you are too high or too low, it is too late to modify your workout. In addition, your finishing heart rate may not be indicative of the intensity of your entire workout.

TIME

Time, or the duration of exercise, is linked with intensity. Together they need to result in the burning of enough calories to meet health, fitness, and weight management goals. The total volume of exercise is important. You can burn the same number of calories by exercising at a low intensity for a longer duration or a high intensity for a short duration.

The ACSM recommends that most adults engage in 30 to 60 minutes of purposeful moderate exercise a day (5 or more days a week), or 20- to 60-minute sessions of vigorous exercise a day (3 or more days a week), or a similar duration of a combination of moderate and vigorous exercise. Less than 20 minutes a day may be beneficial for lower-fit individuals. The length of time can be achieved in more than one way; it can be continuous (all in a row) or broken up into smaller amounts of 10 minutes or more. For example, a 30-minute workout can be done in one 30-minute session or in three 10-minute sessions. Individuals who like the "weekend warrior" pattern of physical activity can also gain some health benefits if they accumulate enough minutes of activity, but this pattern is more prone to injury and less effective for weight loss.

Recent studies show that being sedentary for long periods of time is bad for everyone, fit or not. The solution is to break up long periods of sedentary activities such as watching television or working at the computer by periodically standing or walking. The bottom line is that we need to move to be healthy. Those of us who fidget and can't sit still may have an advantage here!

In addition, Dr. Kenneth Cooper, director of the Institute for Aerobics Research in Dallas, Texas, recommends limiting running to 80 to 90 minutes a week at 3 times a week for 30 minutes or 4 times a week for 20 minutes. He believes that the additional benefits gained by running more (other than additional weight loss) do not outweigh the increased risk of bone, joint, and muscle injury.

Because the impact stress in high-impact aerobic dance exercise is equal to or greater than that of running, it makes sense to limit a high-impact aerobic segment to 20 to 30 minutes per session. If you want to exercise aerobically for a longer duration, you can supplement aerobic dance-style exercise with a non-impact, low-impact, or non-weight-bearing activity. Activities such as a brisk walk can be done for up to an hour with little worry of overuse injury. Individuals, such as competitors and instructors, who choose to perform moderate- to high-intensity aerobics for more than 30 minutes, do so for reasons other than health.

EXERCISE LEVELS

Individuals who have not been exercising regularly, who are returning to exercise after childbirth or an injury, or who are substantially overweight (overfat) should start exercising at the low end of the target zones. For some beginners, even threshold amounts of exercise may be too much of an overload. In this event, start with small, manageable workout segments, 3 to 10 minutes long. Start with walking, cycling, swimming, or easy dance steps, and work up to more formal exercise routines. To overload, first increase the frequency of the short bouts, and then start to increase duration by putting short bouts together. When you can exercise for 20 to 30 minutes, overload by increasing intensity. Longer durations may be advantageous for weight loss. (See Chapter 13 for more information on weight management.) As you become more fit, you will find that you have to use more arm work and larger ranges of motion to challenge your aerobic system. Big movements are recommended, but avoid the use of momentum and do not overextend the limits of your flexibility.

Research has shown that aerobic dance activity results in cardiorespiratory training similar to that of jogging and cycling. However, physiologists have not yet determined whether regular aerobic dance activity can train and maintain very high fitness levels. If you are interested in a competitive level of aerobic conditioning, you may have to combine aerobic dance training with other forms of aerobic exercise. I have had a few highly fit runners in my classes who, even with vigorous movement, were unable to reach the upper ranges of their THR. These individuals used aerobic dance exercise for light workout days and change of pace, while everyone else worked up a heavy sweat! Step aerobics, particularly with power moves, can probably challenge even the most fit. Advanced participants, give it a try!

SUMMARY

Aerobic physical activity is strongly linked to good health and allows you to enjoy many daily activities, recreational activities, and sport activities with good stamina. To obtain the health benefits associated with aerobic activity, the most important factor is to accumulate enough minutes of it. Most adults should build up to a minimum of 150 minutes of moderate-intensity physical activity a week or 75 minutes of vigorous-intensity physical activity, or a combination of moderate and vigorous activity, preferably spread out over the week. Additional health/fitness benefits can be obtained by boosting these numbers to 300 and 150 minutes a week, respectively. The minutes can be accrued in a variety of patterns, but in general, for moderate-intensity activity, the recommendation is 30 to 60 minutes per session on at least 5 days a week. For vigorous activity, the recommendation is 20 to 60 minutes per session on at least 3 days a week. Deconditioned individuals may see improvements even if they do less than these minimums. Either continuous exercise or multiple intervals of 10 minutes or more can be used.

The intensity of activity can be measured several ways. The most direct, but least practical for group fitness, is monitoring oxygen consumption. Heart rate is a useful estimate of oxygen consumption and is a good and practical way to monitor exercise, as long as the heart rate is not being influenced by caffeine, medications, or other factors. Ratings of perceived exertion (Borg scale and OMNI scale) and the talk test are also good tools for monitoring intensity. The more fit you are, the more intensely you have to work out to improve your aerobic fitness. Individuals should first strive to accumulate minutes and only then increase intensity.

For a person engaging in high-impact movements such as running and high-impact aerobic dance, it is suggested that duration be limited to 20 to 30 minutes. Longer aerobic workouts can be safely performed if low-impact or nonimpact activities are used alone, or in combination with, high-impact activities. The bottom line is that any amount of aerobic activity will benefit you, but more is better—within reason, of course.

COMMONLY ASKED QUESTIONS

Is it safe for a fit person's heart rate to exceed the age-related training heart rate zone?

Remember that the THR is calculated based on averages. It is possible that an individual has a higher maximum heart rate than the estimate derived from the formula. If this is true, then it would make sense to raise the THR. Perceived exertion can be considered in this case. As long as the person is healthy and it "feels" right, the zone can be adjusted upward. Recovery rates can also be used to help reestablish a zone.

Can I achieve aerobic conditioning if I am not in the zone?

If you are a low-fit individual, you can achieve aerobic conditioning at the lower intensities, as discussed in the text. Too low a level will not result in aerobic fitness changes but may still provide some health-related benefits. Moderately vigorous physical activity, such as brisk walking, results in health benefits.

I have trouble finding my pulse. What should I do?

Try locating your pulse at the wrist, neck, and temple. Practice this outside class for a couple of days. If you are still unsuccessful, try putting your hand on your chest and counting beats. If you are still unsuccessful, try the talk test and/or ratings of perceived exertion. A heart-rate monitor would also solve the problem.

I am highly fit and can't get my heart rate high in my zone. What can I do?

Use propulsion steps, travel more, raise and lower your center of gravity as much as possible, and use arm movements with every step. Ask your instructor for specific modifications. Also, remember you can achieve a good workout in the middle of the zone.

Other questions pertaining to fat burning can be found in Chapter 8.

KNOWLEDGE TIPS

1. Participants can monitor the intensity of an aerobic workout using heart rate (pulse) counts, ratings of perceived exertion the OMNI scale, or the talk test.

2. To obtain an EHR, the pulse should be counted for 10 seconds using the radial or carotid site within 15 seconds of stopping. If a heart-rate monitor is being used, heart rate can be checked while exercising.

3. Participants should monitor their intensity several times during the workout to make sure they are working in their aerobic target zone.

4. The best measures of oxygen consumption and MHR are obtained through direct measurement during a graded exercise stress test (on a treadmill, stationary bicycle, or other ergonomic device).

5. Heart rate and oxygen consumption have a nearly linear relationship.

6. The Karvonen formula (heart-rate reserve formula) estimates THR using age and resting heart rate. The intensity range is often calculated as 60% to 80% of HRR. However, less fit individuals can use 50% to 60% of HRR.

7. The MHR formula estimates THR by taking a direct percentage of the MHR. The intensity range is often calculated as 70% to 85% of the MHR. However, less fit individuals can use 60% to 70% of MHR.

8. Ratings of perceived exertion can be used to monitor intensity and are particularly useful when heart rate is not a reliable or valid indicator of intensity.

9. The RHR and RecHR are also useful indicators of fitness.

10. Exercise frequency and duration will vary depending on your goal, fitness level, and available time. Minutes of activity can be accrued in short bouts of 10 minutes or in longer bouts. Shorter bouts will need a higher frequency rate to reach the recommended minutes. Higher fit individuals who can do longer (and more intense) bouts will have lower frequencies (i.e., once a day for 3–5 days a week). Athletes add additional training sessions and longer bouts for more extensive conditioning.

THINK ABOUT IT

1. What is the FITT principle for aerobic exercise? Explain how it is adjusted based on fitness level.

2. Identify and explain three methods of estimating (monitoring) intensity during aerobic activity. What is the target zone using each method?

3. Why are there two different heart-rate formulas for estimating the aerobic target zone?

4. Explain how to properly count one's pulse.

5. When should you monitor the intensity of your workout? How often?

6. If weight loss is the primary goal, how does this influence the FITT principle?

7. Explain how a person performing movements at a low level (low amplitude, smaller ranges of motion, low impact) and a person performing movements at a high level (propulsion moves, jumping, etc.) can both be working within their target heart-rate zones.

8. How can two people be performing the same exercise at the same tempo (jumping jacks on a beat) and one person have a higher heart rate than the other person?

9. If a person is over his or her target zone, what kinds of adjustment can be made to get into zone? (*Hint:* There are ways to stay on the beat and still make adjustments.)

10. What are the implications of being below, in, and above your aerobic target zone?

REFERENCES

American College of Sports Medicine. "The Recommended Quantity and Quality of Exercise for Developing and Maintaining Cardiorespiratory and Muscle Fitness in Healthy Adults." *Medicine and Science in Sports and Exercise* 30 (No. 6, 1998): 975–91.

American College of Sports Medicine. "The Recommended Quantity and Quality of Exercise for Developing and Maintaining Cardiorespiratory, Musculoskeletal, and Neuromotor Fitness in Apparently Healthy Adults: Guidance for Prescribing Exercise." *Medicine and Science in Sports and Exercise* 43 (No. 7, 2011):1334–1359.

Åstrand, P. O., and K. Rodahl. *Textbook of Work Physiology.* 2nd ed. New York: McGraw-Hill, 1977.

Bell, J. M., and E. J. Bassey. "A Comparison of the Relation Between Oxygen Uptake and Heart Rate During Different Styles of Aerobic Dance and a Traditional Step Test in Women." *European Journal of Applied Physiology* 68 (No. 1, 1994): 20–4.

Borg, G. *Borg's Perceived Exertion and Pain Scales.* Champaign, IL: Human Kinetics, 1998.

___. "Psychophysical Bases of Perceived Exertion." *Medicine and Science in Sports and Exercise* 14 (No. 5, 1982): 377–81.

Cearly, M., R. Moffatt, and K. Knutzen. "The Effects of Two- and Three-Day-per-Week Aerobic Dance Programs on Maximal Oxygen Uptake." *Research Quarterly for Exercise and Sport* 55 (1984):172–4.

Cooper, K. H. *Aerobics.* New York: Bantam Books, 1968.

Couldry, W., C. B. Corbin, and A. Wilcox. "Carotid vs. Radial Pulse Counts." *The Physician and Sportsmedicine* 10 (No. 12, 1982): 67–72.

Foster, C. "Physiological Requirements of Aerobic Dancing." *Research Quarterly* 46 (1975):120–2.

Garber, C. E., J. S. McKinney, and R. A. Carleton. "Is Aerobic Dance an Effective Alternative to Walk-Jog Exercise Training?" *Journal of Sports Medicine and Physical Fitness* 32 (No. 2, 1992): 136–41.

Gellish, R. L., B. R. Goslin, R. E. Olson, A. McDonald, G. D. Russi, and V. K. Moudgil. "Longitudinal Modeling of the Relationship Between Age and Maximal Heart Rate." *Medicine and Science in Sports and Exercise* 39 (No. 5, 2007): 822–9.

Hooper, P. L., and B. J. Noland. "Aerobic Dance Program Improves Cardiovascular Fitness in Men." *The Physician and Sportsmedicine* 12 (No. 5, 1984): 132–5.

Igbanugo, V. and B. Gutin. "The Energy Cost of Aerobic Dancing." *Research Quarterly* 49 (1978): 308–15.

Jackson, A. S. "Estimating Maximum Heart Rate from Age: Is It a Linear Relationship?" *Medicine and Science in Sports and Exercise* 39 (No. 5, 2007): 821.

Karvonen, M., E. Kentala, and O. Mustalof. "The Effects of Training on Heart Rate: A Longitudinal Study." *Annales de Medicinae Experimentalis et Biologiae Fenniae* 35 (1957): 307–15.

Koltyn, K. F., and W. P. Morgan. "Efficacy of Perceptual Versus Heart Rate Monitoring in the Development of Endurance." *British Journal of Sports Medicine* 26 (No. 2, June 1992): 132–4.

Lind, A. R., and G. W. McNichol. "Cardiovascular Responses to Holding and Carrying Weights by Hand and by Shoulder Harness." *Journal of Applied Physiology* 25 (1968): 261–7.

Mahurin, J., and T. P. Martin. "Anaerobic Threshold: A Trainable Component of Cardiovascular Fitness." *Motor Skills: Theory Into Practice* 6 (1982): 41.

McArdle, W., L. Zwiren, and J. R. Magel. "Validity of the Postexercise Heart Rate as a Means of Estimating Heart Rate During Work of Varying Intensities." *Research Quarterly* 40 (1969): 523–8.

Parker, S. B., B. F. Hurley, D. P. Hanlon, and P. Vaccaro. "Failure of Target Heart Rate to Accurately Monitor Intensity During Aerobic Dance." *Medicine and Science in Sports and Exercise* 21 (1989): 230–4.

Pollock, M. L. "How Much Exercise Is Enough?" *The Physician and Sportsmedicine* 6 (No. 6, 1978): 50–6; 58–60; 63–4.

Reeves., B. D., and L. A. Darby. "Physiological Responses of Female Experienced and Novice Aerobic Dancers During Graded Exercise Tests: Treadmill vs. Dance Exercise." (Abstract). *Medicine and Science in Sports and Exercise* 24 (1992, Suppl.): S97.

Reeves, B. D., L. A. Darby, C. L. Moss, and C. Armstrong. "Energy Costs and Vertical Forces of High-Impact and Low-Impact Aerobic Dance Sequences." (Abstract). *Research Quarterly for Exercise and Sport* 63 (1992, Suppl.): A28.

Robertson, R. *Perceived Exertion for Practitioners: Rating Effort with the OMNI Picture System*. Champaign, IL: Human Kinetics, 2004.

Schaeffer, S. A., L. A. Darby, K. D. Browder, and B. D. Reeves. "Perceived Exertion and Metabolic Responses of Women During Aerobic Dance Exercise." *Perceptual Motor Skills* 81 (No. 2, 1995): 691–700.

Scharff-Olson, M., H. N. Williford, and F. H. Smith. "The Heart Rate VO$_2$ Relationship of Aerobic Dance: A Comparison of Target Heart Rate Methods." *Journal of Sports Medicine and Physical Fitness* 32 (No. 4, 1992): 372–7.

Skinner, J. S., R. Hursler, V. Bergsteinova, and E. R. Buskirk. "The Validity and Reliability of a Rating Scale of Perceived Exertion." *Medicine and Science in Sports* 5 (No. 2, 1973): 94–6.

Tanaka, H., K. D. Monahan, and D. R. Seals. "Age-Predicted Maximal Heart Rate Revisited." *Journal of American College of Cardiology* 37 (2001): 153–6.

U.S. Department of Health and Human Services. *2008 Physical Activity Guidelines for Americans*. U.S. Department of Health and Human Services, 2008.

5

Setting Goals and Reaching Your Dream

"Habit is a cable; we weave a thread of it each day, and at last we cannot break it."

HORACE MANN

- I set goals but don't seem to reach them. What should I do differently?
- How can I track and measure my progress?
- What will keep me motivated?

DO you dream of looking svelte, sporting beautifully toned muscles, living longer, and feeling radiantly full of energy? Millions of people do, and they enroll in exercise classes, buy fancy outfits and expensive equipment, and talk enthusiastically about the fun and benefits. Then, within 6 months, 30% to 70% of these people drop out of their program. Even many former varsity athletes and coaches who have spent most of their lives promoting fitness are overweight (overfat) and out of shape. According to *Healthy People 2020*, more than 80% of adults do not meet the guidelines for both aerobic and muscle strengthening. The irony is that while 80% of adults don't exercise enough (25% don't exercise at all), most have a good attitude about exercise and think it would be a good thing for them to do.

Why, then, do so many people quit exercising or never get started? Physical educators, fitness specialists, and exercise scientists have been trying to answer that question. While there is still much to learn, there is substantial information we can put to work. The reasons that people don't start are usually different from the reasons people quit. You have already conquered all the barriers that keep people from starting (congratulations!), so this chapter will focus on how to keep your commitment to exercise going—for a lifetime.

Now, let's back up for a moment. If you have dreams, the first thing you need to do to turn those dreams into realities is establish some very specific, realistic goals. Many times people have an idea of what they want but don't take the time to nail it down.

And sometimes what we want is media driven rather than realistic. There is not one beautiful body type; there are many. Therefore, individualize your goals to bring your body type to its full potential and to attain personal health. Writing goals will be the first step in reaching your dream. Step two is to find and use sources of motivation. Third, select an activity (or activities) that will help you reach your goals. Because you are already in a group fitness course, let's hope it is the right vehicle for reaching at least some of your goals. Fourth, establish a method for measuring your progress. Fifth, set up a periodic review of your goals and program to make sure they still reflect what you wish to accomplish. And finally, identify barriers, supports, and strategies to prevent relapses and to help you restart if you do temporarily stop exercising.

As you take these steps, you will be using the behavior change strategies introduced in Chapter 1. Reaching a goal usually involves change, and behavior change doesn't happen easily or by sheer willpower alone. These strategies will support your efforts and make success a little easier to reach.

STEP ONE: ESTABLISHING YOUR FITNESS GOALS

THE BASIS FOR YOUR GOALS

A goal is a statement of what you want to happen. Base your fitness goals on what you would like to accomplish through an exercise program. Write down any ideas that come to mind. In addition to basing your goals on personal desire, you can use the five health-related fitness components—cardiorespiratory endurance, muscular strength and endurance, flexibility, and body composition—as guidelines.

Set your goals using personal interest (desire); fitness test results; and knowledge of what is realistic, feasible, and healthy. Guidelines in this chapter, information in other parts of this book, fitness test scores, and guidance from your instructor will help you to refine the goals you identify and to select goals you may not have considered.

This chapter focuses on physical fitness goals. Some very valuable goals cannot be measured by fitness tests or, in some cases, cannot be adequately tested for at all. Your list might also include some of these goals, such as increased social involvement, improvement of self-concept, improvement of self-confidence, achievement of relaxation, and having fun. You can often measure progress toward goals such as these by keeping a journal. For example, if your goal is to have more energy and be more productive, then keeping a journal that tracks your accomplishments and how you feel at the end of a day will give you an idea of how you are progressing.

SPECIFIC GOALS

When asked to write down their goals for the semester, the majority of college students write things such as:

- lose weight
- lose inches
- last longer in the class
- look better
- become more fit
- firm up my body

The ideas expressed provide a good starting point, but they are ambiguous; there are no concrete ways to measure success. For example, does the loss of one pound constitute success? Does looking better mean an attractive appearance or how you look doing the exercises? Does lasting longer mean during the muscle-toning exercises, aerobic exercises, or both? At what point is the body firm?

These goals can be rewritten to be more specific. They might read like this:

- lose 10 pounds (lbs) in the next 10 weeks (a safe 1-lb loss per week)
- lose 1 inch from each thigh, my waist, and my hips by the end of the semester
- complete 20 minutes of aerobics at 60% to 80% of my maximum heart rate by the end of 6 weeks

- tone and firm my legs, as represented by losing 1 inch from my thighs and being able to do 15 leg lifts in a row with a medium-weight exercise band by the end of the semester
- complete all 3 minutes of the step test by the end of 6 weeks
- improve my curl-up score from a poor rating to an average rating in 8 weeks

These very specific goals can be measured, full or partial success can be noted and celebrated, and new goals can be set. Information throughout this book will help you identify specific goals.

REALISTIC GOALS

Beginners and overzealous participants have a tendency to choose unrealistic goals. When you set goals that are too difficult, you set yourself up for failure. Yet, goals that are too easy aren't very motivating. Three guidelines for writing challenging and yet attainable goals are (1) allow enough time to reach the goal, (2) set safe goals, and (3) base goals on correct information.

1. Positive adaptations do not occur overnight. It usually takes 6 to 8 weeks to make significant cardiorespiratory and muscular gains. It can take longer to strengthen ligaments, bones, and tendons. Be patient, and write your goals with time expectations of at least 6 to 8 weeks. People who expect quick results often quit the program before it has had a chance to work. Start with conservative goals so you have success early in the program.

2. To set safe goals, consider your medical history, your present condition, your age, and the amount of time that has passed since you last exercised. Set up a pace and program that are comfortable for you. There is no need to start out too fast and get stiff, sore, or injured. The idea is to have fun and feel good about exercising.

   Many unsafe goals arise from the desire to obtain quick results. For example, people who want very rapid weight loss starve themselves and, at the same time, attempt to attend an exercise class. Without a sufficient intake of carbohydrates, they don't have enough energy to exercise. They may feel listless, tired, dizzy, or even faint during class. Starvation diets result in significant loss of muscle and water, not just fat. The body may even start conserving and storing fat as an energy source because the caloric intake is so low.

3. Misconceptions can wreak havoc on goals. For example, a person with a goal of losing abdominal fat might embark on an intense program of curl-ups. When he or she can do 100 curl-ups a day yet finds the fat still there, discouragement is sure to set in. The problem is that fat is more readily lost through longer-duration exercise, usually aerobic in nature. The result of just doing curl-ups will be strong abdominal muscles hiding under a layer of fat. In addition, fat cannot be taken off in one specific spot (spot reduction); it comes off in a general way from all over the body.

Faulty reasoning can also be dangerous. There have been cases of pregnant women whose reason for exercising during pregnancy was to keep their figures. These women were trying to prevent normal weight gains; if allowed to continue, they would endanger the health of their babies. Pregnant women can benefit from exercise as long as it is done correctly and with the supervision of a doctor.

The best way to avoid making these kinds of mistakes is to read about fitness from reliable sources (books and articles written by professionals and materials published by recognized associations such as the American College of Sports Medicine, the National Academy of Sportsmedicine, the American College of Obstetricians and Gynecologists, the American Alliance for Health, Physical Education, Recreation, and Dance, and the National Strength and Conditioning Association) and to talk with professionals like your instructor.

It is also important to remember the principle of individuality as you try to set realistic goals. Two people on an identical exercise program will respond differently. It can be motivating to compare yourself against norms or averages or even classmates, but remember, the comparison that counts is you against you.

SHORT- AND LONG-RANGE GOALS

Take your dream, your long-range goal, and break it down into short-range goals. If your dream is to lose 3 inches off your waist, make short-term goals of 1/2 inch every 8 weeks. Reaching the short-term goal will give you the confidence and motivation to keep going. One step at a time will take you to your dream.

When you don't establish short-term goals, you set yourself up for total success or total failure: There is nothing in between. If reaching your goal takes a while and you have no intermediate steps of success to celebrate, it is easy to get discouraged and quit. Think of the people who climb Mt. Everest: They are pleased when they establish base camp, and they cheer as they establish each

successive camp up the mountain. Their goal is the summit, but they recognize that success comes in stages.

Fitness professionals can help you set realistic, specific goals, tell you what a realistic rate of achievement is, provide encouragement, and evaluate and adjust your program. These people are service oriented and want to help you. They are your instructor, physical fitness educators in your public and private schools, directors, exercise physiologists, trainers in fitness clubs, owners and directors of private fitness businesses, personal trainers, professors and instructors of fitness and wellness at colleges and universities, health promotions instructors and directors in the workplace, and instructors and coordinators at recreation centers, YMCAs/YWCAs, and corporate programs. Seek them out.

STEPS TO GOAL WRITING

1. In general terms, decide what you want to do.
2. Assess where you are right now.
3. Make your general goal more specific, using information from your assessment (Step 2).
4. Decide how you are going to accomplish your goal.
5. Add a time frame.
6. Write a very specific goal incorporating all the information from the first five steps.
7. Decide how you will evaluate/monitor your progress.

EXAMPLE

General Statement:	I want to lose weight.
Assessment:	Measure (or have a professional measure) my percentage of body fat.
More Specific Goal:	I want to move from 30% body fat to 24% body fat.
Plan (Mode):	I will combine three days of walking and three days of low-impact aerobics with my present weight-loss diet.
Time Frame:	I will lower my body fat by 6% in the next 6 weeks. (For a woman weighing 100 to 200 lbs, this represents a 6- to 12-lb loss, a 1- to 2-lb loss per week.)
Very Specific Goal:	I will lose 6% body fat in the next 6 weeks using 30 minutes of brisk walking on Tuesday, Thursday, and Saturday, and attending a low-impact aerobics class on Monday, Wednesday,

| | and Friday. I will combine this with my present 1,500-calorie balanced diet. |
| Evaluation of Progress: | I will have my body fat measured again in 6 weeks. |

STEP TWO: FINDING MOTIVATION

People usually start exercising to look good, but the main reason habitual exercisers give for continuing is that exercise feels good. Endorphins, hormonelike substances, are released during aerobic exercise; scientists believe that in addition to masking pain, endorphins are responsible for the uplifting feeling that follows a good workout. Unfortunately, many people just starting out have never felt this exercise "high" and can't identify with it. And since it takes 6 to 8 weeks to work into the exercise high, many quit before they experience this wonderful benefit.

In the beginning, you may feel a little stiff, sore, and awkward. The trick is to get past this discomfort so that you can experience the good feelings that come from exercise. When you do experience the exercise high, often accompanied by an increased sense of energy, you'll find it motivates you to keep on exercising.

There are two forms of motivation: intrinsic and extrinsic. **Intrinsic motivation** comes from inside you. If you exercise because you want to look and feel better, then you are intrinsically motivated. When you personally believe in something, you will be more motivated to do it than if someone else is telling you to do it. Find an exercise program that is taught in a style that you like, at a place you enjoy, and at a time and in a location that is convenient for you—aspects that support your intrinsic motivation. If you do this, you will be more likely to stick with your program. Positive talk is also a very powerful tool. Check into the conversation going on inside your head. Is it negative? Are you thinking of bad experiences with exercise? Or previous failures? Try to turn that around and get the little voice inside you to tell you that you can do it, that you are going to enjoy the new feelings that the program will generate. Also, try to picture yourself (visualize) doing the exercise well. During a quiet time, close your eyes and watch yourself (or feel yourself) go through the steps and exercises you've learned. Mental practice can actually make you better at physical activities. Many times, when people begin a new activity, they think that others are watching them and judging them. Get outside of yourself and look around—you will probably be relieved to see that other participants are busy trying to do the exercise and aren't looking at you at all. Be sure to give yourself some positive talk right after the workout. Reaffirm your goals, and congratulate yourself on taking one more step toward them. You can be your own best motivator.

You may already be one of those rare and wonderful people who has the internal desire and discipline to exercise all of your life. If so, fantastic! But if you are like most of us, you need the occasional proverbial "kick in the pants" to keep motivated. Motivation that comes from outside you is called **extrinsic motivation**. Here are a few sources of extrinsic motivation you can tap.

1. Find another person who also wants to exercise, and make a pact to meet at a designated place on workout days. Knowing the other person is waiting for you will get you there. Carpools with rotating drivers also provide an extra incentive to show up, especially if you are the driver.
2. Get the people around you—friends, family, and fellow employees—to support or join you in your exercise endeavors. Plan family outings that involve hiking, swimming, cycling, and other forms of exercise. Organize a college or worksite team to participate in a local road race or walkathon.
3. Find sources of feedback and reinforcement. Get to know your instructor, and find out if you are doing things correctly. A good instructor will be positive and upbeat, will provide feedback periodically, and will miss you when you are not there. It is much more difficult to miss a class when the instructor or participants are going to give you a hard time for not being there.
4. Write down your goals, and look at them periodically. Some people like to post their goals on their bathroom mirror or refrigerator door so they will see them often. Perhaps it will help you to tell someone about your goals, especially if that person is in a position to help you attain them. For example, your instructor may be able to introduce you to someone else with the same goal.
5. Set aside a specific time for your exercise, and let others know so that you won't be interrupted.
6. Do something nice for yourself and others when you reach a short-term goal.

7. Finally, accept that you will have lapses. We are all human. Illness, emergencies, vacation, or even boredom can take you temporarily off your program. It doesn't mean that you are a miserable failure. Just pick a date to begin again, and go forth with new resolve.

STEP THREE: CHOOSING THE ACTIVITY

If your goal is to be aerobically fit, you have a wide variety of activities from which to choose: aerobic dancing, walking, swimming, cycling, rowing, cross-country skiing, stair stepping, jumping rope, and many others. Select an activity you enjoy.

You can select one or more new activities. Using two or more activities in your exercise program is called cross-training. A lot of people find this prevents boredom. Doing things you enjoy will help you stick with exercise and make it a lifetime habit.

STEP FOUR: TRACKING YOUR PROGRESS

To measure progress, you must have a starting point; a good one is your present fitness level. You can measure it using one of the many fitness tests that have been developed over the years. Or if physical activity is your goal, you can use a pedometer to determine your baseline number of steps per day. (See the box Using a Pedometer on the following page.) The tests contained in this text were selected because of their relationship to the health-related fitness components. Table 5.1 is a list of these tests under their appropriate

Table 5.1 Fitness Tests

FITNESS TESTS	
Cardiorespiratory Endurance Tests	
Step Test	Worksheet 5.4
12-Minute Walk/Run	Worksheet 5.5
1.5-Mile Timed Run	Worksheet 5.6
Flexibility Tests	
Trunk Forward Flexion Test	Worksheet 7.1
Quick-Check Flexibility Tests	Worksheet 7.2
Muscular Strength and Endurance Tests	
Partial Curl-Up Test	Worksheet 10.1
Push-Up Test	Worksheet 10.2
Body Composition Tests	
Body Fat Assessments	Chapter 13
Healthy Weight Assessments	Worksheet 13.1

fitness component heading. Each test is described in detail on the designated worksheet available online at www.pearsonhighered.com/bishopaerobics and at the back of the book. The norms provided with these tests should give you a general idea of how well you scored. Don't be too concerned with the norms; it is more important to compare your scores at the beginning of a program to your scores later in the program.

Some fitness tests can be taken right at the beginning of a program. Other, more difficult tests, such as the 12-minute walk/run test and the 1.5-mile timed run test, should be taken only after you've been exercising for about 6 weeks. Retake the tests after about 8 to 12 weeks to see how you are progressing. It is very motivating to see tangible evidence of improvement. (You may even see improvement in 6 weeks, but don't be discouraged if it takes a little longer. Changes in cardiorespiratory endurance can take longer than improvements in muscular strength and endurance.) You may discover that you are very fit in one component and not so fit in another. Follow a program that lets you maintain your strengths and improve your weaknesses.

To track your progress, several worksheets have been provided online at www.pearsonhighered.com/bishopaerobics and/or with this text (in the worksheets section). Worksheet 3.1, available online, provides a place to record your fitness and healthy weight scores over several test periods. Worksheet 4.3, also available online, lets you plot your heart rates over time, including resting heart rate (RHR), so that you can look for trends such as a lowering in RHR over time. Worksheet 5.2, available online, is a fitness log on which you can track all of your physical activity and make comments about how you are feeling during or about the exercise/activity. The latter helps you to evaluate nonfitness but related goals like gaining self-confidence, finding new friends, and so on. Worksheet 5.3, also available online, helps you establish a baseline, set a goal, and track your steps using a pedometer. Keeping track of your progress can be both insightful and motivating.

STEP FIVE: EVALUATING THE PROGRAM AND YOUR GOALS

After you have been exercising for 8 to 12 weeks, it is important to take an objective look at your program to see if it is accomplishing what you intended. Look at your goals and at your most recent fitness test scores. If your goals also included things such as meeting new people, ask yourself how many new friends you have made or read back over your journal to look

USING A PEDOMETER

Pedometers are fun, inexpensive devices that help you track your physical activity by counting the number of steps you take. A popular goal for pedometer stepping is 10,000 steps a day for adults. Although having a 10,000-step goal can be fun to strive for, the best thing to do is find out how many steps you typically take and then challenge yourself to gradually take more. The following baseline and goal-setting approach is recommended:[1]

- A baseline count is determined by wearing the pedometer for 8 days (adults and adolescents) and determining the average number of steps/day.
- When the baseline average is determined, a 10% increase of steps is calculated and added to the baseline number every two weeks with an overall goal of achieving about 4,000 to 6,000 steps above the baseline.
- If your baseline is already 10,000 or more, you can set a higher step goal or simply maintain your baseline amount.
- Use Worksheet 5.3, available online at www.pearsonhighered.com/bishopaerobics to calculate your baseline and your goals and chart your steps.

NOTE: Ten thousand steps may not be the magic number. New research suggests that fewer than 10,000 steps may be enough to meet physical activity guidelines.[2] In addition, walking 10,000 steps does not necessarily mean walking at a moderate intensity, which is the basis for the physical activity guideline of 150 minutes per week. Recent research indicates that 100 steps per minute is a very rough approximation of moderate-intensity exercise.[3] Based on a review of research, ACSM suggests that it may be prudent to use both steps per minute and recommended durations of activity (e.g., taking 100 steps per minute for 30 minutes per session.)[4] To identify this pace, you can time yourself walking for 1 minute and then check your pedometer to see how many steps you have taken. Some pedometers have a steps per minute (SPM) feature that lets you keep track of how many minutes you have exercised at a designated step rate.

TESTING YOUR PEDOMETER

When you get your new pedometer home, give it a test run to make sure it is reasonably accurate.

- Walk or jog 100 steps and then look at the step count; a count within 2–3 steps is acceptable. (This is not an expensive piece of equipment, so it will likely not be "exact.")
- Most pedometer research is done using models with up to 2% error. Some models will have more error, and you can decide what is acceptable to you.

POSITIONING YOUR PEDOMETER

Position your pedometer on your waistline directly above (inline with) the right knee; the pedometer should sit vertically to react to the up and down motion of a step.

- Tilting of the pedometer can interfere with the counting mechanism. Tilt may be the result of a loose waistband or abdominal fat pushing down on the top of the pedometer.
- If the accuracy of your pedometer is more than a few steps off, try wearing it more to the right (slightly in front of, or over the hip); as a last resort, try placing it in the center of your back.
- Fasten the leash, if present, as this will save it from hitting the floor (or falling in the toilet—more common than you'd think!) if it comes off your waistband.

FEATURES

Traditional pedometers can count steps, convert steps to distance using stride length, calculate calories burned, estimate intensity using steps per minute (spm), and keep track of bouts of exercise at designated levels of exertion.

(continued)

---

[1] R. P. Pangrazi, A. Beighle, and C. L. Sidman. *Pedometer Power: Using Pedometers in School and Community.* Champaign, IL: Human Kinetics, 2003.

[2] "Quantity and Quality of Exercise for Developing and Maintaining Cardiorespiratory, Musculoskeletal, and Neuromotor Fitness in Apparently Healthy Adults: Guidance for Prescribing Exercise." *Medicine & Science in Sports & Exercise* 43 (No.7, 2011): 1334–59.

[3] Marshall, S. J., S. S. Levy, C. E. Tudor-Locke, F. W. Kolkhorst, K. M. Wooten, J. MingMing, C. A. Macera, and B. E. Ainsworth. "Translating Physical Activity Recommendations into a Pedometer-Based Step Goal: 3000 Steps in 30 Minutes." *American Journal of Preventive Medicine.* 36 (No. 5, 2009): 410–5.

[4] R. P. Pangrazi, A. Beighle, and C. L. Sidman, *Pedometer Power.*

ACCELEROMETER PEDOMETERS

Accelerometer pedometers are newer technology and have some advantages over traditional pedometers. They use a piezoelectric mechanism to count steps instead of a lever system, which means that they can count steps even when tilted. An accelerometer pedometer can count steps from inside a pocket, on a lanyard around the neck, or clipped on a waistband (the latter being the most accurate). They are quieter than traditional pedometers—no click-click as they count and they are better at not counting incidental movements such as when you cross your legs. Accelerometers can track steps, distance, calories burned and speed, activity patterns over the day, and some even estimate sleep patterns. They can also take input on an activity like swimming and translate it into steps. Depending on the style, the device can store a week or more of data and download information into software and apps. These devices tend to be more expensive than traditional spring or lever-style pedometers. One drawback is that an accelerometer pedometer recording an ongoing tally of movement might not allow you to reset to tally the steps taken for a single event such as a mile run. To get this information, you would have to record steps taken before an event and subtract it from steps taken after the event.

for patterns of improvement. If the results of your program don't indicate achievement toward your goals, something is wrong; change the goals, or change the program.

Sometimes goals change. For example, teenagers often base their goals on a desire to have an attractive body, while adults place more emphasis on weight control and a healthy body. As retirement approaches, people tend to shift their goals again, this time toward sociability and maintaining physical independence.

Keep your goals up-to-date, and adjust your program whenever your goals change.

Sometimes you don't follow your own exercise plan. Here are some examples of how this can happen:

- The instructor and class may have a plan (priorities) different from yours.
- You get injured and have to modify your plan.
- You don't like part of the plan and decide not to do it, or you don't have enough time to work at your whole plan. When these things happen, reassess your priorities and try to create a new exercise plan.

If the class you are in is different from what you expected and you cannot change classes, see if the instructor will let you individualize your workout enough to satisfy you both. For example, if you really want to develop strong abdominal muscles and the class emphasis is on leg work, see if you can do some abdominal exercises while the class continues with leg work.

When you aren't doing something because you dislike it, see if another exercise can accomplish the same thing. For instance, some people don't like or can't do push-ups. An arm-pushing exercise using an exercise band can be substituted. If no substitutes are practical, decide whether an exercise is important enough to you or your health to do it anyway.

In the event of injury, extend the time period on your goal and be patient. If you don't have enough time to work on your entire plan, determine your highest priorities and put time where you need it most.

Sometimes your personal exercise program isn't working. You may be using insufficient overloads or the wrong exercises. Check with your instructor or other fitness professionals for ideas.

In other cases, the program is working, but it is not reflected in the goals. Take, for example, a person whose goal is to lose weight. Eight weeks of aerobics later, she is discouraged because she has gained weight. Upon closer examination, however, she discovers that she has lost inches and has a lower percentage of body fat; she actually lost fat and gained muscle. Because muscle weighs more than fat, she gained weight. The program worked, but the evaluation tool she used (weighing herself versus a body fat measurement) did not reflect the improvement.

Sometimes, a new and better exercise program comes along. If you hear of a new program, find out if it is based on solid information and backed by people with good credentials. Exercise research generates new information, which results in new and sometimes better program ideas. For example, 40 years ago, it was thought that weight training would inhibit strength. Football players were not allowed to lift weights! Today we know that weight training is a good way to improve muscular strength, and it is being incorporated into group fitness classes through the use of dumbbells, bars, weighted balls, exercise bands, and stability balls. Be open-minded when it comes to new ideas, but beware of promises of instant success.

STEP SIX: PROTECTING YOUR COMMITMENT

Starting an exercise program takes initiative; sticking to one requires motivation and a good game plan—one that includes contingency plans. Even the most committed people can find themselves suddenly sidelined by an injury or illness. Other things that can disrupt your normal routine and interfere with an exercise program include vacations, business travel, pregnancy, emergencies, or helping others. Think for a minute and identify the things that could cause you to stop exercising—even for a day. These are called barriers, in this case, barriers toward continued exercise. Now decide how you can break through these barriers. Think about how you can prevent these situations, continue to exercise during certain conditions, or get started again once the disruptive situation has been resolved.

Some examples may make this clearer. When your college or university breaks for a holiday, do you stop exercising until after the break? If yes, how can you prevent this relapse? You could make arrangements to attend an exercise class with a parent at home, use a videotape, or get together with friends to play a sport like tennis. If you travel on business, try taking a brisk walk after checking in or before a meal, or bringing an exercise band and jump rope, or check to see whether the hotel has an exercise room. Some hotels have arrangements with nearby health clubs; you might even be able to take an aerobics class. There are a lot of exciting options for exercise on a vacation, everything from a jog on the beach to a brisk walk down Fifth Avenue. The key is to plan it into the vacation and, if others are involved, plan things you can do together. Try to include two to three fitness activities per week. If you find yourself talking with relatives all day, see if someone would like to walk and talk. If you are planning a pregnancy, look into special exercise programs now for later in the pregnancy. Also, set up a plan for returning to exercise following childbirth. Share these ideas with your physician.

When the flu season catches up with you, you will need to take some time off. Exercise is a stressor; while you are sick or injured, you need to let your body use its resources to make you well. Sometimes, caring for someone else through an illness or crisis can throw you off your exercise routine. In cases like these, you need some strategies for getting started again. When an instructor is marking you absent, that always provides motivation. But when you are no longer enrolled in a course, the motivation must come from within. Some people find that writing down a start date helps them. Others make a pact with someone else, and they start together. Or maybe setting out your exercise clothes is enough to get you going. Decide *now* what you will do if you stop or have to take a break.

Sustaining a wellness behavior like exercise can be difficult at times. Identifying strategies and people who will support you in your efforts gives you somewhere to turn when you feel your commitment wavering. A number of supports have already been discussed under the section on motivation. Positive reinforcement, feeling good about yourself, and having social support for what you are doing go a long way in staying motivated. When you are doing well, look around and see whether someone else needs a word of encouragement!

SUMMARY

Adhering to exercise can be a problem. You can protect your commitment to exercise by taking the time to identify goals, barriers, and supports. With the help of your instructor, determine your fitness goals and set up a plan of action. Make the plan specific and realistic, then stick with it. Check your progress, and celebrate improvement. Update your fitness plan throughout your life, and it will continue to bring you satisfaction and joy.

KNOWLEDGE TIPS

1. The dropout rate in exercise programs is between 30 and 70% within 6 months of beginning the program. Certain strategies may improve adherence.

2. Goals can be based on personal desires, fitness test scores, information from knowledgeable sources, and advice from professional educators.

3. Establish clear, specific, and (whenever possible) measurable goals.

4. For motivational purposes, break long-range goals into a series of short-range goals.

5. Intrinsic motivation comes from within yourself and is the most powerful form of motivation. Extrinsic motivation comes from outside sources. Use both.

6. Select exercise activities that will help you reach your goals. Vary these activities as needed.

7. Use fitness tests to measure your current fitness levels, and continue to check your progress using the same tests. Use journals to track your progress in nonfitness goals such as building self-confidence and making new friends.

8. Periodically evaluate your exercise goals and programs to make sure that they are up-to-date and complement each other.

9. Identify barriers and strategies to break through them. Plan how you will exercise during special situations such as vacations, business travel, and pregnancy.

10. Plan now what you will do to get yourself started again if you stop exercising in the future.

THINK ABOUT IT

1. Why is it so hard for people to attain their exercise goals?

2. Why is it helpful to set goals?

3. What are the qualities of good goals?

4. Give examples of intrinsic and extrinsic motivation. Which kind has the most lasting effect? Why?

5. Why is it important to have baseline information?

6. What are some common barriers to achieving fitness goals and what are some strategies for overcoming these barriers?

7. What are some ways that you can track your progress?

8. If you stop exercising for a period of time, how will you get yourself to start again?

REFERENCES

Crouter, S. E., P. L. Schneider, M. Karabulut, and D. R. Bassett, Jr. "Validity of 10 Electronic Pedometers for Measuring Steps, Distance, and Energy Cost." *Medicine & Science in Sports & Exercise* 35 (No. 8, 2003):1455–60.

Cuddihy, T. F., R. P. Pangrazi, and L. M. Tomson. "Pedometers: Answers to FAQs from Teachers." *JOPERD* 76 (No. 2, 2005): 36–40, 55.

Dishman, R. K. "Exercise Compliance: A New View for Public Health." *The Physician and Sportsmedicine* 14 (No. 5, 1986): 127–43.

Graser, S. V., R. P. Pangrazi, and W. J. Vincent. "Step It Up: Activity Intensity Using Pedometers; If You Think Pedometers Can't Measure MVPA, Think Again." *JOPHERD* 22 (No. 3, 2009): 22–4.

Hatano, Y. "Use of the Pedometer for Promoting Daily Walking Exercise." *International Council for Health, Physical Education and Recreation* 29 (1993): 4–8.

Kravitz, L., and D. Furst. "Influence of Reward and Social Support on Exercise Adherence in Aerobic Dance Classes." *Psychological Reports* 69 (No. 2, 1991): 423–6.

Marcus, B. H., and A. L. Stanton. "Evaluation of Relapse Prevention and Reinforcement Interventions to Promote Exercise Adherence in Sedentary Females." *Research Quarterly for Exercise and Sport* 64 (No. 4, 1993): 447–52.

Marshall, S. J., S. S. Levy, C. E. Tudor-Locke, F. W. Kolkhorst, K. M. Wooten, J. MingMing, C. A. Macera, and B. E. Ainsworth. "Translating Physical Activity Recommendations into a Pedometer-Based Step Goal: 3000 Steps in 30 Minutes." *American Journal of Preventive Medicine* 36 (No. 5, 2009): 410–5.

Martin, J. E., and P. M. Dubbert. "Adherence to Exercise." In *Exercise and Sports Sciences Review*, R. J. Terjung, ed. New York: Macmillan, 1985.

Physical Best and NASPE. *Physical Education for Lifelong Fitness: The Physical Best Teacher's Guide.* 2nd ed. Champaign, IL: Human Kinetics, 2005.

Schneider, P. L., S. E. Crouter, O. Lukajic, and D. R. Bassett. "Accuracy and Reliability of 10 Pedometers for Measuring Steps Over a 400-m Walk." *Medicine & Science in Sports & Exercise* 35 (No. 10, 2003): 1779–84.

Schneider, P. L., S. E. Crouter, and D. R. Bassett, Jr. "Pedometer Measures of Free-Living Physical Activity: Comparison of 13 Models." *Medicine & Science in Sports & Exercise* 36 (No. 2, 2004): 331–5.

Shephard, R. J. "Motivation: The Key to Fitness Compliance." *The Physician and Sportsmedicine* 13 (No. 6, 1985): 88–98.

Tudor-Locke, C., Y. Hatano, R. P. Pangrazi, and M. Kang. "Revisiting 'How Many Steps are Enough?'" *Medicine & Science in Sports & Exercise* 40 (No. 7 Suppl., 2008): 537–43.

Welk, G. J., J. A. Differding, R. W. Thompson, S. N. Blair, J. Dziura, and P. Hart. "The Utility of the Digi-Walker Step Counter to Assess Daily Physical Activity Patterns." *Medicine & Science in Sports & Exercise* 32 (No. 9 Suppl., 2000), S481–88.

U.S. Department of Health and Human Services. Office of Disease Prevention and Health Promotion. *Healthy People 2020* Washington, DC. Available at www.healthypeople.gov/2020/faqs.aspx#g. Accessed June 26, 2012.

6

Posture: A Dynamic Concept

Stand up tall every time you walk through a door-frame; if nothing else, you will always make a grand entrance.

MARIE F. GALEN

- How can I achieve good posture and body alignment during exercise?
- What should I do to take care of my back?
- What is core training?

BODY position can make a big difference in how you feel during and after an activity. For example, good sitting posture during computer use can save neck, shoulder, and back strain. Correct body alignment during exercise ensures the full benefit of the exercise and helps prevent injuries. Correct bending and lifting postures also save your back and let you do more with less fatigue. Good posture and alignment are not just about standing up straight; they are about a dynamic process of repositioning your body segments to produce the best possible mechanical (and sometimes aesthetic) advantage at all times.

The position of your body in space when sitting, standing, and lying down is called **body posture**. **Body alignment** has to do with how the different segments of your body are positioned in relation to each other. Within each posture, different alignments are possible. Sitting posture, for example, can be with a straight or a rounded back. Different alignments within a posture are appropriate at different times. An intentional sway back in the cat stretch (sagging the back before arching it upward) gives a healthy stretch of the back muscles. That same sway back while running in place is a liability that can result in low back pain. This text is packed with descriptions and photographs identifying correct postures and alignments for specific exercises. Careful attention to these and helpful feedback from your instructor can help you attain good exercise alignment.

It should also be noted that yoga, Pilates, the martial arts, and formal dance training have a strong focus on body alignment during a wide variety of body postures. The exerieses included in these programs will the flexibility and strength necessary to hold well-aligned positions. The result—excellent body postures.

FLEXIBILITY AND POSTURE

Poor flexibility can actually pull you out of good alignment. When the hip flexors (muscles that cross the hip joint and attach to the top of the pelvis) are shortened due to muscle tightness, they pull the pelvis forward. This causes excessive curvature of the lumbar (lower) spine, a condition known as lordosis (Figure 6.1). If the hamstrings (the muscles on the back of the legs that attach to the bottom of the pelvis) are tight, they pull the pelvis down and back. This flattens the lumbar curve and rounds the low back. Either condition can cause low back pain and referred leg pain. Good flexibility in both of these sets of muscles allows the pelvis to stay in a neutral position. This becomes even more important during movements like kicks to the front and back, which require hip flexibility in order to prevent low back strain.

MUSCLE STRENGTH AND BODY ALIGNMENT

Strong and long are what you want. Strong muscles provide support and stabilization in addition to performing specific movements. Strong abdominal and

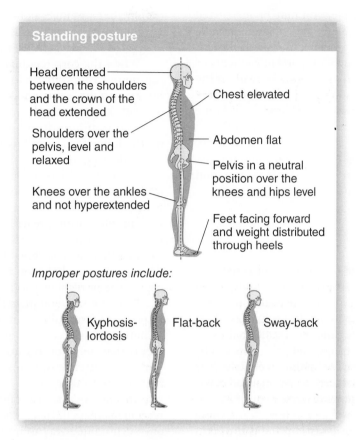

Figure 6.1 A comparison of good and poor standing posture.

spinal muscles are vital to protecting and stabilizing the back. When the body is in proper alignment during muscular strength and endurance exercises, the intended muscles get the proper workout. When the alignment is incorrect, muscles other than the target muscle(s) get recruited. Allowing other muscles to take part of the load defeats the original purpose: strengthening the target muscle(s). It can even lead to unnecessary soreness or injury. For example, a straight-leg sit-up allows the hip flexor muscles to assist the abdominal muscles in lifting the torso. This means that the abdominal muscles do not get as heavy a load as intended. And worse, the iliopsoas (a hip flexor that attaches in the low back), if not countered by strong abdominal muscles, will pull and arch the lower back off the floor—an unhealthy strain on the back. Good alignment becomes even more important when weights or bands are added to an exercise.

Muscular strength imbalances can also compromise posture. Developing the chest muscles without doing corresponding exercises for the upper back can result in rounded shoulders. The stronger chest muscles pull the shoulders forward. Opposing muscles should be exercised equally. Improving the strength and endurance of muscles also helps you maintain good body posture during prolonged exercise or activity. Injuries are most likely to occur when you become fatigued and start to lose exercise technique.

FUNCTIONAL MOVEMENT— FUNCTIONAL FITNESS

The need to maintain good posture and alignment in all our movements *and* to develop strong, supportive muscles has given rise to a way of training that is referred to as **functional fitness.** The goal of a functional fitness workout is to develop strength and flexibility in movements that we use every day. It is often taught using exercise descriptors that match daily activities. For example, the weight-training exercise called "bent-over row" might be referred to in a functional fitness workout as "starting the lawn mower." Alignment is taught so that it will transfer into the real-life setting; for example, you may be instructed to tighten your core to maintain back alignment while you place a box on a shelf. In the past, resistance training has been tied more closely to sports movements or competition; functional fitness focuses instead on the fitness needed to move comfortably and injury-free through a regular day of both work and play. Some ergonomics instructions (body alignment for work and home) are included in this chapter, such as how to sit, sleep, stand, lift, and drive. See Figure 6.2 and the box Your Back and How to Care for It. More information on functional fitness is provided in Chapter 9.

CORE TRAINING

Core training is the use of a variety of resistance exercises to develop the muscles that support and stabilize the middle of the body, especially the spine. The "core" includes the abdominals, back, chest, buttocks, and shoulder girdle muscles. Traditional exercises such as curl-ups, push-ups, and pelvic tilts can be used to strengthen the core, but optimum effectiveness depends on being able to "access" deep spinal and pelvic muscles when you perform these movements. Pilates is a special technique that teaches you how to use these deeper muscles with an emphasis on the connection between the "core," or "powerhouse," and the rest of the body. It accomplishes this using both mat exercises and specialized equipment. Yoga also works the core muscles through special postures called asanas. (See Chapter 12 for more on Pilates and yoga.) Core

training has a number of benefits, including improved posture, greater functional strength, better balance, a lower risk of injury, and improved sports performance.

When the core (center) is strong and stable, we can more easily transfer force and movement out to the extremities, which allows us to move more easily, with less stress and strain. To illustrate how core strength translates into limb strength and stability, try the following: (1) While seated, extend your arm out to the side. Have a partner push it back while you remain relatively passive. (2) As your partner pushes for a second time, react by resisting the movement with your arm and shoulder muscles. (3) This time as your partner pushes, react by resisting the movement using your arm, shoulder, and *abdominal* muscles—contract them as you resist. Using the core (especially if it is strong) can help you maintain good posture and apply force or resistance as needed.

Reactive movement is the idea of a movement response to a stimulus. You do this when you slip on something; you react by quickly employing movements that help you regain your balance. There are some very effective ways to use this idea in core training. Situations that produce an unstable environment require the body to use muscles—core muscles—to react to maintain the body's position. Stability balls offer one such unique way to train. To balance or stabilize yourself on the ball during an exercise, you call into action the core muscles. Stability resistance training can also be done on a Bosu ball, balance disk, or half round foam roller. The Bosu ball looks like a stability ball cut in half. You can put the flat or rounded side down and

Figure 6.2 Good sitting posture promotes a healthy back.

STANDING POSTURE EXERCISES

There are some exercises that help you stand correctly. Since we spend a lot of time on our feet, good standing posture is a must. First, just stand with your back to a wall. and become aware of your alignment. Your head, shoulders, and hips should touch the wall, and there should be natural curves away from the wall in the low back and neck area. Stand tall, with your abdomen pulled in. Be sure to breathe naturally. In this position, try the following three exercises:

- *Abdominal hold:* Pull your abdomen in without moving anything else; in particular, keep your rib cage still. Tighten the abs, as though you were about to take a punch. Breathe naturally, and maintain this isometric hold for 10 to 30 seconds. Repeat 3 to 5 times. You may put your hands on your abdomen to help focus on the muscles to tighten. (You can also do this seated in a chair with good back support.)
- *Pelvic tilts:* This exercise is very similar to the abdominal hold, except that you will tilt your pelvis back and try to bring your low back closer to the wall. Hold this position 10 to 30 seconds 3 to 5 times. You will be flattening a natural curve and then releasing it to its neutral position. This will strengthen the abdominal muscles and stretch the low back.
- *Table wax:* Bend your arms. but keep the elbows close to your sides and touching the wall. Extend your forearms in front of you, with the palms down. Now, as though you were waxing (or wiping) the top of a table, move your arms out and in. Pinch your shoulder blades together, but keep your upper back touching the wall. Repeat 5 to 10 times. (You can also perform this exercise while seated.)
- *Wall angels:* Place your arms overhead, with the elbows bent 90 degrees and with all of both arms along the wall. Moving at the shoulder joint and keeping the arms touching the wall throughout, raise and lower the arms much as you would do for a snow angel. (No snow angel leg movements!)

For more information and exercises, visit: http://ergonomics.ucla.edu/ex_posture.html

Source: Based on exercises from UCLA Ergonomics. Posture Strengthening Exercises. http://ergonomics.ucla.edu/ex_posture.html

perform exercises while balancing on top (See Figure 6.3.) The balance disk (disc) is similar but smaller and less expensive. It looks like an inflated round pillow with a surface of raised bumps (Figure 6.4). (See Figure 9.6 in Chapter 9 for a picture of a half round foam roller.) When the ball, disk, or roller moves, you have to react to that movement by stabilizing your body. Each time you react, you get a little bit stronger! Figure 6.5 demonstrates a fun stability exercise you can perform with a partner. One person slaps the ball at various positions while the other person tries to maintain body position. (See Chapters 7 and 10 for more stability ball exercises.) The unstable environment forces you to use numerous muscles at one time, much as you do when you carry out similar movements in daily life.

Unfortunately, many people are unaware of how to engage their core muscles. You can begin to become aware by lying on your back with your knees bent and feet on the floor. Without moving your back, try to "put your belly button on your back" or think of pulling your abs "in and up." Focusing on your trunk muscles when you cough is another cue teachers use. Now try a curl-up, but first engage the deep muscles and then use the abdominal muscles to pull you up. Kegel exercises (tightening the muscles that would stop urination) also help locate deep muscles. It takes time and often help from an instructor to become good at locating and using your deeper muscles, but once you do, you will be amazed how it changes how you move.

Here are two quick tests you can do to test your core strength. Try to hold these positions for a minimum of 20 seconds without visible shaking.

1. Lie face down. Brace yourself up on your forearms (forearms on the floor). Pull your toes under and lift up your body until you create a straight line from your feet to your head. (see Figure 6.6.)
2. Lie face up. Brace yourself up on your forearms. Lift up your body until you create a straight line from your feet to your head. (see Figure 6.6.)

When performing the following alignment checks, concentrate on stabilizing your posture by using core muscles. These positions are good beginning core exercises.

Figure 6.3 Bosu ball

Figure 6.5 Stability exercise using a partner and a stability ball. One partner pushes the ball in a variety of directions while the other partner uses core muscles to maintain body alignment.

Figure 6.4 Balance disk

Figure 6.6 Two tests of core strength

YOUR BACK AND HOW TO CARE FOR IT

Whatever the cause of low back pain, part of treating it is to correct faulty posture. But good posture is not simply a matter of "standing tall." It refers to correct use of the body at all times. In fact, for the body to function in the best of health, it must be so used that no strain is put on muscles, joints, bones, and ligaments. To prevent low back pain, avoiding strain must become a way of life, practiced while lying, sitting, standing, walking, working, and exercising. When body position is correct, internal organs have enough room to function normally, and blood circulates more freely.

With the help of this guide, you can begin to correct the positions and movements that bring on or aggravate backache. You should pay particular attention to the positions recommended for resting, because it is possible to strain the muscles of the back and neck even while lying in bed. By learning to live with good posture, under all circumstances, you will gradually develop the proper carriage and stronger muscles needed to protect and support your hard-working back.

HOW TO STAY ON YOUR FEET WITHOUT TIRING YOUR BACK

To prevent strain and pain in everyday activities, it is restful to change from one task to another before fatigue sets in. Some people can lie down between chores; others should check body position frequently, drawing in the abdomen, flattening the back, bending the knees slightly.

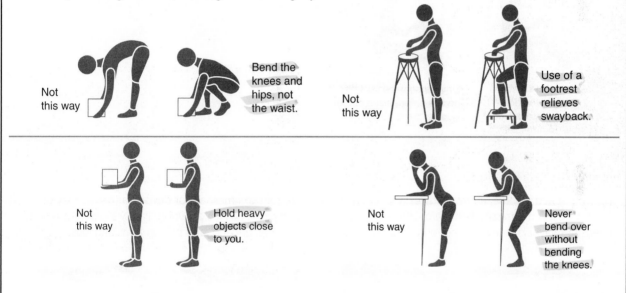

Not this way

Bend the knees and hips, not the waist.

Not this way

Use of a footrest relieves swayback.

Not this way

Hold heavy objects close to you.

Not this way

Never bend over without bending the knees.

WHEN DOING NOTHING, DO IT RIGHT

Rest is the first rule for the tired, painful back. The following positions relieve pain by taking all pressure and weight off the back and legs. Note pillows under knees to relieve strain on spine. For complete relief and relaxing effect, these positions should be maintained from 5 to 25 minutes.

A straight-back chair used behind a pillow makes a serviceable backrest.

HOW TO SIT CORRECTLY

A back's best friend is a straight, hard chair. If you can't get the chair you prefer, learn to sit properly on whatever chair you get. To correct sitting position from forward slump: Throw head well back, then bend it forward to pull in the chin. This will straighten the back. Now tighten abdominal muscles to raise the chest. Check position frequently.

Relieve strain by sitting well forward, flatten back by tightening abdominal muscles, and cross knees.

Keep neck and back in as straight of a line as possible with the spine. Bend forward from the hips.

TV slump leads to "dowager's hump," strains neck and shoulders.

Strained reading position. Forward thrusting strains muscles of neck and head.

Correct way to sit while driving, close to pedals. Use seat belt or hard backrest, available commercially.

Driver's seat too far from pedals emphasizes curve in lower back.

HOW TO PUT YOUR BACK TO BED

For proper bed posture, a firm mattress is essential. Bedboards, sold commercially or devised at home, may be used with soft mattresses. Bedboards, preferably, should be made of 3/4-inch plywood. Faulty sleeping positions intensify swayback and result not only in backache but in numbness, tingling, and pain in arms and legs.

Incorrect:
Lying flat on back makes swayback worse.

Correct:
Lying on side with knees bent effectively flattens the back. Flat pillow may be used to support neck, especially when shoulders are broad.

Incorrect:
Use of high pillow strains neck, arms, shoulders.

Correct:
Sleeping on back is restful and correct when knees are properly supported.

Incorrect:
Sleeping face down exaggerates swayback, strains neck and shoulders.

Correct:
Raise the foot of the mattress 8 inches to discourage sleeping on the abdomen.

Incorrect:
Bending one hip and knee does not relieve swayback.

Proper arrangement of pillows for resting or reading in bed.

EXERCISE — WITHOUT ATTRACTING ATTENTION

Use these inconspicuous exercises whenever you have a spare moment during the day, both to relax tension and improve the tone of important muscle groups.

1. Rotate shoulders forward and backward.
2. Turn head slowly side to side.
3. Watch an imaginary plane take off, just below the right shoulder. Stretch neck, follow it slowly as it moves up, around and down, disappearing below the other shoulder. Repeat, starting on left side.
4. Slowly, slowly, touch left ear to left shoulder; right ear to right shoulder. Raise both shoulders to touch ears, drop them as far as possible.
5. At any pause in the day—waiting for an elevator to arrive, for a specific traffic light to change—pull in abdominal muscles, tighten, hold for the count of 8 without breathing. Relax slowly. Increase the count gradually after the first week. Practice breathing normally with abdomen flat and contracted. Do this sitting, standing, and walking.
6. Sitting in a chair, bend over and grasp your ankles to stretch the low back.

RULES TO LIVE BY — FROM NOW ON

1. Never bend from the waist only; bend the hips and knees.
2. Always turn and face the object you wish to lift.
3. Avoid carrying unbalanced loads; hold heavy objects close to your body.
4. Never carry anything heavier than you can manage with ease.
5. Avoid sudden movements, sudden "overloading" of muscles. Learn to move deliberately, swinging the legs from the hips.
6. Learn to keep the head in line with the spine when standing, sitting, lying in bed.
7. Put soft chairs and deep couches on your "don't sit" list. During prolonged sitting, cross your legs to rest your back.
8. Seek professional/medical advice concerning low back pain.
9. Move heavy objects, such as furniture, using good lifting posture and with help to prevent strain. Lift objects overhead only if you can maintain good back posture throughout (neutral spine, no backward lean). When touching toes, bend knees slightly, or do not arch the back excessively.
10. Wear shoes with moderate heels, all about the same height. Avoid changing from high to low heels as much as possible.
11. Put a footrail under the desk and a footrest under the crib.
12. Diaper a baby sitting next to him or her on the bed.
13. Don't stoop and stretch to take something repeatedly out of a box or laundry basket; instead, raise the box/basket.
14. Beg or buy a rocking chair. Rocking rests the back by changing the muscle groups used.
15. Train yourself vigorously to use your abdominal muscles to flatten your lower abdomen. In time, this muscle contraction will become habitual, making you the envied possessor of a youthful body profile!
16. Don't strain to open windows or doors.
17. For good posture, concentrate on strengthening "nature's corset"–the abdominal and buttock muscles. The pelvic roll exercise is especially recommended to correct the postural relation between the pelvis and the spine.

EXERCISE ALIGNMENT CHECKS

You can perform some alignment checks using a mirror. Some of the following can be checked in a normal full-length mirror. Others will require a larger mirror you might find on campus in a dance room or a weight room. If a mirror is not available, you can work with a partner and evaluate each other. During class, your instructor will also check your alignment and give you helpful suggestions and positive feedback on correct positioning.

During a group fitness class, especially a dance-style class, you will perform a lot of exercises in a standing posture. It is important to maintain good trunk stabilization during these exercises so that the back stays in a healthy position. This can be achieved by pulling in the abdominal muscles and holding the pelvis in a neutral position. "Soft" or slightly bent knees

Figure 6.7 (a) Correct knee lift alignment. (b) Incorrect knee lift alignment.

help relieve pressure on the low back as well. See the Your Back and How to Care for It box on pages 63–65 for more information on standing and other postures. The illustrated information does an excellent job of presenting good body alignment for daily activities such as driving, sleeping, and picking up objects.

Stand sideways in front of a full-length mirror. Assume a good standing posture. Pay special attention to the stabilizing effect your abdominals have. Now try the following moves while watching in the mirror to see whether you are able to maintain good back and neck alignment.

- Raise both arms overhead without arching your back. Now, one at a time, extend your legs to the back, side, and front and see if you can maintain a good back position.
- Perform knee lifts, first with the right and then the left leg. (See Figures 6.7a and 6.7b for examples of good and bad alignment.)
- Kick straight legs (one at a time) to the front. (See Figures 6.8a and 6.8b for examples of good and bad alignment.)
- Bend your right knee, and touch your right foot behind your back with your left hand. Then try touching your left foot with your right hand. (See Figures 6.9a and 6.9b for examples of good and bad alignment.)
- With your feet shoulder width apart, stretch directly to the side. (See Figures 6.10a and 6.10b on page 68 for examples of good and bad alignment.)

- Jog in place. (See Figures 6.11a and 6.11b on page 68 for examples of good and bad alignment.) In addition to a neutral back, you want to keep your arms and legs moving forward and back without angling away from your body or crossing over your body.

Back stabilization is also very important in exercises performed on the hands and knees. Position yourself sideways to a mirror or partner. This will allow you to turn your head to look in the mirror rather than look up, which will arch your back. Your back and head should form a straight line, and your weight should be balanced between both hands and knees. Now try the following while checking back and neck/head alignment:

- Pick up one arm at a time and extend it straight forward.
- Extend one leg at a time directly to the back.
- Starting with the leg extended straight back, raise the leg until it is even with your back. Be sure the leg stays close to the midline. To raise your leg higher, lower down onto your forearms. (See Figure 6.12a for correct alignment and Figures 6.12b and 6.12c on page 69 for *incorrect* alignment.)

OTHER INFLUENCES ON POSTURE

Poor posture is not always born of a lack of attention to alignment or to weak inflexible muscles. In some cases, posture or muscular tension reflects a

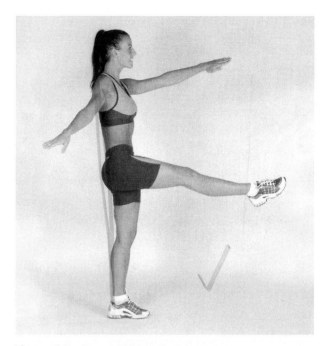

Figure 6.8a Correct kicking alignment

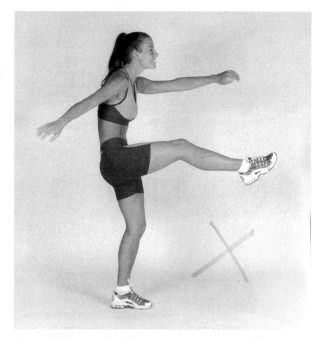

Figure 6.8b Incorrect kicking alignment

Figure 6.9a Correct back toe touch alignment

Figure 6.9b Incorrect back toe touch alignment

psychological state, an emotional issue, and/or physical pain from injury or a chronic condition. While stretching exercises may be helpful in identifying and lengthening tight muscles, other approaches such as finding the source of the stress and releasing tension may also be highly beneficial. Sometimes we don't

need to "do" something like stretch or strengthen, but rather we need to *stop* doing something like worrying or looking up at a movie screen or computer monitor that is too high. When a lot of time is going to spent in one position, such as viewing a computer, it is critical that the equipment is positioned correctly and fits

Figure 6.10 (a) Correct side stretch alignment. (b) Incorrect side stretch alignment.

Figure 6.11 (a) Correct jogging alignment—back neutral, knees forward. (b) Incorrect jogging alignment—back arched, knees down, feet to the side.

your body, and that you take regular breaks to stretch your muscles and increase circulation (see Figure 6.2 on page 60)

Another source of muscle tension is a cold environment. When people are chilled, they usually pull up their shoulders and drop their chin. All the strength and flexibility exercises in the world will not remove this tension, but turning up the heat or putting on more clothing will. Also, exercise will not improve poor posture brought on by self-consciousness or shyness. Other times, we try too hard and tense too many muscles. A beginning swimmer tenses many unnecessary muscles in an attempt to stay afloat.

The experienced swimmer uses only the muscles needed for buoyancy and movement. It may be that identifying and relaxing muscles that are not needed during an activity can bring relief. The next time you walk somewhere, see if your upper body is fully relaxed. How about your inner thigh muscles? Your hip

muscles? Your gait will become much easier when you learn to release unnecessary tension. The important thing is to look for the source of muscle tension and detrimental postures, and work to change or relieve the root cause. If the source is disease or injury, be sure to consult the proper medical authority before embarking on posture-correcting exercises.

POSTURE AND SPORTS AND DANCE

Sometimes we elect to use postures and body alignments that are stressful to the body but helpful for sport or dance movements. For example, the flat back position (Figure 6.13) is used in dance to create an aesthetic line. Deep knee bends, the hurdler's position, and back arching are just a few of the movements used in athletics that are not recommended for normal health and fitness. If you participate in activities that

POSTURE QUICK TIP

If you regularly carry out posture checks and realignments, over time they will become unconscious habits. Misalignments will start to "feel" wrong, and you will automatically make adjustments. To build

good standing and walking posture, try standing up tall every time you walk through a doorway. You will always make a grand entrance!

Figure 6.12a Correct leg and back alignment.

Figure 6.12b Incorrect alignment. Raising the leg too high results in back arch.

Figure 6.12c Incorrect alignment. When the working leg is lifted out to the side instead of directly upward, the body's weight has to shift away from center to maintain balance. This poor alignment can stress the back as well as interfere with the toning effect of the exercise.

use these types of movements, it is even more important to develop strong, long muscles to help ease the strain to your body. Dancers and athletes also try to minimize their use of such positions because they, too, want healthy, pain-free bodies.

Figure 6.13 The flat back position stresses the muscles and ligaments of the lower back. It may, however, be used in dance for aesthetic reasons.

SUMMARY

The word "posture" conjures up images of a mother or army sergeant barking out orders to "stand (or sit) up straight!" It is easy to dismiss posture as something you should do for the sake of appearance and as something you need worry about only during static sitting and standing activities; in fact, posture is a dynamic concept. Every movement we make should be done with the best possible body alignment. This reduces strain to unneeded muscles and applies mechanical force to its best advantage. Whether you are removing boxes from the trunk of the car, cleaning, sleeping, or exercising, it is smart to pay attention to, and make automatic, good body postures. And, of course, someone with good body mechanics, strong core muscles, and nice alignment looks good moving.

COMMONLY ASKED QUESTIONS

Can good posture feel "wrong"?

Yes. We are creatures of habit, and if you have held a posture incorrectly for a long time—probably years—a new posture may feel odd. Awareness is the first step to obtaining good posture, and the key is to keep finding the right position until it becomes habit. At this point the good posture will feel "right."

Is it true that your feet can throw off your posture?

Yes, if you roll your feet in (over pronate) or roll them out (over supinate), the position will affect your knees, which will affect your hips and consequently your spine. It's like the old song, "Your ankle bone is connected to your shin bone…"

Why does my back hurt after an aerobics class or a run?

Backs can hurt for many reasons, and you may need to consult a doctor. Any of the following may lead to back pain after a group exercise class or run. If you hold your back in a swayback (lordotic) position, the natural curves of the spine cannot dissipate the impact forces as they normally would. Old shoes without enough support and misaligned knees and hips during exercise may also play a role. Poor leg and trunk alignment is another possible cause, so pay special attention to that while running and during a class. Also be careful not to hold your head too far forward or raise your rib cage out of alignment.

KNOWLEDGE TIPS

1. Posture is a dynamic process whereby individuals try to select the posture and body alignment best suited to the activity in which they are engaged.

2. Posture is the position of the body in space.

3. Body alignment refers to how the body segments relate to one another.

4. Inflexibility can cause postural misalignments.

5. Muscular strength imbalances can result in postural misalignments.

6. Strengthening the "core" muscles will enhance posture and make you a better, stronger mover.

7. Proper exercise alignment during muscle strengthening ensures maximum benefit to the target muscle(s) and prevents injuries.

8. Awareness exercises can help correct postural problems that are due to inattention.

9. Poor posture may be the result of physical injury or disease.

10. Poor posture may be the result of a psychological or emotional state.

11. Seeking and eliminating sources of physical and psychological muscle tension can relieve tension and enhance posture.

THINK ABOUT IT

1. What is dynamic posture?

2. What is the difference between body posture and alignment? Give an example of each.

3. What kinds of things influence posture and alignment?

4. Give two examples of how strengthening and lengthening opposing muscles can improve body alignment.

5. In terms of posture and alignment, identify a stationary position (i.e., sitting) that you would like to improve. What changes would you make?

6. In terms of posture and alignment, identify a dynamic movement (i.e., leg kick) that you would like to improve. What changes would you make?

7. Which muscles make up the core and what are some exercises you can do to develop the core?

8. What are some exercises one can do to help build or maintain a healthy back?

9. Describe three abnormal curvatures of the spine and how development of these curvatures can be prevented. (The prevention part of this question is referring to functional curvatures that are the result of poor posture and alignment vs. structural curvatures with which a person may be born.)

10. Describe an activity that might encourage development of an imbalance in musculature and/or posture. Describe how to prevent and correct this.

REFERENCES

Barr K. P., M. Griggs, and T. Cadby. "Lumbar Stabilization: Core Concepts and Current Literature, Part 1." *American Journal of Physical Medicine and Rehabilitation* 84 (No. 6, 2005): 473–80.

Chiu, Loren Z. F. "Are Specific Spine Stabilization Exercises Necessary for Athletes?" *Strength and Conditioning Journal* 29 (No.1, 2007): 15–7.

Clippinger, K. S. *Dance Anatomy and Kinesiology.* Champaign, IL: Human Kinetics, 2007.

Hodges, P. W., and C. A. Richardson. "Inefficient Muscular Stabilization of the Lumbar Spine Associated with Low Back Pain. A Motor Control Evaluation of Transversus Abdominis." *Spine* 15 (No. 21, 1996): 2640–50.

McGill, S. *Ultimate Back Fitness and Performance.* Ontario, Canada: Wabuno Publishers.

Segal, D. D. "An Anatomic and Biomechanic Approach to Low Back Health: A Preventive Approach." *Journal of Sports Medicine* 23 (1983): 411–21.

Thompson, C. W., and R. T. Floyd. *Manual of Structural Kinesiology.* 12th ed. St. Louis, MO: Mosby, 1994.

7

Flexibility: Warm-Up/Cool-Down

"A muscle is like a car. If you want it to run well in the morning, you have to warm it up."

FLORENCE GRIFFITH JOYNER

- Why do I need to warm up and cool down?
- I've heard there is more than one way to stretch. Is that true?
- Are some stretches bad for you?
- Can you be too flexible?

A group exercise class consists of three components (parts): (1) the warm-up, (2) the workout, and (3) the cool-down. Although opposite in purpose and at opposite ends of the class, the warm-up and cool-down are actually very similar in content and technique. The warm-up starts off with low-intensity movements and easy stretching and builds to moderately vigorous activity. The cool-down begins as the moderate to vigorous activity of the workout segment ends and slowly reduces the intensity, finishing with stretches and relaxation exercises. Both activities are composed of two similar parts: the first increases or decreases overall body activity, while the second stretches the muscles. Stretching during the warm-up helps prepare your muscles for action, and stretching during the cool-down helps increase flexibility.

This chapter teaches you general techniques for warming up and cooling down. It explains the principles of flexibility, provides examples of recommended stretches, and indicates stretches that may be harmful or cause unnecessary soreness for the "average" participant. Discussions for the workout component of class (aerobic workout and muscle strength and endurance exercises) are presented in subsequent chapters.

WARM-UP

The purpose of the **warm-up** is to prepare your body and mind for activity. Most people arrive at class after a relatively inactive day. Muscles can be tight from sitting in class, driving, working at a computer, or bending over machinery. You need to ease into a workout, and a good warm-up is the way to do it. If you exercise early in the morning, the warm-up is even more important, because your muscles have been inactive all night. The warm-up is also a time to prepare mentally, increase your body awareness, concentrate on posture and movement technique, and rehearse, at a slower speed, some of the movements you will be using during the workout segment.

The first step in a warm-up is to literally make your body warm. This is the **general warm-up.** It may also be referred to as the standing warm-up. Easy, active movements to energizing music get your blood circulating and raise your body's internal, or core, temperature 1 to 2 degrees. This increase makes most people break a sweat.

The second part of the warm-up consists of stretching exercises. There is some professional debate about how much and what type of stretching should be included in the warm-up. This will be discussed in more detail shortly. When warm-up stretches are performed, they are usually done standing, but they may include floor work, and they are usually held for less time (about 10 seconds) than those performed during the cool-down. Stretches may be performed in combination with active warm-up movements, such as inserting a calf stretch between some jogging in place, as long as enough general warm-up has occurred prior to this to fully warm the muscles. A warm-up generally takes 5 to 10 minutes. More time may be needed if you are a beginner, are an older adult, or have a medical condition such as asthma.

GENERAL WARM-UP

It is important to start your workout slowly and easily and build up to a moderate pace. Warming up your muscles allows them to:

- become more elastic
- execute more forceful, rapid movements
- receive more oxygen because of increased blood flow
- increase metabolism
- become less vulnerable to injury

Starting slowly also gives the cardiorespiratory system a chance to adjust to the increasing oxygen demand of the muscles. Sudden, vigorous activity is hard on your body, and the quick shunting of blood to the muscles can leave you light-headed. Think about how you feel when you sprint to catch a closing door or leap out of the way of danger. To prevent this jarring feeling, start gradually and give your heart and muscles a chance to adjust.

Warm-up activity stimulates the secretion of synovial fluid. This fluid, secreted into the joints, acts as a lubricant. Much like the Tin Man in *The Wizard of Oz*, you need to "oil up" your joints. Start out with small movements, and as the joints and muscles respond, work up to bigger ones. Wearing high heels keeps the Achilles tendon in a shortened position all day. The transition from high heels to flat-soled athletic shoes should be made carefully. Too often, people who are late to class skip the warm-up and jump directly into vigorous activity. If you are late, take a few extra minutes to warm up. Your heart, muscles, and tendons will all benefit.

The warm-up is a good time to mentally prepare yourself for exercise. Set aside the worries of the day, and release yourself to a fun-filled hour of invigorating exercise. Concentrate on the following five technique tips during the general warm-up:

1. *Move from general to specific.* Start with general whole-body movements such as walking, marching in place, light jogging, or easy dance steps with light arm work. When space permits, add traveling steps. After you are warmed up, you can move on to more specific movements such as new steps for class, sports movements, or dance isolations.
2. *Start with smaller ranges of motion, and work up to bigger ones.* For example, start a shoulder warm-up by just lifting and rotating your shoulders while your arms hang relaxed at your sides.

Next, do a circling motion with your arms, letting your elbows draw the circle. Last, work the circles with straight, but not locked, arms. Start with low arms and eventually use above-the-shoulder arm movements. Start with step touches, and work up to stepping wider and using a deeper squatting position.

3. *Use movements that stay in a comfortable range of motion.* Wait until your muscles are warmed up before you put a lot of stretch and pull on them. For example, reaching one arm overhead and then the other is good, but stretching your arm way up and as far across your body as possible is too much right away. Similarly, use easy knee lifts and kicks as opposed to higher leg movements until your muscles are warm.
4. *Work with smooth movements.* This is not a time for bouncing or jarring your muscles and joints. Use flowing, sustained movements, and allow your body to make the transition from a sedentary day to an active class.
5. *Start slowly, and work up to a moderate pace.* This will gradually increase your heart rate, raise your core temperature, activate the synovial fluid, and increase metabolism.

A **dynamic warm-up** consists of a series of exercises that include general mobility exercises, dynamic stretching, and balance and coordination movements. A typical dynamic warm-up progresses through some stationary general body warm-up movements such as jogging in place and jumping jacks, to low-intensity transit movements such as skipping and jogging across the floor, then to muscle activation exercises such as squats and arm presses, followed by dynamic flexibility exercises such as walking (single) knee hugs and straight-leg marches, and finally moderate- and high-transit movements such as butt kicks and power skips. If the participants are preparing for a sporting event, sport-specific movements can be added at the end of a dynamic warm-up. The advantages to this kind of warm-up are that they are similar to everyday movements that occur in more than one plane and that they prepare you neuromuscularly for a dynamic workout. They also improve coordination and balance when they include movements such as standing on one leg and bending down to touch the ground.

WARM-UP STRETCHING: STATIC OR DYNAMIC

Stretching is an important part of warming up. You may have heard that stretching before an exercise is bad. This comes from a misunderstanding. The question is not whether stretching is good or bad, but rather which type of stretching should be used during the warm-up. Traditionally, static stretching (holding one position without movement) has been used. However, a growing body of research suggests that dynamic flexibility exercises more effectively prepare the body for dynamic movements. There is also some research evidence, stemming from running and weight-training studies, that static stretching calms the muscle rather than exciting it, and that in so doing may diminish the amount of force a muscle can exert in the activity following the stretch. This calming effect may also result in less muscular stabilization of joints, which could then lead to soreness or injury. Based on this, some professionals feel that dynamic stretching should be used in warm-ups and that static stretching is best left to the end of class. Dynamic flexibility research is still in its infancy, and as a result, there is not enough evidence yet to say that dynamic stretching is the best way to warm up for all individuals and for all sports events. Considerably more research is needed before we can reach definitive conclusions. In the meantime, knowing about the two types of stretching will allow you to understand the debate and perhaps try different types of warm-up stretches to see how they feel to you.

Dynamic stretching is using the pull of a muscle or group of muscles and the body's momentum to move through a full range of motion. **Dynamic flexibility** is how much range of motion you have at a joint during a dynamic movement. This is different from static flexibility, which is the stretch obtained in a held position. It differs from traditional ballistic stretching, in which the momentum of the body is used, but in a way that accentuates the endpoint of the movement, and the stretching is more "ballistic" or "bouncy" in nature as opposed to dynamic flexibility stretches that are done using smooth controlled and fluid movements. Dynamic stretches are also designed to move the body through functional (typical daily) movements, such as reaching for something on the shelf or bending to pick something up, and if desired, through sport-specific movements, such as throwing or striking a ball. It is fairly easy to see how certain aerobic dance warm-up movements can be dynamic flexibility exercises. Here are a few examples:

- The front lunge stretch can become dynamic by stepping into the lunge and then either returning to a stand or walking forward into a front lunge with the opposite foot forward.
- A knee-up (lifting one knee up in front while standing), which is dynamic to begin with, can become a dynamic stretch by lifting the knee high, hugging it with your arms, lowering it, and step hugging the opposite leg.
- The shoulders can receive a dynamic stretch by performing controlled arm circles forward and backward and by swinging both arms across the front of the body at chest height to one side and then the other.

As with all aspects of exercise, it is important to start off easy and progress gradually with dynamic flexibility exercises. For some individuals, high knee skips and a series of squats can feel like a workout, not a warm-up.

For dance-style aerobics, special consideration is usually given to warming up and stretching out the calf and leg muscles. There is lots of agreement that performing longer, sustained stretching is best done at the end of class, when the muscles are really warm and flexibility can be developed. Static, ballistic, proprioceptive neuromuscular facilitation (PNF), active, and passive stretching will be explained in more detail later in this chapter, followed by a number of flexibility exercises.

COOL-DOWN

Like the warm-up, the **cool-down** has two sections. The first part, sometimes called the standing cool-down, is done right after aerobic exercise to reduce the body's exertion level gradually. The second portion of the cool-down is the developmental stretch, which follows either the standing cool-down or a final set of muscle-toning exercises. The purpose of this stretch is to elongate the muscles and improve range of motion. The standing cool-down usually lasts 3 to 5 minutes, and the developmental stretch about 5 to 10 minutes. If time permits, some instructors will follow the stretch with a few minutes of quiet relaxation.

STANDING COOL-DOWN

During exercise, a large portion of the blood (usually 30% to 50%, but it can be as much as 70%) is shunted (circulated out) to the limbs to supply the big working muscles with oxygen. At the end of a workout, it is important to keep moving so the blood is returned to the heart and lungs to be reoxygenated instead of being pooled out in the limbs. If you stop exercising suddenly, you may find yourself feeling light-headed because of a lack of oxygenated blood in the brain. If the lack of oxygen in your brain is significant enough, you will faint. This is your body's way of bringing you horizontal so that oxygenated blood can travel to your head more easily. There is no need to feel light-headed or faint in a group class; simply keep moving and gradually reduce your activity level.

When you move the big muscles of your arms and legs during the standing cool-down, the muscles contract around the veins and help push or massage

Table 7.1   Summary of Warm-Up and Cool-Down

ACTIVITY	PURPOSE	DURATION
Warm-Up		
Core Warm-Up: Start with easy, active, whole body movements; move from small to larger ranges of motion.	• Raise core temperature 1–2 degrees • Increase blood circulation • Stimulate secretion of synovial fluid • Prepare mentally	5–10 minutes total
Warm-Up Stretch: Hold static stretches 10–30 seconds or perform a series of dynamic flexibility exercises.	• Prepare muscles for action and prevent injury	
Cool-Down		
Standing Cool-Down: Start with big, active movements, and slowly wind down to smaller, easier movements.	• Reduce the body's exertion level • Return blood to the heart and lungs	3–5 minutes
Developmental Stretch: Hold static stretches for 15–30 seconds, 2–4 times for a total of 60 seconds.	• Increase flexibility • Prevent muscle soreness	5–10 minutes

the blood upward. This aids the **venous pump,** the system of moving blood up through the veins against gravity. Blood is pumped up the **veins** by the pressure created from the heart's contractions. Between heartbeats (contractions), blood is held in its newly elevated position by one-way valves inside the veins. Muscle contractions added to the heart's contractions help move the blood more quickly, which, in turn, helps you recover from exercise more quickly.

When you first start exercising, your aerobic system takes about 3 minutes to reach a point where it is producing as much energy as you are using. During this time, the anaerobic systems produce energy without the use of oxygen. At the end of exercising, you have to replenish these systems. During the post-exercise time, you continue to operate at a high level of oxygen consumption— that's why you continue to breathe hard and sweat after you finish exercising. As everything gets caught up and reset, your breathing and heart rate slow down, and you begin to cool off.

The actual movements and technique required for the cool-down are just like the warm-up, only you reverse the process. Start with big, active movements, and slowly wind down to smaller, easier movements. The cool-down can be as simple as a light jog that winds down to a brisk walk and, finally, normal-paced walking. The cool-down should continue until your heart rate is below 120 bpm.

DEVELOPMENTAL STRETCH

The end of class is the best time to work on developing flexibility because your body temperature is high and muscle tissue is elastic. In addition to standing stretches, this final stretch often includes stretches sitting or lying down. The closing stretch differs from the opening stretch in the opportunity to hold stretches longer. See Table 7.1 for a summary of the warm-up and cool-down.

PRINCIPLES OF FLEXIBILITY

Flexibility is defined as the range of movement you have around a joint or group of joints. Sometimes this flexibility is taken for granted, and it's not until you lose flexibility that you realize how much it affects your daily life. Flexibility is required to raise your arms to take off a shirt, to throw a ball, or to do the tango. These movements are effortless when you have good range of motion, painfully difficult when you don't. To appreciate flexibility, imagine that you have a stiff neck and try to go a few hours without turning your head independently of your body.

As you get older, your independence is, to a large degree, dependent on your flexibility. (I recently cringed while I watched one of my older relatives try, and fail, to bend over far enough to pick up her purse from the floor.) Regardless of your age, you can always improve your flexibility. However, it is easier to develop and maintain flexibility when you are young than to start to develop it when you are older. Now, let's look at how the principles of exercise introduced in Chapter 3 are applied to flexibility.

PRINCIPLE OF SPECIFICITY

Flexibility is specific to a joint or group of joints. This means that you can't perform just one exercise to develop body flexibility; you must select a variety of exercises for all of the body's major muscles and joints. This is also true for assessing your flexibility. On Worksheets 7.1 and 7.2, available online at www.pearsonhighered .com/bishopaerobics and also at the back of the book, you will find a series of tests to determine the flexibility of your shoulders, back, hips, and so forth.

PRINCIPLE OF INDIVIDUALITY

Flexibility of a joint depends on a combination of factors, including bone shape, muscle and connective tissue properties, aging effects, the presence of disease such as arthritis, and other factors. Some individuals are born with looser joints than others. What is a healthy stretch for one may be injurious for another. For example, a loose joint would benefit more from strengthening of the muscle, which stabilizes the joint, than more stretching. People will also progress at different rates as they attempt to increase muscle flexibility. The one thing we all have in common is that (except for some rare cases involving specific diseases or disabilities) we can all improve the flexibility of muscles and the range of motion of joints that need it.

PRINCIPLE OF REGULARITY

If you do not perform flexibility exercises on a regular basis, you will gradually become less flexible. Aging has some effect on the elasticity of tissues, but overall much flexibility can be retained through a regular stretching program.

FITT PRINCIPLE

The flexibility target zone is described by four variables: frequency, intensity, time, and type of stretch (FITT). The American College of Sports Medicine (ACSM) recommendation is to perform a general stretching routine that exercises the major muscle and/or tendon groups using static or PNF (proprioceptive neuromuscular facilitation) techniques:

Frequency: at least 2–3 days a week with the greatest gains from daily stretching.

Intensity: stretching to a point of tightness or slight discomfort

Time: a total accumulation of 60 seconds as a combination of time held and number of repetitions

Static Stretch: 10- to 30-second hold, repeat 2-4 times. The accumulated 60 seconds can be achieved in a variety of ways including 4 repetitions of a 15-second hold or 2 repetitions of a 30-second hold.

PNF Stretch: 3–6 second isometric contraction followed by an assisted stretch for 10-30 seconds, repeat 2-4 times

PRINCIPLES OF PROGRESSION AND OVERLOAD

A progressive overload is achieved in stretching by manipulating the variables in the FITT principle. You can increase your frequency until you are stretching 5 to 7 days a week. You can increase the intensity by stretching a little further than normal, but remember to back off if you feel pain. And you can hold stretches for longer periods of time or increase the number of times you hold a shorter stretch (a 15-second hold, repeated 4 times). Whether you are adding frequency, time, or intensity, be sure to add on slowly to what you are presently doing.

TYPES OF STRETCHING

Types of stretches include static, ballistic, and PNF. Another way to classify stretching yields two additional ways of stretching: active and passive (or assisted) stretching. These may be used in combination with the first. For example, one can perform an active static stretch. You may want to build several different methods of stretching into your program. Each type of stretch facilitates flexibility in a different way. See Table 7.2 for the benefits and drawbacks of the different types of stretches, including previously discussed dynamic stretching.

In Chapter 1, you were introduced to special sensors located in the muscle tissue that monitor muscle tension. In the following discussion on stretching, you will see the roles these sensors and the nervous system play in flexibility development. Here is a quick review of these mechanisms. When a muscle is rapidly stretched, the muscle spindle sends a message to contract; this is called the "stretch reflex." The inhibitory Golgi tendon organ (GTO) reflex tells the muscle to relax when it feels too much tension from either a strong contraction or a rapid, forceful lengthening of the muscle. And finally, "reciprocal innervation" is the neuromuscular message to relax the muscle(s) opposite the one(s) being stretched. Now let's look at how the different types of stretching are affected by these mechanisms.

Table 7.2 Types of Stretching

TYPE OF STRETCH	ACTION	BENEFITS	DRAWBACKS
Static	Move slowly into stretch position, and hold for at least 15 seconds. Performing a series works best.	Easiest safe way to increase flexibility	Possible muscle soreness May result in less force production in movements following the stretch May decrease joint stability
Ballistic	Place the muscle rapidly in and out of stretch position by bouncing or pulsing.	Increases flexibility Recommended after static stretching for those performing quick, explosive movements	Increased potential for injury May cause muscle to contract during the stretch Possible muscle soreness
PNF	Contract–relax (CR): isometrically contract muscle then passively stretch it.	Most effective type of stretching	Possibility of increased muscle soreness Requires a partner and more time
Dynamic	Move the muscle(s) and joints through a full range of motion using controlled active movements.	Increases dynamic flexibility; helps maintain joint stability Prepares body for dynamic movement	Many of the exercises require a degree of fitness (muscular endurance) to do repetitiously (e.g., squats or lunges). Primarily for warm-up; more research needed to assess overall effectiveness.

ACTIVE AND PASSIVE (ASSISTED) STRETCHING

Passive stretching is when something or someone else creates a stretch in your muscles. Because an outside force is helping you stretch, this is often referred to as **assisted stretching.** If you are the one being stretched, it is important to relax your muscles as your partner, gravity, or another part of your body creates the stretch.

A partner creates a static passive stretch by moving your muscles into a stretch position and holding you there. While the partner does the holding, you can relax and let the muscle lengthen. This works well if you have a trustworthy partner. Passive ballistic stretching is not recommended, as it carries a much greater risk of injury.

You can assist your own stretch using muscles that aren't the one(s) being stretched. For example, you can create a passive calf stretch by wrapping a towel around the ball of your foot and using your arms to pull your toes toward your shin. Gravity can also supply the assist. For example, a passive calf-muscle stretch is achieved when you stand on your toes on the edge of a platform and allow your heels to drop below the platform surface. Machines that put you in traction also provide a passive stretch.

In an **active stretch,** you are required to contract one muscle in an effort to stretch another. This type of stretch takes advantage of reciprocal innervation. This works well as long as the contracting muscle is strong enough to pull the other muscle through a full stretch. If it is not, additional stretching can be achieved by adding a passive assisted stretch. For example, an active stretch of the hamstring is achieved by lying on your back and contracting your quadriceps muscle to pull your leg toward your head. If your quadriceps muscle is too weak to create an effective stretch, maintain the quadriceps contraction and add an assist by pulling gently with your hands. Some people also like to follow an active stretch with a passive one.

STATIC STRETCHING

To perform a **static stretch,** move slowly into the stretch position and then hold (without moving) for 10 to 30 seconds. Holding a stretch position "quiets" the stretch reflex and elicits the Golgi tendon organ reflex. This combination relaxes the muscle and allows it to stretch with little risk of injury. The stretch should be held at a point of mild discomfort but not pain. If you feel pain, either release the stretch entirely and begin again, or ease back on the stretch until the pain is relieved. Performing a series of static stretches works even better because the GTO's thresholds are reset at a less sensitive level following the first stretch. This allows you to stretch further before encountering resistance. These relaxation effects are purposely elicited during developmental stretching and are avoided in dynamic stretching.

BALLISTIC STRETCHING

A **ballistic stretch** is one in which you put the muscle rapidly in and out of a stretch position by bouncing or pulsing during the stretch. Ballistic stretching may improve flexibility but has a couple of significant drawbacks. First, the rapid lengthening of the muscle elicits the stretch reflex, thus causing the muscle to contract—the opposite effect desired in a stretch. Second, because the movement is more forceful, it has more potential to injure the muscle and connective tissue. Thus, static stretching is generally recommended over ballistic stretching.

There is a time, however, when ballistic stretching may be beneficial. If you are going to be involved in an activity that requires quick explosive movements, then you need a final warm-up that is specific to that movement. After you have warmed up and done some dynamic stretching, you can start gently with ballistic stretching and build up to performance-level ballistic movements. For example, a softball player uses an explosive movement to throw the ball. After warming up and doing some dynamic stretches, the athlete can perform a series of bounce stretches, pulling the arm backward in the arm preparation position (elbow up, hand behind head). This is an example of an active stretch as the shoulder muscles pull the arm backward. For the full throw, easy throwing (dynamic action) precedes harder more ballistic throwing. Before a player takes the field, the athlete should practice all-out throwing for at least several repetitions.

PNF Stretching

Proprioceptive neuromuscular facilitation (PNF) stretching was originally developed as a rehabilitation tool. PNF stretching is a very effective type of stretching, but it requires a trustworthy and patient partner and considerably more time, and can result in more muscle soreness. Static stretching is almost as effective and is usually easier to perform. PNF stretching might be worth trying if you feel you are at a sticking point in your flexibility. Or you may want to include a few PNF stretches in a predominantly static stretching routine. There are a number of ways that PNF can be performed. The easiest one to incorporate into a group exercise class is called contract–relax (CR). You must first isometrically contract the muscle you want to stretch for 3–6 seconds. Then, using a passive assisted stretch, stretch the previously contracted muscle. For example, place your left hand on your left cheek and then try to rotate your head to the left. Hold this isometric contraction for 3 to 6 seconds. (During an isometric contraction, nothing moves. Your left hand does not allow your head to rotate.) Then relax and gently push your head through rotation to the right. To use CR with a hamstring stretch, lie on the ground and raise one leg up in the air. Have a partner place his or her hands on the back of your leg and resist you

when you try to push your leg toward the ground. Hold this isometric contraction for 3 to 6 seconds and then, while you relax, have your partner gently push your leg toward your head. To do this same exercise by yourself, push your raised leg against a door jamb or use your own arms to resist the downward push of your leg. Then relax your leg and pull with your arms.

Stretches to Avoid

Someone once said that "a weed is a flower out of place." So it is with some exercises; they are "weeds" in a health/fitness program but "flowers" in certain sports settings. A back bend is a good example. Gymnasts need a lot of hyperextension flexibility for tumbling stunts and to accent dance moves. But for most people, back bends place an unnecessary amount of stress on the back, particularly on the vertebral discs. The hurdler's stretch is another example. In track and field, hurdlers must use this position to clear the hurdles, but stretching in this position places an unhealthy torque on the knee. Because there are other exercises that effectively stretch the same muscles, even hurdlers limit their use of this position. Similarly, some positions that are performed in yoga and Pilates classes can cause injury when attempted without the guidance of a well-trained instructor and preparation through lead-up exercises. Some exercises that are *not* recommended for general fitness are pictured in this chapter, along with healthier alternatives.

There is often more than one way to stretch (and strengthen) a muscle. If one particular exercise does not feel good to you, select a second one that will achieve the same effect. Sometimes simply doing a stretch lying down instead of standing can make it more comfortable. There are also some stretches that can be performed with the back supported against a wall to relieve back strain. Certain exercises, such as a seated straddle stretch, are difficult when you are inflexible but become more comfortable as you develop flexibility. If you do not see an alternate stretch in this text, consult your instructor, physical therapist, or a stretch-specific text. If the class is performing an exercise that you know will hurt your body, don't do it; modify the exercise or perform a different one. It is tempting to want to look like the rest of the class, but it is important to listen to your body and individualize your exercise to suit it.

FLEXIBILITY EXERCISES

The following is a series of stretches for the body's major muscle groups. These stretches are appropriate for the warm-up and cool-down. Only the major muscles being stretched are listed; however, a number of smaller muscles will also be stretched during these exercises. The stretches are described for one side only (the side pictured), but they should be done on both sides. Emphasis is placed on body alignment. When performing standing stretches, be sure to maintain good abdominal tone, a neutral spine (natural curves), and slightly flexed knees. It takes practice to develop good exercise technique. Use the help of instructors, classmates, and mirrors to check your alignment and technique. When you change your technique, it may

feel funny or awkward at first, but after a while you will feel better. Be sure to learn both the look and the feel of correctness.

To make the following stretches active, contract the muscles opposite those you are trying to stretch. You can add a passive assist by pulling with your hands or by having a partner work with you. For more ideas on PNF stretching, talk to your instructor or consult a more in-depth text.

Neck Stretches

Muscles stretched: sternocleidomastoi-deus, trapezius, and numerous smaller neck muscles

1. Rotating or holding the head to the sides and front provides a nice stretch of the neck muscles (Figures 7.1a, 7.1b, 7.1c). Rolling or laying the head to the back (Figure 7.1d) places pressure on the cervical vertebrae, so avoiding this position is probably healthier over the long run. (However, it may be necessary to stretch and strengthen the neck in hyperextension for certain sports.)

Trapezius; various neck muscles

VARIATIONS

a. Lifting the chin after fully rotating the head adds a little extra stretch to the neck muscles.
b. Dropping the chin and then looking to the right shoulder adds another angle to the stretch. Repeat to the left.

2. Pull the chin from a protruding position (Figure 7.2a) in toward the centerline of the body as if to create a double chin (Figure 7.2b). Hold for 2 to 3 seconds and release. Do 5 to 10 neck glides. This exercise helps counter the tendency to let the chin protrude and can be performed throughout the day to improve posture and prevent neck fatigue.

Scan to view video ◄

Figure 7.1a

Figure 7.1b

Figure 7.1c

Figure 7.1d Hyperextending the neck places unnecessary stress on the cervical vertebrae.

Figure 7.2a

Figure 7.2b

Arm and Shoulder Stretches

Muscles stretched: triceps, posterior deltoid (Figure 7.3), triceps, anterior deltoid (Figure 7.4)

Muscles stretched: biceps brachii, forearm flexors (Figure 7.5)

Deltoids   Triceps brachii

Biceps brachii   Forearm flexors

1. Stretch the left arm across the front of the body vparallel to the floor. Place the right hand above the left elbow and gently apply pressure across and in toward the chest (Figure 7.3). Be sure to keep the shoulder down away from the ear.

2. Reach the right arm straight up. Bend at the elbow, and try to touch the right hand to the middle of the back. Place the left hand just above the right elbow, and push the arm into a stretch position (Figure 7.4a). Drop the head forward slightly for comfort.

Variation: A towel can be used behind the back between the two hands when flexibility is limited (Figure 7.4b).

3. Extend the arm you wish to stretch in front of you with the palm facing the ceiling. Hyperextend the wrist of the extended arm by pulling down and back on the fingers with the opposite hand (Figure 7.5). Maintain good back alignment and soft knees during the stretch.

Variation: Extend both arms back behind the body with elbows extended and shoulders rotated backward so that the palms face forward and upward. Hands are at about waist level.

Scan to view video ▶   Scan to view video ▶

Figure 7.3   **Figure 7.4a**   **Figure 7.4b**   **Figure 7.5**

Shoulder and Chest Stretches

Muscles stretched: pectorals, anterior deltoids

Pectoralis
major

Deltoids

1. Grasp the hands behind the back, interlacing the fingers or holding a towel or strap (Figure 7.6). Pull the shoulders back without arching the back.

2. Place your hands by your ears with the elbows extending to the side. Press the elbows backward. Lift and open the chest but keep the shoulders down (Figure 7.6).

3. Extend your arms behind you, and have a partner grasp your upper arms very gently and smoothly pull your arms together and slightly upward (Figure 7.7a). Your palms can be facing each other or rotated outward for more stretch through the chest and front of the shoulder. Be sure the partner grasps your arms between elbows and shoulders to avoid putting pressure on your elbow joint.

4. Bend your arms and have a partner pull them backward gently (Figure 7.7b).

Scan to view
video ▲

Figure 7.6

Figure 7.7a

Figure 7.7b

Shoulder and Upper Back Stretch

Muscles stretched: deltoid, rhomboids, trapezius

Deltoids   Rhomboids   Trapezius

Stability ball: Kneel down with the ball in front and slightly to the left of your body. Place the back of your right hand on top of the ball. Roll the ball out to your left using the right arm. As your arm extends, bend forward at the waist (Figure 7.8). Keep your head facing front. Your chin may touch your upper arm. Keep your lower body stable with the hips square.

Figure 7.8

Back Stretches

Muscles stretched: erector spinae (Figures 7.9a, 7.9b, 7.10a, 7.10b)

1. Stand with feet shoulder width apart and knees bent. Tuck the pelvis under by contracting the abdomen. Grasp the hands in front of the body with palms facing outward. Try to cave in or hollow out the chest and abdominal areas (Figure 7.9a). The back should appear rounded. Allow the head to follow the natural line of the curve.

Erector spinae

VARIATIONS

a. You can also perform this standing exercise with the hands on the knees, rounding and flattening (or slightly arching) the back.

b. In an all-fours position (on hands and knees), alternately round and arch the back (Figure 7.9b). This is commonly referred to as the "cat stretch."

Scan to view video ▲

Figure 7.9a   **Figure 7.9b**

2. Lie on the ground and draw both knees toward the shoulders, grasping underneath the knees (Figure 7.10a). This exercise specifically targets the lower back. The "plow" position should be avoided because of the pressure it places on the neck (Figure 7.10b).

AVOID

Figure 7.10b The "plow" position puts the weight of the entire body on the cervical vertebrae. This is very stressful to the upper spine. See the discussion concerning yoga positions in the Stretches to Avoid section on page 77.

Scan to view video ▶

Figure 7.10a

Muscles stretched: lattisimus dorsi (Figure 7.11a, b)

3. Stand with the feet shoulder-width apart and knees softly bent. Reach both arms upward directly overhead with the palms facing forward. Touch the thumbs together or grasp the hands. Maintain a neutral back position. Lift the arms upward, lifting through the rib cage to create a stretch through the upper arm, armpit, rib and lower back. (Figure 7.11a) This stretch can be performed in a sitting position or lying on your back with your knees bent (arms overhead with thumbs touching the ground). For an

Latissimus dorsi

additional stretch when sitting or standing, you can bend to one side (See the side stretch, Figure 7.14b).

4. Perform a similar stretch in a horizontal position using a stability ball and one arm at a time. Kneel on all fours with the ball in front of you. Lift one arm and place the wrist and hand on the ball with the thumb facing up. Maintaining good back alignment, roll the ball away from you by extending your arm. (Figure 7.11b)

5. On all fours (without the ball), sit back onto your heels and touch your forehead to the floor to take the position known as the child's pose in yoga. Your arms will be extended overhead.

Figure 7.11a

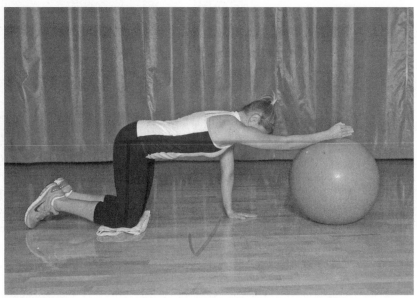

Figure 7.11b

Abdominal Stretches

Muscles stretched: rectus abdominus (Figure 7.12a)

1. Lie face down with hands up by the ears. Gently press up, supporting your weight on the forearms. Elbows should be under or slightly in front of the shoulders (Figure 7.12a). Hold for 5 to 10 seconds. If you experience pain, discontinue this exercise and consult a physician. Hyperextension of the spine to the extent involved in a back bend is not recommended for normal health and fitness (Figure 7.12b).

Rectus abdominis

2. *Stability ball:* Sit on the ball. Walk your feet forward until the natural curve of the low back is over the ball (Figure 7.13a, on page 83). Hands can be by the ears with elbows out and laying on the ball or extended sideways. Press your feet into the floor and extend the legs, causing the ball to roll backward (Figure 7.13b). The farther back the ball rolls, the greater the stretch. If dizziness occurs, try holding this stretch for a shorter time or select a different stretch.

Figure 7.12a

AVOID

Figure 7.12b Hyperextension of the back is stressful to the spine. See the discussion on yoga positions in the Stretches to Avoid section on page 77.

Figure 7.13a

Figure 7.13b

Side Abdominal Stretch

Muscles stretched: obliques, latissimus dorsi

External Obliques

Latissimus dorsi

1. Place the feet shoulder width apart. If you are stretching to the right, be sure that the right foot is angled outward and the right knee is bent. This keeps the torso, knee, and foot all going in the same direction and decreases the chance of knee soreness. Bend directly to the right side. The left arm can be relaxed by your side or extended for balance (Figure 7.14a) or, for a more advanced stretch, extended up by the left ear (Figure 7.14b). Incorrect alignment is shown in Figure 7.14c. For added support, place the right hand on the thigh of the bent right leg. If this position is held for an extended amount of time, pressure is put on the vertebral discs. Controlled movement into and out of the position is recommended.

2. *Stability ball:* Sit with one hip on the ball. Move your inside leg forward and outside leg backward for stability. Lay your torso down sideways

Scan to view
video ▲

AVOID

Figure 7.14a

Figure 7.14b

Figure 7.15 Poor back alignment.

on the ball. Keep one hip directly over the other. One arm is placed on the ball for stability; the other reaches overhead to add stretch. It may be necessary to place your feet against a wall to prevent yourself from rolling forward.

3. Lie on the floor, with the knees bent and feet on the floor. Arms can be extended out to the side

for stability. Slowly lower the legs to one side while maintaining a neutral back position. (Do not do this exercise if it causes low back pain.) Turn your head away from the knees. Exhale and relax into the position.

Abdominal and Buttocks Stretch

Muscles stretched: external obliques, gluteus maximus, erector spinae

External
Obliques

Gluteus
maximus

Erector spinae

Scan to view
video ▶

To do the pretzel stretch, first sit with your right leg extended forward and your left leg bent. Now lift and place your left foot against the outside of your right knee. Turn your torso gently, and position your extended right arm so that the back of your right elbow is against the outside of your left knee. Place your left

hand on the floor comfortably behind your buttocks. Gently press your right arm against your right leg, and turn your body to the left. Look over your left shoulder (Figure 7.16).

Figure 7.16

Buttocks Stretch

Muscles stretched: gluteus maximus

1. Lie on the floor on your back with knees bent. Place the left foot on the right knee. Grasp the right thigh, and gently pull the right thigh toward the chest (Figure 7.17).

Gluteus
maximus

Scan to view video ▶

Figure 7.17

Thigh Stretches

Muscles stretched: quadriceps

Stand on the left leg. Bend the right leg, and grasp the ankle (not the foot) with the same arm. Keep the knee pointed downward. Allow a comfortable knee bend, and pull gently backward at the ankle. (The right foot should not be forced to the right buttock.) Maintain good posture and alignment by pulling in the abdomen and keeping the pelvis stretch. Avoid arching the back

Quadriceps

or leaning forward. More stretch is not achieved by leaning forward, but a slight forward lean may relieve back pressure for some individuals. To keep your balance, extend the free arm to the side or overhead, look at something stationary, and keep the abdomen pulled up (Figure 7.18a). You can also place the extended hand against a wall or on a partner's shoulder. This same stretch can be performed lying on your side on the floor (Figure 7.18b). Stretching the thigh by leaning back in the hurdler's position (Figure 7.18c) is not recommended.

Scan to view video ▲

Figure 7.18b

AVOID

Figure 7.18c Leaning back in the hurdler's position stresses knee ligaments on the bent leg and may irritate the lower back.

Figure 7.18a

Back-of-the-Leg Stretches

Muscles stretched: hamstrings (Figures 7.19, 7.20, 7.21, 7.22), gastrocnemious (Figure 7.23)

Hamstrings   Gastrocnemius

Exercisers have traditionally stretched the muscles at the back of the legs by performing a standing toe touch (Figure 7.19). Today, sports medicine professionals are concerned that hanging in this position stresses the ligaments that support the back, which could result in lower back pain. When the knees are straight, most of the major muscles in the hip and lower back area cannot function effectively to support the back. Bending the knees helps relieve the pressure on the lower back and allows the muscles to aid the ligaments. But, like the side stretch, hanging in one direction for an extended amount of time places stress on the intervertebral discs. Rather than hang in forward flexion, the toe-touch position, you can use some alternative methods of stretching the hamstrings. Some of these alternatives include the following.

1. Sit on the floor with the legs extended forward. Bend the left knee, and place the left foot flat on the floor. Hold the bent leg, and pull yourself gently forward (Figure 7.20a). If this is uncomfortable, place the hands behind the buttocks for support and try sitting up straight. This sitting position is good for inflexible people. (More flexible people may not feel a stretch in this position.) This stretch is preferable to the hurdler's stretch, which strains the knee (Figure 7.20b).

Scan to view video ▲

Figure 7.20a

Figure 7.19 The straight-leg toe touch (standing or sitting) places stress on the ligaments in the lower back region. Bending the knees will take some pressure off the low back.

Figure 7.20b Stretching forward in the hurdler's stretch stresses the knee ligaments of the bent leg.

2. Lying flat on the back, extend the right leg straight out, bend the left leg, and place the left foot flat on the floor. Lift the right leg up until you feel the hamstring stretching. Keep the knee facing the chest; don't turn it out (Figure 7.21a). For an active stretch, use the thigh and hip muscles to pull the right leg toward your head. By contracting the quadriceps muscle, you are allowing the hamstrings to relax. The hands should assist as needed. In a passive stretch, the hands pull and the leg muscles are relaxed.

Use a towel if you have difficulty reaching the leg (Figure 7.21b). Assisted stretching can also be achieved by having a trustworthy partner push slowly and steadily against the leg. Partners must listen carefully to each other and push the leg only to a point of mild discomfort. The lower leg can also be straightened along the floor as long as this does not cause the lower back to strain or lift up off the floor.

3. Stand with the right leg bent and the left leg extended forward with the heel resting on the floor, stability ball, or step (bench). With hands on the thigh of the right leg, bend forward at the waist (Figure 7.22).

Figure 7.21a

Figure 7.22

Figure 7.21b

4. *Stability ball:* Sit on the ball with one foot close to the ball and the other extended farther out in front. Put both hands on the knee of the close foot, and curl the body down over the knee (Figure 7.23). This stretches the calf muscles (gastrocnemius, soleus) of the near leg. Then push backward extending the front leg until only the heel is touching. This stretches the back of the leg (hamstrings) of the extended leg.

5. *Stability ball:* Lie down near a wall. Place the ball up on the wall, and hold it there with the bottoms of your feet. Your knees are bent and your torso flat on the ground. Roll the ball up the wall by slowly extending your legs. The closer your bottom is to the wall, the greater the stretch. Keep the hips square and the pelvis flat throughout (Figure 7.24).

Figure 7.23

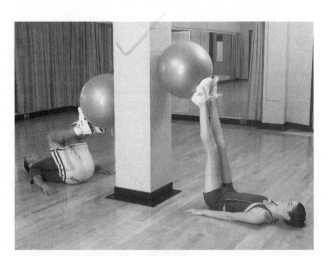

Figure 7.24 A pillar is used here to allow the reader to see both positions simultaneously. A flat wall is recommended for this exercise.

Inner Thigh Stretches

Side Lunge Position (Legs to the Sides)

Muscles stretched: adductors (gracilis)

1. With your body facing forward, assume a lunge position with right knee bent and left leg extended. Both feet should be comfortably aligned with the knees. Hands are placed on the upper thighs (Figure 7.25a). Hands can also

Adductors

be placed on the floor in front of the body for support (see Figure 7.25b on the next page). Try to lower hips. When a bench (step) is used, straddle the bench and place hands on top. Less flexible individuals may find this position more comfortable (Figure 7.25c). This stretch can also be performed with the trunk upright (standing) and hands on thighs. The bent right knee should not extend beyond the right instep (Figure 7.25d).

Figure 7.25a

Figure 7.25b

Figure 7.25c

AVOID

Figure 7.25d Extending the knee beyond the instep results in stress to the knee ligaments.

Butterfly Position

Muscles stretched: adductors, gracilis

1. Sit on the floor with the soles of the feet together. Grasp the ankles. (Grasping the toes and pulling may stress the ligaments of the feet.) It is usually most comfortable to grasp the right ankle with the left hand and the left ankle with the right hand. Sit up tall, and lean forward until you feel a stretch in the groin area (Figure 7.27). Touching the head to the feet stresses the lower back instead of stretching the groin area.

2. *Stability ball:* Sit on the ball with legs apart and feet flat on the floor. Your respective feet and knees should be pointing in the same direction. Place your hands on your knees. Roll the ball to one side while extending the opposite leg to the side (Figure 7.26).

Figure 7.26

Scan to view video ▲

Figure 7.27

Modified Straddle Position

Muscles stretched: adductors, gracilis

Sit on the floor with the left leg extended and the right leg bent in front. Stretch forward from the base of the spine (Figure 7.28). Think of putting your nose on the floor as far in front of you as possible.

You can also use this exercise to stretch the back of the legs by turning the hips to face the extended left leg and stretching forward. This is called the modified hurdler's stretch.

Scan to view video ▶

Figure 7.28

Combination Leg and Hip Stretch

FRONT LUNGE POSITION (ONE LEG FORWARD, ONE BACK)

Muscles stretched: quadriceps, hamstrings, hip flexors

Quadriceps   Hamstrings   Hip Flexors

1. Pretend you are straddling a straight line. Place the left foot out in front of your body just to the left of the imaginary line. Bend the left knee. Extend the right leg straight back with the right big toe just to the right of the line. Keep the hips absolutely square. Place your hands on the floor (or bench), one on each side of the bent leg, to support your weight. Try to lower the hips toward the ground (Figures 7.29a, 7.29b). This stretch can also be performed with the trunk upright (standing) and the hands on the front thigh. The bent front knee should stay above or behind the instep. (When the knee is pushed forward and the heel of the front foot lifts, stress is placed on the knee ligaments [Figure 7.29c].) When you want more stretch, move the rear foot back.

2. *Stability ball:* Take a front lunge position on the ball. Sit down on the ball. Place your hands on the ball on either side of you. Place the front foot far enough forward to maintain a 90-degree

Figure 7.29a

Figure 7.29b

Figure 7.29c When the knee is pushed beyond the instep, pressure is placed on the knee ligaments.

Figure 7.30

Figure 7.31a

Figure 7.31b

Scan to view
video ▲

angle in the knee. Allow the heel to lift on the back foot (Figure 7.30). For additional stretch, roll the ball forward (move the front foot forward as needed). Keep the hips square throughout.

HIP STRETCHES

Muscles stretched: hip flexors, quadriceps, hamstring

1. Place the legs in a front lunge position with the right foot in front. The back toes face straight ahead. The front foot may be turned slightly inward for balance. The back heel is off the ground. Keeping the hips square and the pelvis tucked under, try to lower the hips. Be sure the front foot is far enough out in front to do this comfortably. To avoid ligament stress, the bent front knee should stay directly above or behind the instep. The hands can be placed on the hips or on the front leg (Figure 7.31a). This same stretch can be achieved in a kneeling position (Figure 7.31b). You may want to pad the knees with a towel or mat.

2. *Stability ball:* Take the same position as described in Step 1 but with the hip resting on the side of the ball.

3. You can also stretch the hip flexors while lying on your back. Grasp under the knee, and pull one leg to the chest while keeping the other leg straight along the floor (Figure 7.32a). The extended bottom leg results in a greater stretch to the iliopsoas muscle (versus the quadriceps) than the previous two positions. Both the quadriceps and iliopsoas are hip flexors. Even more iliopsoas stretch can be achieved using a bench (Figure 7.32b).

Figure 7.32a

Figure 7.32b

Scan to view video ▲

Figure 7.33a

Figure 7.33b

Figure 7.33c

CALF STRETCHES

Muscles stretched: gastrocnemius, soleus

Gastrocnemius   Soleus

1. Stand in the same front lunge position used for the hip stretch, but adjust the stance so that the back heel touches down. Support or balance yourself by placing hands on the forward knee. Be sure to keep the back foot facing directly front, and keep the abdomen pulled in. A straight back leg stretches the calf muscle called the gastrocnemius (Figure 7.33a). When you bend the back leg but keep the heel on the ground, you provide a deeper stretch for the underneath calf muscle called the soleus (Figure 7.33b).

To perform a calf stretch using a bench (step), stand on top of the step. Put weight on the right foot, bending the right knee slightly. Place the left foot so that the ball of the foot is on the step but the heel is over the edge. Gently press the heel down (Figure 7.33c).

Variation

You can also stretch the calves in a sitting position. Extend one leg forward, keeping the knee slightly flexed. Reach forward, grasp the ball of the foot, and gently pull back. If you can't reach your foot, loop a towel around the ball of your foot and pull.

2. *Stability ball:* See Figure 7.23 on page 88.

Shin Stretches

Muscle stretched: tibialis anterior

1. Stand tall on one leg, and extend the other leg directly behind the body. Point the toe on the extended leg, and place the back of the toes on the ground. Keep the knee and foot facing forward. Press the ankle forward and downward, encouraging extension in the ankle. Feel the stretch through the shin and ankle (Figure 7.34, right)

Tibialis anterior

2. Stand on one leg. Cross the other leg in front, and place the back of the toes on the ground on the far side of the standing foot. Keep the feet close together. Bend the standing leg to create a stretch through the ankle and shin (Figure 7.34, left)

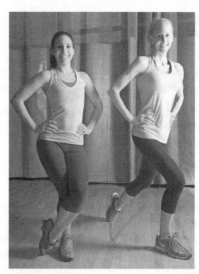

Figure 7.34

SUMMARY

A well-planned 50- to 60-minute class should include the following segments: a 5- to 10-minute warm-up, a 20- to 30-minute aerobic workout, a 5-minute standing cool-down, a 10- to 15-minute muscle-toning workout, followed by a 5- to 10-minute final (developmental) stretch. If you are late to class, take the time to prepare your body for vigorous exercise. If you must leave early, step out of class with enough time to cool down. The warm-up and cool-down are similar in the exercises and movements they incorporate, even though one is preparing the body for exercise while the other is bringing the body back to a resting state. Both the warm-up and cool-down promote flexibility. There are a number of ways to stretch, each with its advantages and disadvantages. A combination of methods may be the most effective. Finally, flexibility adds to the quality of your life and is something that can be maintained throughout your life.

COMMONLY ASKED QUESTIONS

Is warming up bad for some sports?

Warming up is always good. Your body needs to gradually move into more intense activity. What you may have heard is that some forms of stretching during the warm-up are "bad" for sports. There is some research evidence that static stretching may relax muscles in such a way that it is difficult to get the same amount of contraction for explosive movements. Dynamic stretching can be used instead. In some running studies, it was found that static stretching resulted in more muscle soreness. This may be due to a small amount of destabilizing of the joint. More research needs to be done to determine definitively how different types of stretching affect different activities.

Is there such as thing as being too flexible?

Yes. If a joint has too much flexibility it is less stable and more susceptible to injury. Acrobats who are very flexible use very strong muscles to maintain joint integrity. When ligaments that connect bones are overstretched, a joint can become loose. A sprained ankle, for example, results in overstretched ligaments. If not rehabilitated properly the ankle will be more apt to roll and get hurt again. Ligaments are slow to heal when overstretched and may never regain their original length. Sometimes muscles can support the loose joint and sometimes surgery is needed to "tighten" it back up. Pregnant women experience greater flexibility around joints due to hormone changes in the body. This is needed to allow the pelvic bones to spread for delivery. However, other joints are also affected by this hormonal change so a pregnant woman needs to be careful not to overstretch when exercising. "Double jointed" individuals are born with more joint laxity and will benefit from building muscle strength to surround and protect loose joints.

How long should you hold a stretch—10, 15, 30, 60 seconds?

The American College of Sports Medicine (ACSM) recommends accumulating 60 seconds of stretch per muscle. During a warm-up, a 10-second hold may be enough to prepare the muscles for activity. When the muscles are really warm (usually at the end of class) and stretches are being done to increase flexibility, you should hold for 15 to 30 seconds, with enough repetitions to reach 60 seconds. This is a change from ACSM's 2010 recommendation of two 30-second holds. Older adults may benefit from holds that last more than 60 seconds. Yoga often uses long holds for building both strength and flexibility.

KNOWLEDGE TIPS

1. The warm-up prepares the body and mind for physical activity. Warm-up movements raise the body's core and muscle temperature.

2. Warm-up movements work within comfortable ranges of motion, move from general to specific exercises, and raise the heart rate gradually moving from slow to moderate intensity activity.

3. The standing cool-down is used to bring down your activity level gradually. This activity helps bring blood shunted to the limbs back to the heart.

4. The developmental stretch, which occurs at the end of class, develops flexibility and helps prevent muscle soreness.

5. The ACSM guideline for flexibility is to stretch a minimum of 2 to 3 days a week, or even better, daily, at an intensity best described as holding to a point of tightness without discomfort, holding the stretch for 10 to 30 seconds for a static stretch; a 3–6 second contraction followed by 10 to 30 seconds of assisted stretch for PNF, with 2 to 4 repetitions for each stretch. Accumulate 60 seconds of stretch.

6. A stretch can be active (using contraction of the opposing muscle) or passive (using an outside force like a partner to elongate the muscle).

7. There are four types of stretches: static (sustained hold), ballistic (bounce stretch), dynamic, and PNF (combination of muscle contractions and stretches).

8. Good technique during a stretch ensures that you will receive the full benefit of the exercise.

9. Some exercises are appropriate in sports settings and inappropriate in health/fitness settings.

10. The step (bench) and stability ball can be used as effective tools for stretching.

THINK ABOUT IT

1. Why is it important to perform a warm-up? cool-down?

2. When in a group fitness class is the best time to work on developing flexibility? Why?

3. Each type of stretching has advantages. Explain the advantages associated with static, dynamic, and PNF stretching.

4. Describe the FITT principle for flexibility.

5. A static stretch can be passive or active. Explain the difference and give an example.

6. What is the stretch reflex and what role does it play in each of the types of stretching (static, ballistic, dynamic, and PNF)?

7. Identify a range of motion you would like to improve and identify a stretch you can use to achieve this goal.

8. What are some stretches that are considered unhealthy for normal health-enhancing activity?

REFERENCES

Alter, J. *Stretch & Strengthen*. Boston: Houghton Mifflin, 1986.

____. *Surviving Exercise*. Boston: Houghton Mifflin, 1983.

Alter, M. J. *Science of Flexibility*. 2nd ed. Champaign, IL: Human Kinetics, 1996.

American College of Sports Medicine. *ACSM's Guidelines for Exercise Testing and Exercise Prescription*. 8th ed. Media, PA: Lippincott Williams & Wilkins, 2010.

American Council on Exercise. *Aerobics Instructor Manual: ACE's Guide for Fitness Professionals*. San Diego, CA: American Council on Exercise, 2000.

Åstrand, P. O., and K. Rodahl. *Textbook of Work Physiology*. 2nd ed. New York: McGraw-Hill, 1977.

Barnard, R. J. "The Heart Needs a Warm-Up Time." *The Physician and Sportsmedicine* 4 (No. 1, 1976): 40.

Corbin, C. B., and M. L. Noble. "Flexibility." *Journal of Physical Education and Recreation* 51 (No. 6, 1980): 23–6; 57–60.

Faigenbaum, A.D., M. Bellucci, A. Bernieri, B. Bakker, and K. Hoorens. "Acute Effects of Different Warm-Up Protocols on Fitness Performance in Children." *Journal of Strength and Conditioning* 19 (No. 2, 2005): 376–81.

Gerson, R. "Point-Counterpoint: Calisthenics Before Aerobics." *Dance Exercise Today* (May/June 1985): 26–8.

Holt, L. E., T. M. Travis, and T. Okita. "Comparative Study of Three Stretching Techniques." *Perceptual and Motor Skills* 31 (1970): 611.

Jones, A. "Point-Counterpoint: Aerobics Before Calisthenics." *Dance Exercise Today* (May/June 1985): 27–8.

Paraskevi, M., S. Rokka, A. Beneka, G. Mavridis, and G. Godolias. "Reducing Risk of Injury Due to Warm Up and Cool Down in Dance Aerobic Instructors." *Journal of Back and Musculoskeletal Rehabilitation* 20 (No. 1, 2007): 29(7).

Schultz, P. "Flexibility: Day of the Static Stretch." *The Physician and Sportsmedicine* 7 (No. 11, 1979): 109–14, 117.

Shellock, F. G. "Physiological Benefits of Warm-Up." *The Physician and Sportsmedicine* 11 (No. 10, 1983): 134–9.

Silvestri, L., and J. Oescher. "Use of Aerobic Dance and Light Weights in Improving Measures of Strength, Endurance, and Flexibility." *Perceptual and Motor Skills* 70 (April 1990): 595–600.

Taylor, D., J. Dalton, A. Seaber, and W. Garrett. "Viscoelastic Properties of Muscle-Tendon Units: The Biomechanical Effects of Stretching." *American Journal of Sports Medicine* 18 (No. 3, 1990); 300–9.

Wiktorsson-Moller, M., B. Oberg, J. Ekstrand, and J. Gillquist. "Effects of Warming Up, Massage and Stretching on Range of Motion and Muscle Strength in the Lower Extremity." *American Journal of Sports Medicine* 11 (No. 4, 1983); 249–52.

8

Rhythmic Aerobics: Variations and Styles

The sound of many sneakers dancing ...

- I tried to sign up for a class but got confused by all the different names (styles). What do they mean?
- Do I have to do high-impact, running, jumping moves to get or stay fit?
- Will one style of aerobics make me more fit than another?
- Can I use interval training to train aerobically?
- Is the target heart-rate zone different for water aerobics?

GROUP fitness has grown to encompass a wide variety of classes—everything from spinning to Latin dancing. This chapter and the next explore some of the many trends in group fitness. This chapter focuses on the variations of the activity that kicked off the whole group fitness movement—aerobic dance. The first aerobic dance classes in the 1970s were highly choreographed high-impact dance routines created and franchised by Jackie Sorenson. Since then, many styles have evolved. Because there are so many styles, some that are more dance-like than others, the phrase "rhythmic aerobics" may be a better way to describe these exercises as a group. It is, after all, the matching of the rhythms of music to aerobic movement that is at the core and appeal of all the styles. The rhythmic aerobic scene includes high-impact, low-impact, step, interval, and circuit aerobics. And that doesn't even begin to describe all the styles that have become popular—everything from funk to Latin to combat aerobics.

If you have the opportunity to choose from among these different types of rhythmic aerobic programs, first watch the one(s) you are thinking of joining, or take a free trial class. Make sure the class suits your fitness level and that the instructor is knowledgeable. You may find that one style feels right for you, or with all these possibilities (and more), you may decide to mix it up using a variety of styles. Maybe high-impact or step aerobics gets you in shape for some fall hiking, a low-impact class gives you a change of pace and a workout with less impact stress on your legs for the winter, a salsa aerobics gets you set for that spring vacation to Cancún, and water aerobics keeps you cool and fit during the hot summer.

DANCE EXERCISE AEROBICS

Founders Jacki Sorensen (Aerobic Dancing—workout) and Judi Sheppard Missett (Jazzercise) have both drawn on their dance backgrounds to choreograph dancelike routines that have had great appeal for three decades. Following their lead but definitely in their own style are Victoria Johnson and Christy Lane, both well known for their funky fitness routines done to pop-funk and rap music. Funk is a mixture of ballet, jazz, modern dance, street dancing, maybe some line dancing, and a whole lot of "attitude." You can perform funk steps in a style that gets "down and into the floor" or in one that is up, light, and bouncy, called hip-hop. Funk can be fast moving and thrilling when you start picking up the moves. (Usually, moves are taught at a slower pace and then performed at a fast pace.) Country line dancing, upbeat and widely popular, has also expanded into the aerobic arena. You can get fit doing the Tush Push and the Electric Slide or the Achy Breaky. Salsarobics and Zumba are just two of the many companies exploring Latin moves on the aerobics floor. These forms of dance aerobics use steps from the merengue, cha-cha, rumba, samba, lambada, and more. If it's African you like, or Gospel ... you

95

can find that, too. Instructors are pulling from their strengths and producing all kinds of specialty classes.

For those who want to jump less, at least two companies have developed nonimpact aerobic styles. Debby and Carlos Rosas introduced NIA (nonimpact aerobics), a flowing, undulating, rising-and-falling form of dance that sustains training zone heart rates with nonimpact changes of feet on the floor. Another company, called Yogarobics, has used yoga and tai chi to develop a style that involves moving from a state of quiet or stillness to one of chaotic (vigorous) movements and back to stillness. And, of course, there is step aerobics, started by Gin Miller, which is more comfortable for individuals who prefer a class with less dance emphasis.

THE AEROBICS PORTION OF CLASS

All aerobics classes, regardless of type or style, use continuous, rhythmic, large-muscle movements to condition your cardiorespiratory system. The training strengthens your heart, reduces the risk of coronary heart disease, reduces your percentage of body fat, and provides you with a sense of well-being. Some evidence even suggests that aerobic training can lengthen your life, and it definitely can improve the quality of it. (For a complete discussion of the benefits of aerobic dance exercise, refer back to Chapter 1.)

The aerobic part of class follows the warm-up and/or any muscle-toning exercises that follow the warm-up. The most commonly used cardiorespiratory workout uses a sustained aerobic approach. The first part of the routine is 5 to 10 minutes of moderately paced activity to gradually bring you up to a training intensity. Instructors often use low-impact aerobics for this. Once in your training zone, you sustain this level of exertion for 20 to 30 minutes and then taper down as you reach the end of the workout. (The aerobic portion of class may be slightly longer in a low-impact or nonimpact style of rhythmic aerobics or advanced classes.) The aerobic section is followed by the standing cool-down (postcardial section) during which the activity level continues to decrease until you are well below your training zone and sufficiently recovered (a heart rate of 120 beats per minute [bpm] or lower) to go on to muscle-toning exercises or a cool-down stretch. A cardiorespiratory workout may also be obtained using short segments of high-intensity exercise alternated with lower intensity (but still in the training zone) recovery exercise periods. See Circuit and Interval Training for Aerobics on page 107 for more information. Many people do not find this type of workout as comfortable and, as a result, more people drop out. Highly fit, highly motivated individuals, however, may enjoy it.

TECHNIQUE TIPS

1. Maintain good standing or sitting posture. Pull your chin back to prevent jutting the head forward. Pull back gently on your shoulders, pull in your abdomen, keep your hip joints released (relaxed) and vertically aligned, soften your knees, and avoid unnecessarily rounding or arching the back. Pretend you are being pulled up by a string that attaches to the top of your head. Good alignment relieves pressure in your lower back and prevents unnecessary exercise stress.

2. Breathe! Some people have a tendency to hold their breath when they pull in their abdomen. Breathe normally. This means breathing more deeply and quickly as the oxygen demand increases.

3. Keep your feet and knees going in the same direction to prevent rotation soreness, and bend the knees when landing from a jump. Try to absorb the impact of a jump or step by bending your knees instead of arching your back. (Some people lose their alignment by arching their backs when they land.)

4. Maintain good neutral spine back alignment during straight-leg kicks. Enthusiastic aerobicizers tend to exceed the limits of their flexibility by kicking too high. To compensate, the lower back will round. Kick only as high as your hamstring flexibility allows. Correct and incorrect kicking alignment are shown in Chapter 6, Figures 6.6a and 6.6b, on page 62.

5. Limit repetition of a movement to a healthy number. This concept is discussed more as it applies to each type of aerobics. For example, in step aerobics, you switch lead legs after 1 minute, and in high-impact aerobics, you should limit yourself to four consecutive hops. Repetitions should be limited anytime overuse is a concern. If you are recovering from an injury, the number of repetitions may need to be fewer than normal.

6. Control your arm movements. Momentum from flinging an arm can carry the arm beyond its normal range of motion and hurt the joint. Arm movements can and often should move above shoulder level, but the arms should not be held above the shoulders for extended periods of time. The isometric contractions performed by the shoulder muscles will increase blood pressure and may add to unnecessary

soreness. Instead, arms should frequently move between low, middle, and high positions.

7. Do not wear ankle weights during the aerobic portion of class. Extra weight attached to the ankle increases the risk of impact injury to the lower leg.

8. Handheld and wrist weights are generally not recommended during the aerobic phase of class. Even small weights can pose a risk in a fast-moving activity.

9. Use an intensity that is high enough to create an overload but low enough to allow oxygen delivery and let aerobic metabolism dominate.

10. Elevate or lower intensity by increasing or decreasing range of motion, arm movements, the amount or height of jumps (high-impact aerobics, step), or the amount of knee bend (low-impact aerobics).

When your movements demonstrate good positioning, alignment, and control, you are said to have "clean lines." It is always fun to watch people with clean lines because they make the movements look crisp and effortless. Strive for this in whichever form of aerobics you select.

HIGH-IMPACT AEROBICS

High-impact aerobics (HIA) classes consist of large-muscle movements such as jogging, jumping, hopping, skipping, knee lifts, dance steps, and calisthenics. Some routines are highly choreographed; others are improvised. Choreographed routines are not necessarily more dancelike but are planned routines that closely follow the music and can be repeated exactly the same way each time. Because they are planned, well-choreographed routines usually provide a more balanced workout. The advantage of freestyle routines is their spontaneity and easy adjustment to class ability (Figure 8.1).

Planting the foot is probably the most important skill to perfect, since many HIA steps require you to land on the balls of your feet. A dancer counts four different positions between being on the ball of the foot and standing flat. Although you don't need to be able to identify the four positions, you do need to learn how to roll down through all of them as you land from a jump. To land, roll down through the balls of your feet (Figures 8.2a and 8.2b), and bend your knees as you touch down your heels (Figure 8.2c). When you forget to touch your heels down, your calf muscles remain contracted. Constant contraction for 20 to 30 minutes makes for very tight calf muscles. Rolling your feet all the way down will also help prevent shin splints.

Figure 8.2a

Figure 8.2b

Figure 8.1 Aerobics with "attitude."

Figure 8.2c

ON THE BEAT!

Understanding the way music is organized and used can help you know what to expect in a routine. For example, most movements are done an even number of times. If an instructor works with songs in their original form, there may be musical irregularities (such as bridges) that result in odd numbers of steps or some recovery marching while waiting for the chorus. If, however, the instructor is working with music produced for exercise classes, the music is much more predictable. There are advantages to working with both kinds of music.

UPBEATS AND DOWNBEATS

The strong beat of the music is the downbeat; the softer one that follows is the upbeat. Most aerobic dance exercise movements will start on the downbeat. For example, during a jumping jack, you move your arms and legs outward on the downbeat and back to center on the upbeat. Funk and hip-hop movements often emphasize the upbeat, which makes them a little trickier for people to learn. Putting the accent off the beat like this is a form of syncopation. But when you get the hang of it, it is a lot of fun.

TEMPO

Tempo is how quickly the beats are played, usually expressed in beats per minute. Different styles of aerobics use different tempos. Low-impact and step require slower tempos than high-impact aerobics.

TIMING

Regular or single timing means to make one movement per beat. To jog in single time means to land on the right foot for one beat and then the left foot on the next beat. When you perform a step in double-time, you must make two movements per beat. To double-time the jog, you must land on the right and then left foot within one beat. To half-time the same movement means to take twice as long. So with our jogging example, you would land on the right foot and hold there for a second count before jumping to the left foot. Half-timed movements are slower; double-timed movements are faster. In a routine, you might do single-time marching, double-time marching or jogging, and then half-timed squats.

RHYTHM

Rhythm is the pattern of the music. Much of the music used today is created for exercise classes and uses a very strong and regular beat pattern. Different rhythmic step patterns can be put to the beat pattern.

Three typical rhythm patterns, each with an example of a corresponding step pattern, are shown on the opposite page. Note that all of them use 4 beats. When an "and" is used, the movement must occur quickly between the beats.

Moderation is the key. Since you are bringing about 3 times your body weight down on your foot each time you hop, it is a good idea to limit the number of consecutive repetitions on one foot to four hops. This moderation will help prevent overuse injuries such as **shin splints** and **tendinitis.** Similarly, overdoing two-footed movements can be hard on the lower legs. Switch off two-footed steps with steps that involve alternate feet. Lateral leg movements, such as jumping jacks, press the knee and ankle in an outward direction. They are good exercises, but you should limit the number you perform in a row, and you should bend your knees as you land. If at any time you feel overuse occurring, modify the routine you are doing. Most instructors will be glad that you took the initiative to individualize your workout.

A forward running stride results in less impact stress than more vertical movements such as hopping or jumping. Therefore, whenever there is enough room, high-impact choreography should include use of the regular running (jogging) stride. Jogging with heel-toe mechanics also stretches and therefore provides relief to the calf muscles. Instructors will often have the class jog in place while working on arm movements. During this time, pay special attention to foot plant and leg position. Letting up on technique— kicking your heels out to the side or letting your knees turn out—is easy. Instead, concentrate on technique—lift your knees directly to the front and roll down through your foot with each step.

HIA is exciting and upbeat. Faster music (150 to 170 bpm) can be used with it than with step aerobics

---

ON THE BEAT! (*continued*)

1, 2, 3, 4 (STEP TOUCH)

Count 1: Step sideways to the right onto the right foot.

Count 2: Touch the left foot next to the right foot.

Count 3: Step sideways to the left onto the left foot.

Count 4: Touch the right foot next to the left.

1 AND 2, 3, AND 4 (PONY)

Count 1: Step forward or sideways onto the right foot.

Count and: Move the left foot next to the right instep, and briefly place weight on the ball of the left foot.

Count 2: Return the weight to the right foot.

Count 3: Step forward or sideways onto the left foot.

Count and: Move the right foot next to the left instep, and briefly place weight on the ball of the right foot.

Count 4: Return the weight to the left foot.

1, 2, 3, AND 4 (MAMBO, CHA-CHA)

Count 1: Step forward onto the right foot.

Count 2: Shift the weight back to the left.

Count 3: Step right.

Count and: Step briefly on the left foot.

Count 4: Step right.

PHRASING

Music is grouped into units called phrases. The most common phrase length for aerobic dance exercise is 32 beats. During these 32 beats, the instructor can build choreography in a variety of ways. One way is to introduce a step for 8 counts, such as a march/jog. Keep the step going for another 8 counts but add an arm movement such as biceps curls to it. Then change to another step, such as a grapevine, for 8 counts (4 to the right, 4 to the left), and finally add upright row arms to this movement during the last 8 counts. A new 32-count pattern may then be started or may simply be added on to this one. Movements are generally repeated 2, 4, or 8 times in a row. Instructors often count backwards to let you know how many steps you have left to go. They reserve the last couple of beats in an ongoing pattern to call out the next move. For example, "8 more, 7, 6, 5, 4, 3, grapevine right." The instructor may also count up and not voice 7 and 8 so that he or she can call the next move.

---

or low-impact aerobics. When fast-paced music is used, however, use smaller movements so that you stay with the beat comfortably, or you can perform movements to every other beat. Conversely, slow music can be double-timed.

LOW-IMPACT AEROBICS

Low-impact aerobics (LIA) is designed to provide an aerobic experience without the risk of impact injury that may result from the stress of high-impact movements. To accomplish this goal, one foot must touch the floor at all times. Keeping one foot on the ground effectively cuts the impact stress in half. In place of the jumping movements of HIA, LIA substitutes bending movements that lower and then raise the body's center of gravity.

Because it lessens impact shock, LIA is a good activity for people who are prone to shinsplints, but both the bending and the lateral steps often associated with LIA may irritate a knee joint that is prone to injury.

LIA is low-impact but not necessarily low-intensity. Participants can increase their workout intensity by moving their body's center of gravity upward against gravity. When you jump, you move your center of gravity up the number of inches you jump. In LIA, you bend your knees, lowering your center of gravity, and then lift it upward by returning to your starting position or perhaps higher by rising up on the balls of your feet. The sinking and rising motions of LIA are one way in which work is created. Large, controlled arm movements also increase intensity. Extended limbs (long levers) are also more challenging to move than are bent limbs (short levers). For example, swinging the arms out to the side and then overhead is more difficult when the arms are extended than when they are bent at the elbow. Finally, large moving patterns are effective for raising the heart rate. Think of the energy expended in long, striding steps such as those used in power walking. Traveling moves can go side to side, forward and back, on the diagonal, or in a circle. The larger the space in which you work out, the more you can take advantage of traveling steps. Traveling steps help LIA achieve similar intensities and benefits as HIA. Stationary choreography with a lot of overhead arm movements appears to reach the same intensities, but the arm work elevates heart rate without a corresponding rise in oxygen consumption and metabolic costs. In other words, your circulatory system works harder, but you don't get corresponding aerobic benefits.

The following will help you prevent injuries:

1. Turn your feet and knees out during large (wide) steps to the side—this placement helps maintain hip, knee, and foot alignment.
2. Make sure knee flexion does not exceed 90 degrees.
3. Avoid too many steps that cross the foot in front while moving to the side (such as that which can occur in "grapevine" step), because this type of movement can promote foot pronation. This can be prevented in the grapevine by crossing the foot behind.

The music for LIA is moderately paced (120 to 140 bpm) to allow sufficient time to execute larger movements. Occasionally, instructors use slightly faster music for which they may increase the speed of dance steps and decrease the size of steps or movements. LIA choreography should follow natural movement patterns and be performed with good muscle control.

One of the advantages of LIA is its emphasis on arm work. Most women lack good upper-body strength, as is evident by the small percentage of women who can perform just one pull-up. LIA and some good upper-body resistance exercises can improve upper-body strength. However, the arms should not remain raised above the shoulder for too long. This results in a sustained isometric contraction for the shoulder muscles, which, in turn, can result in pain, fatigue, and a sharp increase in blood pressure.

Another advantage of LIA is that more people can do it than HIA. LIA is ideal for people who are overweight, because it does not involve jumping, which in overweight people can place excessive strain on joints. It is also good exercise for older people who no longer enjoy jumping and for those who experience incontinence with jumping. Large-breasted women and women in a

prenatal or postnatal condition may also prefer this less bouncy exercise. People who tend to have chronic impact stress injuries as well as people returning to exercise after an injury may prefer LIA. In addition, HIA exercisers may enjoy LIA for a change of pace. It is also a less stressful class for individuals who demonstrate poor biomechanical technique or who have poor structural leg alignment. And it provides a comfortable way for beginners to start exercising, because LIA is easy to adapt to a low-intensity workout. Under a physician's care, people with high blood pressure, heart problems, orthopedic problems, or physical disabilities can enjoy an LIA class, although participants with a special medical condition should check with their physicians before beginning a class. LIA may also be a good way for people with diabetes and asthma to start exercising, because it can enable them to increase their workout intensity gradually.

When these individuals know how exercise will affect them, they can work up to a high-intensity LIA or HIA class. Because LIA is so adaptable, it appeals to people of all ages, often bringing together one, two, or even three generations.

COMBINATION HIGH-/LOW-IMPACT AND MODERATE-IMPACT AEROBICS

Combination high-/low-impact aerobics (also known as **combo-impact, CIA,** and **hi/lo-impact aerobics**) is a form of aerobic dance exercise that uses both LIA and HIA in one class, with a tempo range of 130 to 170 bpm. This can be done three different ways. One whole song can be LIA and another HIA. Or a set of movements (a phrase) within a song can be LIA, and another sequence HIA. Or each sequence of steps can contain both LIA and HIA steps. These combinations add some terrific variety, eliminate some of the impact stress, and produce routines that are easily adjusted to people's fitness levels.

Moderate-impact aerobics (MIA) keeps one foot on the floor at all times like LIA, but it moves the center of gravity by emphasizing going up and down on the ball of the foot. The emphasis is not on getting lower to rise up like LIA, but rather on moving upward from a normal bend of the knees onto the ball of the foot. For example, march, and as your right knee goes upward, rise up on your left toe. Or rise up and down on the ball of your left foot as you move your right leg in and out of a side lunge position. MIA is less "bouncy" than HIA and can cut down the impact stress by about a third. MIA can constitute its own class, but more often MIA movements are incorporated into higher-intensity (or power) LIA classes and used to gradually increase or taper down intensity during HIA classes.

STEP AEROBICS

Step aerobics (also called bench), a form of aerobics that involves stepping up and down on a bench using a variety of step patterns, was invented and popularized by Gin Miller in the late 1980s. It became very popular when she teamed up with Reebok to create the Step Reebok program. Stepping up and down on a bench, however, dates much further back. Bench stepping has been used for rehabilitation purposes and for screening individuals for cardiovascular fitness for many years. In fact, it was when Miller was recovering from an injury and prescribed therapeutic bench stepping that she conceived the idea of using a variety of stepping patterns for general fitness. It caught on, not only with the regular aerobics crowd, but also with those who had been uncomfortable with some of the "danciness" of aerobic dance.

Step aerobics uses a bench or "step" that is between 4 and 12 inches high. Bench height is adjusted according to the participant's fitness level: lower for beginners and higher for more advanced students. Higher platform heights are associated with knee discomfort. A person's height, particularly leg length, should be considered in this decision. In general, most people should use a bench height that results in knee flexion of 60 degrees or less when the foot is placed on the bench. The 60-degree angle provides a good workout and limits knee soreness. A 30-degree knee angle provides the most comfort and the least impact stress, but the corresponding step height may be insufficient to produce the desired training intensity. For safety and injury prevention reasons, the knee angle should never be more than 90 degrees. Bench heights of 4, 6, and 8 inches work for most people.

One of the biggest advantages to step training is that people of different fitness levels can perform the same steps to the same tempo side by side—the bench height, the amplitude at which steps are performed, and arm movements determine the intensity. This is one of the most popular forms of aerobic dance exercise for men. Some instructors use very linear, almost military-looking movements, while others use more dancelike movements. Stepping patterns start out very simple and build in complexity. Some instructors even use two or more benches per person and take the steps up and down across both. Although this practice adds a lot of fun variations, it does not increase the aerobic effect, and it often requires more equipment and space.

Step aerobics can be performed on the floor (lowest intensity), on a low step, or on a higher step for higher intensity (Figure 8.3). Step aerobics use a range of tempos, from 118 to 122 bpm (beginners) to a maximum of 128 (advanced). Combination bench mixes patterns

Figure 8.3

of steps on and off the bench with patterns that stay on the floor or stay on top of the bench. This combination lowers the number of step (up and down) repetitions, which will reduce knee discomfort and overuse for some people. For advanced students, higher intensities can be achieved by adding power moves. The use of weights and step is still somewhat controversial. The existing evidence indicates that it is preferable to restrict the use of weights to a separate muscle training segment of class during which slow, controlled movements with the proper technique can be ensured.

BASIC STEPS FOR STEP AEROBICS

The leg you step with first is referred to as the "lead leg." Usually, you begin a new step with the right leg. Because it's best not to lead off with the same leg for more than 1 minute of stepping, you can use a "tap change" to change from one lead leg to the other. The tap change is explained and diagrammed on page 102.

Tapless step is a version of step aerobics that doesn't use tap changes. The choreography is designed to use steps that naturally change the lead leg rather than inserting numerous tap changes. This allows the routine to flow more, but in some cases it also makes the routines more complex. After you have learned the basic steps presented in the next section, try performing the two routines in the Step Aerobic Routines box on page 106. One is a traditional-style step routine, and the second is tapless. Often instructors use a combination that uses some tap changes but also takes advantage of other transition steps.

In these diagrams, all steps are presented with an initial right-leg lead. The right foot has been shaded to help you distinguish between right and left legs. When necessary, an aerial view of the step has also been included. Most steps are performed in 4 counts, although positions between counts are also shown for clarification. The positions you should be in on the count are labeled. The names for the steps are fairly standard, but there may be some variation between instructors.

Classes begin with an off-the-bench warm-up and then slowly bring up the intensity. The progression pattern most often used is one of learning the step pattern, adding arms, and then adding a direction change. For example, you might begin with a basic pattern of stepping on and off the bench, add arm curls with each step, and then turn the stepping so that you are stepping on the diagonal (corner to corner). Depending on the level of the class, the instructor may stop the arm motion until the new direction is established

and then may restart the arm motion or begin a new arm motion. The stepping portion of class is followed by an aerobic cool-down, which finishes with off-the-bench steps and then some strength and flexibility work. The bench is a useful tool for strength and flexibility moves such as the triceps push-ups (Figure 11.20 on page 151) and hamstring stretch (Figure 7.22 on page 87).

A visual and written description of a sampling of the basic movements for step aerobics follows. More can be found online; a good source is the website www.turnstep.com, which offers an excellent dictionary of step aerobic steps with animated step patterns that make step aerobics easy to learn. Individuals can also post their routines, but be aware that they are not professionally screened for correctness.

Basic Step

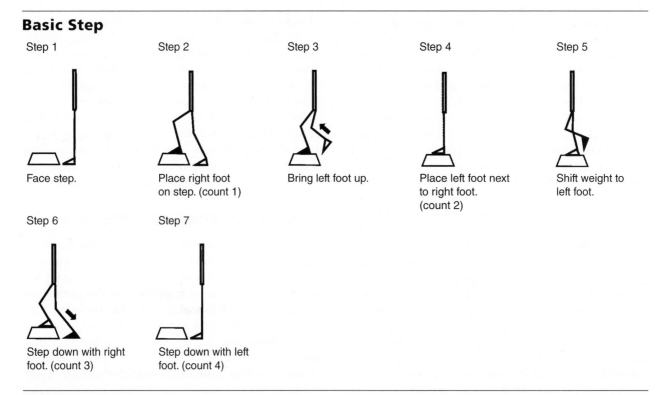

Step 1 — Face step.

Step 2 — Place right foot on step. (count 1)

Step 3 — Bring left foot up.

Step 4 — Place left foot next to right foot. (count 2)

Step 5 — Shift weight to left foot.

Step 6 — Step down with right foot. (count 3)

Step 7 — Step down with left foot. (count 4)

Tap Change

The basic step above was performed with a right-foot lead. To change to a left-foot lead, perform the tap change with this alternate Step 7. This tap allows you to lead with the left foot for the next basic step. Tap changes may be used to change the lead leg after one step or after a series of different steps.

Step 7 alternate

Tap left toe on floor without putting weight on it, then lead with left foot in next step.

V-Step

The V-step step is the same as the basic step, but the feet are positioned further apart on the bench and closer together on the floor. An aerial view helps demonstrate this.

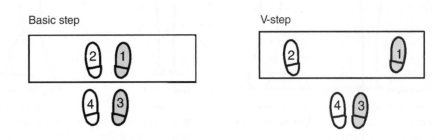

Note: A Turnstep can be accomplished by turning one-quarter to the right as you step off the bench. This will put you sideways to the bench.

Knee-Up

The basic step can be performed with a knee-up as shown, or a leg curl, a forward leg kick, or a side leg lift.

Note: To make this a Repeater step, only touch the ball of the foot down in Step 6, then draw the knee back up. Repeat twice more and then perform Steps 5 and 6 as normal. (8 counts)

Over the Top

▲ = Right foot
△ = Left foot

Stand sideways to step. | Step up with right foot. (count 1) | Step up with left foot and shift weight onto it. (count 2) | Step down with right foot. (count 3) | Step down with left foot. (count 4)

Straddle Down

Step 1   Step 2   Step 3   Step 4   Step 5

▲ = Right foot
△ = Left foot

Stand on step facing end. | Step down to right with right foot. (count 1) | Step down to left with left foot, straddling step. (count 2) | Step up with right foot. (count 3) | Step up with left foot. (count 4)

Note: To make this a Lunge step, perform Steps 1 and 2 and then step the right foot back up onto the bench. Repeat to the right or perform alternating left and right lunges.

Corner-to-Corner

Perform Steps 1–7 with a right-foot lead. To continue the corner-to-corner pattern, use the opposite corner (right) and a left-foot lead as follows: Count 1, place the left foot diagonally on the corner of the step. Count 2, draw the right leg into a knee-up position. Count 3, step down with the right foot. Count 4, step down with the left foot and turn toward the left corner of the step. (The knee-up can be substituted with a leg curl or leg kick.)

Step 1   Step 2

Face left corner of step. | Lift right (inside) leg.

Step 3   Steps 4 and 5   Step 6   Step 7

Place right foot diagonally on corner of step. (count 1) | Draw left leg into knee-up position. (count 2) | Step down with left foot. (count 3) | Step down with right foot and turn toward right corner of step. (count 4)

Hop Turn (Pivot Turn)

Starting position can be facing the bench or from a sideways position with the bench on the right. You can execute the rotation of the turn (1) while in the air during the hop or (2) by pivoting with the foot in contact with the bench.

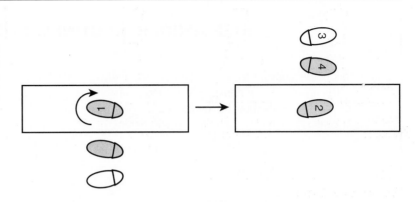

Step 1 Step the right foot up on the bench. (count 1)

Step 2 Hop and turn (pivot) to the right until you are facing the opposite end of the bench.

Step 3 Land the hop on the right foot. (count 2)

Step 4 Step the left foot down off the bench (opposite side from the starting position). (count 3)

Step 5 Step the right foot down. (count 4)

AROUND THE WORLD

This pattern can be accomplished by performing two hop turn steps using the same lead foot. This will result in a 360-degree turn in the same direction.

Step training is fun and easy to do. Here are some technique tips to get you started.

1. Place your whole foot on the bench. Be careful that the heel of your foot is not hanging over the near edge.
2. Lean from your ankles, not your waist. (This helps keep the pressure off your lower back.)
3. Step down near to the bench. (This helps prevent Achilles tendinitis.)
4. Roll down through your foot (toe, ball, heel) unless you are doing lunge steps or repeaters, in which case touch only the ball of your foot down. (This helps prevent tight, sore calf muscles, and plantar fasciitis.)
5. Look where you are stepping by keeping your head up and using your eyes to look down.
6. Wear shoes that have a heel notch to avoid irritation of the Achilles tendon.
7. Before stepping, warm up calf muscles well.
8. Adjust the step height to match your fitness level. Never use a step that bends your knee more than 90 degrees.
9. Adjust workout intensity by increasing or decreasing arm use and extension and the number of propulsion or power moves.
10. Decrease intensity by performing steps off the bench if you become fatigued.
11. Change lead legs after a maximum of 1 minute.
12. On repeater steps, perform a maximum of 5 repetitions. Here is an example of a repeater step: Step onto the bench with the left foot, draw the right knee up in a knee-lift, touch the ball of the right foot to the floor, draw the right knee back up in a knee-lift, touch the right ball of the foot to the floor, knee-lift again, step down right, step down left. The 3 knee-lifts constitute 3 repetitions.
13. If you are working at an advanced level and are using power/propulsion moves, perform

STEP AEROBIC ROUTINES: TWO STYLES

Try to follow the steps for these two types of routines. You can use an actual step bench or a rectangle on the floor to simulate the bench. The number of counts (musical beats) required for each pattern is in parentheses.

STEP ROUTINE: TAP TRANSITIONS

3 basic steps with a right-foot lead.
1 basic step with a right-foot lead finishing with
   a tap change.   (16)

3 basic steps with a left-foot lead.
1 basic step with a left-foot lead finishing with
   a tap change.   (16)

3 V-steps with a right-foot lead.
1 V-step with a right-foot lead finishing with a tap
   change.   (16)

3 V-steps with a left-foot lead.
1 V-step with a left-foot lead finishing with a tap
   change.   (16)

1 turnstep (V-step turn) with a right-foot lead.
   Finish with a tap change.
1 turnstep (V-step turn) with a left-foot lead.
   Finish with a tap change.   (8)

Repeat above turnstep pattern 2 more times.
(You will finish with the bench on your right.)   (8)

4 over-the-top steps alternating right- and
   left-foot leads.
   Use a tap change to change the foot-leads.   (16)

*A mambo-cha-cha-cha pattern may be substituted.

STEP ROUTINE: TAPLESS TRANSITIONS

4 basic steps with a right-foot lead.   (16)
1 cha-cha step to transition to a left-foot lead.
(Step right for count 1; step left and right more
quickly for count 2.)   (2)

4 basic steps with a left-foot lead.   (16)
1 cha-cha to transition to a right-foot lead.
(Step left for count 1; step right and left more
quickly for count 2.)   (2)

4 V-steps with a right-foot lead.   (16)
2 jumping jacks.   (4)
4 V-steps with a left-foot lead.   (16)
2 jumping jacks.   (4)

4 knee-lifts with alternating right- and
   left-foot leads.   (16)

4 corner-to-corner knee-lifts starting with a
   right-foot lead to the left corner and transitioning
   to a left-foot lead to the right corner. Repeat right
   and left. Finish facing square to the bench.   (16)

1 hop turn with a right-foot lead and turning to the
   right. You will end on the far side of the bench,
   weight on the right foot.
4 marches in place, turning 180 degrees to the right,
   starting with the left foot (LRLR).*
1 hop turn with a left-foot lead and turning to the
   left. You will end on the original side of the bench,
   weight on the left foot.
4 marches in place, turning 180 degrees to the left,*
   starting with the right foot (RLRL).   (16)

the moves for approximately 1 minute (or less) and then alternate with a less stressful step.

14. When performing a kick or a lunge to the back, be careful about placing your arms high overhead, because this movement may lead to back arching.

15. Step quietly. Stamping or stomping on the step will increase impact stress—unless, of course, you are so mentally stressed that the release is well worth the added leg stress!

Caution: Step aerobics is *not* recommended for people with knee joint problems unless prescribed by a physician.

CIRCUIT AND INTERVAL TRAINING FOR AEROBICS

Circuit training is the use of a series of exercise stations through which an individual progresses in a specified order. The participant progresses from one station to the next, with or without a rest, depending on the type of training desired. The circuit can consist of stations of any type: aerobic, anaerobic, flexibility, muscular strength, or endurance. If the purpose of the circuit is to train the aerobic system, then an all-aerobic circuit is desirable. This way, continuous, large-muscle, rhythmic activity occurs throughout. Such a circuit might have in it an exercise cycle, a rowing machine, a stair machine, a jump rope, a mini-trampoline, a dance mat, and a treadmill. Or it might be composed completely of aerobic dance exercise step patterns. For example, one station might be knee-lifts, the next might be four jumping jacks and four kicks, and the next might be a series of steps onto a bench.

A mixed circuit might consist of resistance training (muscle-toning) stations such as lunges and squats interspersed between aerobic stations. Although this can be effective training, be careful that the resistance exercises do not require you to drop your head below your waist after vigorous aerobic work, because lowering your head may cause light-headedness. You should also be careful that fatigue from previous stations does not result in poor technique, especially if you are using weights or other resistance equipment. Muscle strength and endurance can also be increased using a circuit composed of resistance training stations. At one time, it was believed that moving through a series of stations composed of weight-training equipment with only 30-second intervals between stations would result in aerobic fitness gains. Research has shown that while the heart rate may be in the training zone, oxygen consumption does not increase proportionately. Although all individuals receive muscular strength benefits, only low-fit individuals will increase their aerobic fitness using this type of circuit.

Interval training consists of a series of short bouts of high-intensity activity alternated with rest intervals or lower-intensity activity. Interval training that alternates activity intensities between the high and low ends of the heart-rate target zone will develop aerobic fitness and may be referred to as interval aerobics. Intervals that use intensities that exceed the target heart-rate zone will emphasize anaerobic work. This type of training will improve the cardiorespiratory system but does not target the aerobic system. Anaerobic training is uncomfortable for most people, increases the risk of injury, and results in a greater exercise drop-out rate.

For this reason, anaerobic interval training is recommended for advanced students who like this kind of demanding workout.

AEROBICS VIDEOS

Some excellent videos are on the market, but some that promote ineffectual or even harmful exercises are also available. Ask your instructor for guidance in selecting one. Also, please be aware that an instructor on a screen can't see and correct your body position and technique, whereas live instructors can provide you with this valuable feedback. A combination of live and taped instructors may be the best solution.

SUMMARY

Aerobic dancing has expanded into a family of rhythmic aerobic activities. Some of the newer variations have made it possible for a greater variety of people to get involved. Other variations have resulted in more coeducational classes, and still others have enabled friends of varying fitness levels to exercise together.

COMMONLY ASKED QUESTIONS

Am I working hard enough if I don't sweat much?

Sweat is not a good measure of exercise intensity. Different people sweat different amounts and in different places. Some sweat profusely before they even cross the training threshold. Others hardly sweat at all. Heart rate and ratings of perceived exertion are better indicators of intensity.

Men usually sweat more than women because they have more sweat glands and more muscle. When muscle is working, heat is generated—the more muscle, the more heat. Sweat is a good thing. The evaporation of sweat cools the body.

Is it good to "go for the burn"?

The burn is the feeling you get when your muscles are working so hard that oxygen cannot be supplied to them fast enough to produce energy. This ischemia (lack of oxygen) and the accumulation of lactic acid make your muscles feel heavy and sometimes cause a burning sensation. If you are trying to work aerobically, the burn is counterproductive because it is a product of heavy anaerobic exercise. Muscle-toning exercises are anaerobic, and it is during these exercises that you are most likely to feel the burn. If you feel the burn during the aerobic portion of the class, you should reduce the intensity or change the exercise until you no longer feel it. For example, if your arms are burning in an overhead position, bring them down and do an easier motion at or below waist level. When you have recovered, you can return to the original exercise or intensity or continue with the modification.

Sometimes I get bored with aerobic dance exercise. Is that normal?

Yes; everyone can experience burnout. You can take a break from aerobic dancing by getting involved with another kind of aerobic exercise. The important thing is to continue exercising!

What is cross-training, and should I do it?

To cross-train is to use two or more types of exercises to train. For example, you can train aerobically using both swimming and aerobic dance exercise. Because each activity uses your muscles differently, you will get a more complete workout. But you do not need to cross-train to achieve health-related fitness—each activity by itself provides a good aerobic workout. Cross-training can help combat boredom and prevent overuse injury, two reasons that people drop out of programs. Cross-train if it appeals to you and if you want to increase your skill and ability in more than one activity.

To avoid confusion—or add it!—be aware that cross-training can also refer to using different types of activities to make up a complete workout, such as combining stretching, dumbbell exercises, and step aerobics.

I don't feel like I'm getting a workout when I exercise in my training heart-rate range (THR). Why?

There may be several reasons for this. You may have calculated your THR incorrectly. Check your figures. Or you may not be counting your pulse accurately. Have someone else take your pulse, and compare it to your count. If you have calculated and counted correctly, it might be that the formulas are not working for you. Remember, they are based on the average person. If you have the opportunity, run a treadmill or cycle test to find out your true range. You can also try working with the rating of perceived exertion scale (Chapter 4). It is also possible that you are used to competitive levels of training and need time to adjust to the feel of exercise just for the health of it. Discuss your situation with a health/fitness professional.

KNOWLEDGE TIPS

1. There are many excellent forms of aerobic exercise. Select one or more activities (styles or variations) that appeal to you.

2. Precede aerobic activity with a good warm-up, and follow it with a good cool-down.

3. Perform all aerobic movements with good alignment and control.

4. Aim to sustain a target heart rate throughout the aerobic portion of class.

5. The risk of injury in all forms of aerobic dance exercise is low; however, some forms have lower impact stress than others.

6. Handheld and wrist weights are better reserved for muscle-toning. Ankle weights are not recommended for use during the aerobic portion of class.

7. High-impact aerobics consists of large-muscle movements like jogging, jumping, hopping, skipping, knee lifts, dance steps, and calisthenics.

8. Low-impact aerobics is similar to high-impact except that jumping-type moves are not used, as one foot must always be in contact with the floor. There is also usually a greater emphasis placed on arm work and movements that involve lowering and then raising the center of gravity.

9. Step aerobics involves stepping up and down on a bench with a variety of step patterns.

10. Circuit aerobics training involves a series of stations through which the participant moves either with no break or short breaks while sustaining a target heart rate.

11. Interval training consists of high-intensity bouts of work alternated with short rest periods or low-intensity activities.

12. Aerobic intensity can be increased or decreased by increasing/decreasing arm movements; by raising the step height in step aerobics; or by increasing speed, amplitude, or lever length in water or high-impact aerobics.

THINK ABOUT IT

1. Why are there so many different styles of "aerobic dance"?

2. Describe the differences between low- and high-impact aerobics.

3. What are some key technique points to remember while performing aerobic moves?

4. What are some key technique points to remember while performing step aerobics?

5. How can you make aerobic movements easier (less intense) and harder (more intense)?

6. What are some advantages to water (aqua) aerobics?

7. What type of group exercise appeals to you? Why?

REFERENCES

American Council on Exercise. *Aerobics Instructor Manual: ACE's Guide for Fitness Professionals.* San Diego, CA: American Council on Exercise, 2000.

Berry, M. J., C. C. Cline, C. B. Berry, and M. Davis. "A Comparison Between Two Forms of Aerobic Dance and Treadmill Running." *Medicine and Science in Sports and Exercise* 24 (No. 8, 1992): 946–51.

Blessing, D. L. "The Energy Cost of Bench Stepping With and Without One and Two Pound Hand-Held Weights." *Medicine and Science in Sports and Exercise* 23 (No. 4, 1991): S28 (abstract).

Bonelli, S. *Step Training.* San Diego: American Council on Exercise, 2000.

Bricker, K. *Traditional Aerobics.* San Diego, CA: American Council on Exercise, 2000.

Brooks, G. A., T. D. Fahey, and K. Baldwin. *Exercise Physiology: Human Bioenergetics and Its Applications.* 4th ed. New York: McGraw-Hill, 2004.

Brown, D. *Dawn Brown's Complete Guide to Step Aerobics.* Boston: Jones and Bartlett, 1992.

Calarco, R. M., J. Wygand, J. Kramer, M. Yoke, and F. D'Zamko. "The Metabolic Cost of Six Common Movement Patterns of Bench Step Aerobic Dance." *Medicine and Science in Sports and Exercise* 23 (No. 4, 1991): S140 (abstract).

Carroll, M. W., R. M. Otto, and J. Wygand. "The Metabolic Cost of Two Ranges of Arm Position Height With and Without Hand Weights During Low Impact Aerobic Dance." *Research Quarterly for Exercise and Sport* 62 (No. 4, 1991): 420–3.

Copeland, C., L. Francis, P. Francis, and G. Miller. *Power Step Reebok.* Boston: Reebok International, 1992.

Darby, L. A., K. D. Browder, and B. D. Reeves. "The Effects of Cadence, Impacts, and Step on Physiological Responses to Aerobic Dance Exercise." *Research Quarterly for Exercise and Sport* 66 (No. 3, 1995): 231–8.

Elder, D. "Cardio Combat." *Women's Sports and Fitness* 14 (January–February 1992): 55–6.

Francis, L., P. Francis, and G. Miller. *Introduction to StepReebok.* Boston: Reebok International, 1991.

Francis, L., P. Francis, and G. Miller. "Teaching Step Training." *Journal of Physical Education, Recreation, and Dance* 64 (March 1993): 26–30.

Francis, L. L. "Improving Aerobic Dance Programs: The Key Role of Colleges and Universities." *Journal of Physical Education, Recreation, and Dance* 62 (September 1991): 59–62.

Garber, C. E., J. S. McKinney, and R. A. Carleton. "Is Aerobic Dance an Effective Alternative to Walk-Jog Exercise Training?" *Journal of Sports Medicine and Physical Fitness* 32 (No. 2, 1992): 136–41.

Garrick, J. G., and R. K. Requa. "Aerobic Dance: A Review." *Sports Medicine* 6 (1988): 169–79.

Giddens, S. "Yogarobics." *Women's Sports and Fitness* 14 (January–February 1992): 54.

Gordon, J. "Jam Up for Jelly Bellies: Street Dancing Pumps New Life into Aerobics." *Newsweek* 117 (April 29, 1991): 57.

Grant, G. *Technical Manual and Dictionary of Classical Ballet.* New York: Dover, 1967.

Harste, A. "Bench Aerobics: A Step in the Right Direction?" *The Physician and Sportsmedicine* 18 (No. 6, 1990): 25–6.

Hooper, P. L., and B. J. Noland. "Aerobic Dance Program Improves Cardiovascular Fitness in Men." *The Physician and Sportsmedicine* 12 (No. 5, 1984): 132–5.

Hopkins, D. R., B. Murrah, W. W. K. Hoeger, and R. C. Rhodes. "Effect of Low-Impact Aerobic Dance on the Functional Fitness of Elderly Women." *The Gerontologist* 30 (April 1990): 189–92.

Hovell, M. F., M. M. Mulvihill, M. J. Buono, S. Liles, D. H. Schade, T. A. Washington, R. Manzano, and J. F. Sallis. "Culturally Tailored Aerobic Exercise Intervention for Low-Income Latinas." *American Journal of Health Promotion* 22 (No. 3, 2008): 155(9).

Hufhand, D., L. Crowe, M. Whaley, and P. Banning-Schaffner. "Metabolic Responses to Low-Impact Aerobic Dance." *Medicine and Science in Sports and Exercise* 20 (1988, Suppl): S88 (abstract).

Kennedy-Armbruster, C. K., and M. M. Yoke. *Methods of Group Exercise Instruction.* 2nd ed. Champaign, IL: Human Kinetics, 2009.

Koszuta, L. E. "Low–Impact Aerobics: Better Than Traditional Aerobic Dance?" *The Physician and Sportsmedicine* 14 (No. 6, 1986): 156–61.

Kravitz, L. "Getting in Step." *Women's Sports and Fitness* 12 (April 1993): 18.

Kravitz, L., V. H. Heyward, L. M. Stolarczyk, and V. Wilmerding. "Does Step Exercise With Handweights Enhance Training Effects?" *Journal of Strength & Conditioning Research* 11 (No. 3, 1997): 194–99.

Malanka, P. "Aerobics Rebound! From Sports Drills to Step Training, New Techniques Are Transforming the Way America Works Out." *Health* 22 (March 1990): 59–65.

Martin, K. "Soft Aerobics: Gain Without Pain?" *Ms* 14 (May 1986): 52, 54, 113.

Michaud, T. J., J. Rodrigues-Zayas, C. Armstrong, and M. Hartnig. "Ground Reaction Forces in High Impact and Low Impact Aerobic Dance." *Journal of Sports Medicine and Physical Fitness* 33 (No. 4, 1993): 359–66.

Neporent, L. "Aerobics: Watch Your Step." *Women's Sports and Fitness* 14 (September 1992): 71–2.

Nethery, V. M., and P. A. Harmer. "The Energy Cost of Slideboard Training and Cycle Ergometry." Unpublished ms. Department of Physical Education, Health Education, and Leisure Services, Central Washington University, Ellensburg, WA; and Exercise Science, Willamette University, Salem, OR, 1994.

Olson, M. S., H. N. Wiliford, D. L. Blessing, and R. Greathouse. "Cardiorespiratory Responses to 'Aerobic' Bench Stepping Exercise in Females." *Medicine and Science in Sports and Exercise* 23 (No. 4, 1991): S27 (abstract).

Otto, R. M., C. A. Parker, T. K. Smith, J. W. Wygand, and H. R. Perez. "The Energy Cost of Low Impact and High Impact Aerobic Dance Exercise." *Medicine and Science in Sports and Exercise* 18 (No. 2, 1986): 523 (abstract).

Pahmeier, I., and C. Niederbaumer. *Step Aerobics for Schools, Clubs, and Studios.* Meyer & Meyer Sport (UK) Ltd., 2001.

Paul, L. "Funky Fitness: Victoria Johnson's Technifunk Aerobics Mixes Exercise and Expressive Dance." *Women's Sports and Fitness* 14 (No. 1, 1992): 68–9.

Reebok International, Ltd. *Slide Reebok™ Professional Training Manual.* Los Angeles: Reebok University Press, 1993.

Reeder, S. "The New Aerobics: Now You Can Bop to the Beat Without Jarring Your Joints." *Women's Sports and Fitness* 7 (December 1985): 27–9.

Reeves, B. D., L. A. Darby, C. L. Moss, and C. Armstrong. "Energy Costs and Vertical Forces of High-Impact and Low-Impact Aerobic Dance Sequences." *Research Quarterly for Exercise and Sport* 63 (1992, Suppl.): A28 (abstract).

Seabourne, T. *Complete Guide to Cardio Kickboxing.* Boston: YMAA Publication Center, 1999.

Sekulic, D., N. Rausavljevic, and M. Zvan. "Characteristics and Differences in the Heart Rate and Blood Lactate Concentration Values Measured During Hi-lo and Step Aerobic Classes." *Kinesiology* 33 (No. 1, 2001): 27–36.

Smith, T. "Swing into Salsa." *Women's Sports and Fitness* 13 (March 1991): 60.

Stanforth, D., C. Hamman, and C. Senechal. "Relationship of Heart Rate and Oxygen Consumption During Low Impact Aerobic Movements." *Medicine and Science in Sports* 20 (No. 2, 1988): S88 (abstract).

Stanforth, D., K. Velasquez, and P. R. Stanforth. "The Effect of Bench Height and Rate of Stepping on the Metabolic Cost of Bench Stepping." *Medicine and Science in Sports and Exercise* 23 (No. 4, 1991): S143 (abstract).

Wilson, B. R., D. C. Nirwtsu, J. M. Lindle, and C. Winters. "Doing the Two-Step." *American Health* 12 (May 1993): 92.

Yoxall, P. "All the Right Moves." *Current Health 2* 20 (November 1993): 16–7.

9

Group Fitness Exercise

"A great sense of self-worth comes from sharing important experiences with good friends."

UNKNOWN

- What falls into the category of group fitness exercise?
- Do I need any special equipment or training to join a group fitness class?
- Is one kind of group fitness exercise better than another?

INTRODUCTION

The idea of exercising to motivating music in a group setting has taken hold and expanded in all kinds of directions. Group fitness classes range from cycling classes, to pumping weights together, to exercising with friends in the pool. Chapter 8 explored the many varieties of rhythmic aerobics that have grown out of the aerobic dance movement, and Chapter 10 focuses on yoga and Pilates. This chapter captures some of the other popular trends in group fitness, including cardio machine group classes, water aerobics, functional training, kickboxing (martial arts), cross training, and high-intensity interval training.

CARDIO MACHINE GROUP FITNESS

The aerobics movement jumped off the exercise floor and landed on the cardio equipment. You can go "spinning" on a stationary cycle, "stomp" on a stair stepper, or go "trekking" or "treading" on a treadmill. Even rowing machines are getting into the act. What all these group fitness classes have in common is an instructor who leads, educates, and motivates participants through a shared event. Music is used to energize and, in most cases, set a cadence for the workout. These classes appeal to both men and women and can span a range of ages and fitness levels. Because they are low-impact to nonimpact, they can be excellent choices for people prone to impact-stress injuries, people who are rehabilitating after an injury, or overweight individuals who want a class that is easy on their joints.

Some classes include the use of small weights to promote upper-body muscle development, but usually muscular fitness is best done before or after the cardio workout so that participants can be sure to concentrate on technique. (Some research suggests muscular fitness is better done after the cardio segment, but the evidence is not definitive at this time.) When possible, concentrating on cardio one day and muscle fitness a different day allows for total focus and eliminates the fatigue factor that can influence technique. A range of fitness levels can be incorporated into one class, but as these activities have grown in popularity, more classes are being offered for specific fitness levels and fitness objectives. The intensity of classes can range from a high-level athletic workout to a health-fitness endurance workout.

GROUP CYCLING

Indoor group cycling became a popular form of group exercise when John Baudhuin and Johnny G. (John Goldberg) founded Mad Dog Athletics Inc. in 1994 as a result of the growing bike-building business that they had started in their garage. They launched their group cycling program and dubbed it Spinning®. While Spinning® is a registered name, it is often (albeit incorrectly) used to refer to any group cycling program (Figure 9.1). Over the years, a number of other companies have developed their own programs and/or instructor certification programs, including, but not limited to, the Indoor Cycling Group (ICG®), Cycling Fusion, Keiser, and Cycle Reebok. Group cycling classes are filled with camaraderie as an instructor leads you through a ride together in a special room that often has an ambience of its own. Some cycling

Figure 9.1

rooms are big and bright, others smaller; some dim the lights, use black lights, or even candles. Some clubs even provide a movie-like visual of a riding path and scenery. On campuses, sometimes the stationary bikes are moved outside on good weather days for a fresh-air ride. The sound of the other bikes, the beat of the music, and the encouragement and tips from the instructor are all highly motivating.

An instructor will direct your focus to technique points to keep you injury free and to get the most out of your ride and will motivate you by describing hills and flat stretches as though you were on a real outdoor ride. You may also be asked to focus on how your body feels with cues such as "Feel the circle you are drawing" as you drive your legs.

GETTING STARTED

Arrive early to class so that the instructor can guide you through the bike set-up. You will learn how to set the seat and handlebars at the right height and the correct distance apart and how the flywheel operates. (The flywheel is the "wheel" on the front of the bike. It differs from a road bike wheel in that it doesn't touch the ground and whenever it is turning the attached pedals always move; you can't coast.) Here are some quick tips for orienting yourself to the bike:

- *Seat height:* When you sit on the seat to pedal and one foot is at the bottom of the cycle, that leg should be slightly bent. If not, raise or lower the seat accordingly. When off the bike, the seat should be roughly hip height.
- *Handlebar height:* Handlebars should be set even with the seat height or slightly higher for beginners. Let comfort be the guide.
- *Saddle to handlebars:* When you sit on the saddle (seat) and bring one leg to a position where the thigh is parallel to the floor, you should be able to

see the toes on that foot. If you are too far forward, the toes disappear under the knee. You can also think of centering the knee over the pedal when both pedals are side by side (3 and 9 o'clock).

- Keep your feet on the pedals, and keep them moving; there is no "coasting" feature to these bikes. If you do need to take your feet out, hold them out to the sides so they do not get hit by the pedals. Most bikes have a red emergency stop button that will stop the flywheel. This is safer than pulling your feet off the pedals.

Wear clothing made of fabrics that dissipate heat, stay in place, and don't chafe. Consider purchasing specialty cycling shorts with high-density foam padding to enhance sitting comfort. Alternatively, you can buy a seat cover that is gel-padded and slip it on the bike when you arrive. These will ease "saddle soreness," but you should still expect to feel sore for a few days.

There are special shoes for serious cycling, but you can easily get started with a cross trainer. Running and aerobic shoes are not advised. Be sure the sole is stiff, because a flexible shoe will result in greater foot fatigue. You also want the power of your leg motion to transfer through the stiff-soled shoe to the pedal. If you are purchasing shoes, look for a good retaining system on the shoe—these are the straps or laces that hold your feet securely in place and are particularly helpful during the upward pedaling motion. You will also want a shoe with good ventilation. Place the shoe so that the ball of the foot is directly over the pedal. Some pedals have clips you slide your shoe into; other pedals are clipless. The latter work with shoes that come with a system that allows the sole of the shoe to cleat directly into the pedal. Before purchasing shoes, see what kind of system is used where you intend to cycle.

A water bottle is a must, and most bikes have a place to keep it within easy reach. A towel, or two, is also nice for wiping the sweat off you and the handlebars.

RIDING—BASIC POSITIONS

There are three arm positions. The first is with your hands resting on either side of, and near, the center bar (Figure 9.2a). The second is a wider grip farther out from the center post but still on the horizontal bar. If there is a second set of horizontal bars on the bike, the ones more forward are used for position 2 (Figure 9.2b). The third is on the part of the handlebars that extend forward from the bike. This grip will include having the thumbs off and bent over the ends (Figure 9.2c).

There should never be significant weight on the hands. In position 1, the hands rest lightly on the handlebars; in position 2, on or lightly gripping the bars; and in position 3, the grip is as described above. The arms should remain soft (lightly bent). There are short periods of time when you are moving from a seated to standing position when the grip will tighten and the arms pull backward on the bars to assist the position change.

Body positions work in concert with the hand positions and are determined by the kind of ride you are doing. Some basic movements and the correct positioning for each follow:

- *Seated flat:* The rider is seated, with a forward lean from the hips that maintains the natural curves of the back. The arms rest comfortably on the handlebars in position 1. The elbows should be slightly bent, with very little pressure on the hands. This position is used with a light to moderate resistance for warming up and cooling down and for flat terrain riding (80 to 110 RPM).
- *Seated climb:* The rider stays seated but moves back in the saddle. Hand position 2 is used. The back continues to maintain its natural curves. Resistance is increased, and the pedaling rate (60 to 80 RPM) is lower than for the seated flat (Figure 9.3a).
- *Standing flat:* The rider stands up, keeping the weight over the pedals. The arms are in position 2, and the resistance light to moderate (80 to 110 RPM). The body is nearly vertical, which is markedly different from the seated position.
- *Standing climb:* The rider is out of the saddle and in a nearly vertical body position. The hands are in position 3, which means the body will have more forward lean. The rider keeps the majority of the weight over the feet, not over the arms (Figure 9.3b).
- *Jumping:* The rider moves smoothly from a seated to standing position and back. This is an advanced move used for short bursts that use gravity and body weight to accelerate quickly.

A class will consist of a ride orchestrated by the instructor but during which you are free to adjust the tension of the flywheel to your fitness level at any time. You can also remain seated and not perform sprints to lower the intensity. The amount of time spent on flat terrain versus hills will depend on your fitness level. All-out sprints followed by recovery pedaling are used once participants have a good endurance base.

RIDING—TIPS

- When you are standing, keep enough resistance on the flywheel to support your weight. Too little resistance can result in sudden leg extension and possible injury to the knee.

Figure 9.2a Hand position 1

Figure 9.2b Hand position 2

Figure 9.2c Hand position 3

- Think of keeping yourself streamlined and avoid side-to-side motion.
- Keep the buttocks near the saddle even when standing. Think of it as "hovering" over the saddle. This keeps the body balanced so that the arms and hands don't receive too much pressure.

Figure 9.3a Seated climb, left, and seated flat, right

Figure 9.3b Standing flat, left, and standing climb, right

- Maintain a steady breathing pattern. Try not to take shallow breaths. Don't hold your breath, even on a steep climb or during a sprint.
- Keep the elbows "soft," meaning slightly bent.
- Be sure to finish by performing stretches, especially for the legs, buttocks, and chest.
- Perform upper-body strength exercises off the bike to balance the lower-body workout. Also include additional hamstring exercises, because riding works the quadriceps more than the hamstrings.

MARTIAL ARTS GROUP FITNESS

There are many martial arts-based aerobic programs. The first, Cardio Kickboxing, started in 1992 by Frank Thiboutot, set out to promote the sport of kickboxing through kickboxing for fitness. His objective has been

Figure 9.4

to safely mainstream the workout of a fighter to the general public for its fitness and self-defense benefits. Other types of martial arts group fitness classes include Cardio-karate, Karatics, Kempocise, Tae-Bo, and TKO Aerobics.

This style of group fitness uses jogging; calisthenics; rope jumping; a number of punches, jabs, and kicks, alone and in combination; shadow boxing; and self-defense moves (Figure 9.4). When equipment is available, these programs use a variety of hanging or free-standing bags, focus pads, and punch mitts. The philosophy behind the workout will vary depending on the particular type of martial art from which the program draws.

GETTING STARTED
When the class does not involve contact hitting, all you need is a good pair of cross trainer shoes, comfortable clothing, and water. Some fitness classes use such equipment as a bag, boxing gloves, and focus mitts.

BASIC MOVEMENTS
Although the specific technique of the leg kicks, arm punches, and avoidance moves will vary a little depending on the form of martial arts being adapted for group exercise, the following descriptions will give you a sense of what to expect in this type of class. The descriptions are intended to familiarize you with the basic movements; they are not detailed enough to teach all of the important technique. It can take years to perfect kicks, punches, and defensive moves for fights. For fitness, basic technique proficiency is needed to keep the joints in healthy positions while getting a good muscular and cardiovascular workout. Like all group fitness, the class will start with a warm-up, which should include low-intensity versions of the movements that

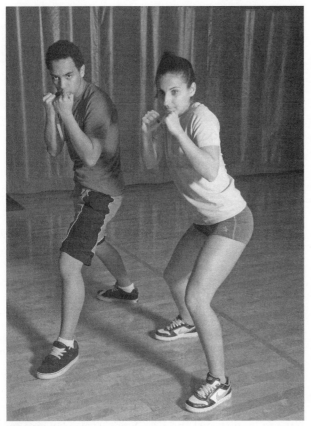

Figure 9.5

will be used later in the class. This gives you an opportunity to rehearse the movements at a slower tempo.

The first thing you need to know is the on-guard, or defensive, position (Figure 9.5). Start with feet shoulder width apart, with a staggered (one foot in front of the other) stance. The knees are bent a little, and you can do "rocking," or bounce steps, moving the weight from one foot to the other. The arms are bent at the elbow so that the fists cover the chin. The arms are close to the body.

Whenever kicking is involved, it is very important to protect the back by maintaining good posture throughout the execution of the kicks. Chapter 6 discussed correct and incorrect kicking with illustrations of how the kick should be only as high as can be performed with the spine in a natural position. As soon as the low back has to round to compensate for leg flexibility, the back is at risk. Don't try to follow others; make sure that you participate within your flexibility range. If you want to do higher kicks, work on increasing flexibility.

There are four basic types of kicks: front, side, back and round (turning kick or roundhouse, depending on the leg used). All these kicks have two technique points in common. The first is to maintain the neutral spine

(as previously discussed). The second is to do a concentric contraction in both the kick and the recovery from the kick. This means to extend the leg by using the knee and hip extensor muscles and bend the leg by pulling in with the knee and hip flexors. If you don't do this during aerobic kickboxing where there is no target to hit, the leg ends up being flung outward into the air, possibly hyperextending the knee. This can have repercussions for the knee, hip, and back. It is also important to rotate the feet on the ground during many of the kicks to prevent rotational torque on the knee. Remember that power comes from the legs. Just extending a knee or elbow will not provide power; a tight core and push from the legs is needed for power. Finally, as you kick or punch, breathe out. This is similar to resistance training, where you breathe out upon exertion.

Arm blocking techniques, ducks or slips used to dodge a hit, and foot drills also can be added to the workout. Once you establish technique, you can perform combinations of kicks, punches, and defensive moves. Multiple repetitions of movements at pace can provide a great workout. Before you start a martial arts group exercise class, review the instructions for safe kicks, jabs, and other movements found in Worksheet 9.1, provided online at www.pearsonhighered.com/bishopaerobics.

FUNCTIONAL TRAINING GROUP FITNESS

Although not a new concept, the application of functional training to group fitness is relatively new. The idea is rooted in physical therapy, where exercises are selected to help an individual better perform daily tasks. **Functional training**, therefore, is training that focuses on improving fitness that supports movements we use in everyday life to function as healthy human beings. It involves a variety of exercises, some which you would find in a more traditional program, and some which look quite different. In a functional fitness class, the focus is on making sure you are strong enough, flexible enough, and have enough endurance to carry you through a typical day. Instructors teaching these classes make a point of connecting the exercise being performed to the daily movement it is helping. For example, a shoulder press becomes "placing a box on the top shelf," lunges and squats are used to "pick up something from the floor," and bent-over row is "starting the lawn mower."

When we move in life, we seldom move one muscle at a time. Even with a task as simple as taking a casserole out of the oven, we use our legs, back, and arms. Carrying a suitcase upstairs requires leg, hip, and arm strength and abdominal strength to counterbalance the one-sided weight of the bag. It makes sense then, that functional fitness exercises will mostly involve multiple joints and multiple muscles.

Life's movements don't usually happen in one direction at a time, either. Movement can happen in three planes: vertical, horizontal, and diagonal. When we open a heavy door, for example, the arm starts in front of the body, pulls back, and then moves along an arc out to the side. Yet traditional weight machines allow us to move only in one plane. To strengthen this motion with weight machines, you would first strengthen the pull back with a seated row and then strengthen the lateral movement with reverse fly movements. During functional training, you use equipment that allows you to incorporate multiple planes in one motion, thus making it more "lifelike." Cables, bands, medicine balls, dumbbells, smartbells, and kettlebells all allow this kind of multi-planar movement.

But before we throw out traditional weight machines, there are a few considerations. These machines allow us to perform valuable stabilization exercises, especially for the scapula, hips, and abdominals. For example, it is unwise to add weight to a throwing motion unless the core (abdominal) muscles are strong enough to maintain good posture during the throw. Therefore, stabilizing exercises to strengthen the abdominals may be considered functional exercises, depending on how you define them. In addition, a single-joint exercise, such as a leg extension, can be used to correct a weakness or imbalance. Machines also allow you to perform high-resistance loads safely while you learn how to control the movement. Considering again the example of taking the casserole out of the oven, to do this you have to lean forward and lift the weight of the dish with a flexed spine. Bending the knees and good arm strength will assist this movement, and strong abdominals will help the back in what can be a vulnerable position. However, it is not advisable to do a functional exercise with a heavy load in this position because it compromises the back and can result in injury. Instead, by using the machine, you can strengthen the back in a safer manner and still contribute to the movement. So while the aim is strength in everyday activities, rehearsing with the exact same motion may not always be a good idea.

Recall that the principle of specificity advises us to train in a way that matches the desired outcome. Additionally, there is a motor learning concept called the **transfer of learning**. A transfer of learning occurs when something learned in one activity is able to result in learning in a related but different activity. The more similar the two activities are, the greater the transfer. For example, someone who has learned how to hit a tennis serve can transfer this motion into a badminton smash fairly easily. Walking up and down stairs (or up and down on a step bench) with dumbbells or a weighted vest is very similar to, and can prepare one for, carrying a sleeping child to bed. To facilitate the transfer of learning, a good portion of what is important is the neuromuscular training, meaning that the coordination of muscles by the nervous system must be trained. Strong muscles on their own are not enough to aid movement—you want strong and coordinated muscle movement. A good example is how people can press quite a bit of weight with their legs on a leg press machine, but standing on a stool and slowly stepping down can be difficult. Practicing one-legged squats will prepare you for stepping up and down on stools, and performing a squat with a medicine ball that you lift overhead at the end of the squat prepares you for lifting and placing objects.

One kind of functional training involves balance and coordination exercises. One of the simplest balance practices can be done by standing on one leg. You can bend down and try to touch the ground, rise up on the ball of your foot, or tip your body forward until it is parallel to the ground, like a skater. Balance doesn't have to involve just the legs. You can also balance on one arm in a side plank position (see Figure 11.45 in Chapter 11) or perform inverted balances, such as a handstand or other advanced yoga poses. Balance can also be challenged by using such equipment as balance boards, half foam rollers, balance discs, pillows, pads, Bosu, and stability balls (Figure 9.6). Standing, sitting, or lying on this equipment makes you unstable and forces a lot of muscles to work together to maintain balance. Some fun outdoor activities that require balance include roller blading, cycling, and skiing.

Figure 9.6

Another kind of functional training involves band systems that connect to the walls or immovable frames that allow a lot of multiple-muscle and multiple-planar exercises to be done using body weight. Wall-mounted cable/strap systems (e.g., TRX suspension training, Perform Better systems) use positioning and body weight in a way that can challenge beginners and advanced individuals. Given that we perform many of our daily motions while we are standing, these systems allow for a lot of exercises to be done on the feet leaning backward or forward to create more resistance. Cable machines that are often available in weight rooms also offer quite a bit of flexibility. They work on a pulley system, have multiple attachments to hold onto (bar, triangle, ankle wrap), and can be used to create a multiple-planar workout.

In life, we often do things in a one-sided manner. In order to keep our bodies in good alignment during these activities, we need a strong core. For example, when you carry a suitcase in one arm, it is the core that keeps you from twisting or falling sideways toward the suitcase. A new way of functional training purposely challenges one side of the body to bring in that subsequent core strengthening. For example, cable exercises using one limb, and squats or lunges with a weight on one side, challenge one side of the body and transfer well to real-life activities. It is also important to train muscles through rotating movements. Twisting curl-ups can also be done for other muscle groups with cables or bands and a bar with a cable attached (e.g., Rip Trainer by TRX).

In summary, the main tenet of functional training is to gain strength and neuromuscular control using fitness-enhancing activities that translate to coordinated strength and balance in real-life activities. Functional fitness can be used for rehabilitation, for making life movements easier, for decreasing movement fatigue, for preventing injury, and for improving sport or recreational activities (sport-specific training).

CROSS TRAINING GROUP FITNESS

There are two definitions of **cross training**. One is the use of different modes of exercises to achieve the same goal. For example, both cycling and step aerobics can be used to develop cardiorespiratory endurance. A second definition of *cross training* is the use of a variety of activities to achieve total fitness—all the health-related components of physical fitness. In this case, an example is swimming for aerobic fitness and performing yoga for strength and flexibility. One big benefit of cross training is that it can eliminate boredom or staleness in a workout. It changes how the body is worked, which helps stimulate continued improvement, and it challenges improvements in neuromuscular coordination.

Fusion classes, which are group fitness classes that combine two modes of training, can fall into either of these definitions. For example, a Pilates/yoga combination will promote muscular fitness, whereas a spinning/yoga fusion will develop both cardiorespiratory and muscular fitness. Programs such as Bootcamp, CrossFit, Insanity, and P90-X, discussed in the next section, promote exercise regimens that use cross training to achieve overall fitness.

MILITARY-STYLE TRAINING

Programs such as Bootcamp and British Military Fitness offer a combination of group fitness and personal training. This type of program is group fitness, but usually with a smaller group of people, and thus offers a more personalized training approach. Because the class size is small, it can meet in a variety of settings, including outdoors (Figure 9.7). The leader puts the group through a series of demanding body weight exercises, jump roping, and footwork drills. A typical workout will include a dynamic warm-up; body weight exercises to build muscle strength and endurance; cardiovascular work, usually using intervals (higher-intensity movements such as jumping jacks, sprints, etc., followed by lower level movements for recovery); a cool-down; and flexibility work. Some examples of typical exercises are climbers, burpees (squat thrusts) followed by a vertical jump, moving under a rope while holding a push-up position, agility runs (basketball shuffle, karaoke step, etc.), and a variety of challenging positions for such exercises as push-ups and squats. Rope climbing (cargo nets) and obstacle courses that include going over and under objects and through tunnels may also be used.

Figure 9.7

One of the advantages to this style of training is the support of the group. Just as in the military, the instructor works to forge camaraderie between group members. In addition to cheering each other on, activities that require group or partner cooperation, such as back-to-back squats, build a sense of togetherness. Another advantage is that the workout is not tied to a set location or musical beat, so the instructor can take advantage of natural surroundings and change the pace to meet the needs of the class. A creative instructor can introduce a lot of variety, which helps keep the workout fresh.

HIGH-INTENSITY TRAINING (HIT)

HIT or **HIIT** (high-intensity interval training) is a training technique that has become popular for several reasons. One reason for its popularity is that it operates at such a high intensity level that it allows you to expend a lot of calories. This can aid in weight loss if you can sustain the workout. It also uses demanding muscle exercises that promote the building of new muscle tissue. Some people thrive psychologically on the intensity of the workout. It is empowering, and finishing a workout provides a sense of achievement. And along with the high number of calories, it burns up the stresses of the day.

What needs to balance the enthusiasm for this type of workout is the idea of readiness. Although people may be enthusiastic about high-intensity workouts, these workouts are not for beginners. Some of the programs offering high-intensity workouts try to reach a broader market by encouraging participants to "do only what you can do with good form," but the workouts are demanding; and if you are out of shape, your body may not be ready for this level. Entering into this type of exercise too quickly, without some base conditioning, poses potential risks. These include stress on tendons and ligaments, whose strength adaptations occur more slowly than muscular strength gains; impact stress from jumping with extra body weight; and the possibility of pushing the cardiovascular system to too high a level. If, however, you are free of injury and disease and have some base level of health-related fitness, then pushing into this higher level of fitness may be something that is right for you.

The author does not endorse any particular commercial program, but included here is a brief overview of some of the popular programs currently on the market.

CrossFit, founded by Greg Glassman in 2000, operates in what is referred to as "box" gymnasiums (no-frills workout spaces independently owned and run) and/or through on-your-own WODS (workouts of the day). The aim is to provide a comprehensive broad fitness program that targets cardiovascular and respiratory endurance, stamina, strength, flexibility, power, speed, coordination, agility, balance, and accuracy. The workouts incorporate a variety of free-weight equipment, including barbells, dumbbells, chin-up bars, and kettle bells. The workouts include competitive Olympic lifts that emphasize power and strength, such as the snatch and the clean and jerk. Workouts also include activities in other venues, such as swimming, biking, and rowing. The emphasis is on demanding workouts and includes exhortations to leave "sweat angels" on the floor and work so hard you feel like throwing up. This image has been modified somewhat as the program has grown and is trying to reach more of the marketplace.

Workout ideas are shared on the company's website. One caution is that many of these workouts are not screened by anyone, and not all the videos that are posted show exercises done with good form. The workouts are generally short—20 minutes—but include nonstop sets of exercises. An example is the very demanding FRAN workout which consists of 21 thrusters (a front squat followed immediately with an overhead press of a weight) and 21 pull-ups. This is followed by 15 thrusters and pull-ups, then 9 more of each. All of this is done as quickly as possible. It is the continuous nature and combination of exercises that makes CrossFit workouts very different from a traditional weight workout. CrossFit has also broadened from fitness workouts to competitions. The Reebok CrossFit Games involve a variety of activities and build from submissions of videotape entries to live regional and national competitions.

Beachbody Inc. is pumping out high-intensity workouts to be performed at home via a series of videos using HIIT. Driven by Shaun T (Insanity), Tony Horton (P90X), and Charlene Johnson (Turbofire), these videos promise quick results if you put in the high-intensity work. The cardio workouts range from low-impact (but high-intensity) to high-impact with lots of jumping. The muscle workouts, depending on the program, include body weight exercises, bands, stability balls, dumbbells, medicine balls, and a foam roller. A pull-up bar is also used. The beginning level is aimed at basic strength, core work, balance, and some plyometrics (jumping with preloaded stretching of the muscle). Advanced workouts use HIIT and more complex and challenging combinations of exercises. Cardio and muscle fitness are both part of the program, making it a cross training program.

The Tabata protocol was created by Izumi Tabata in Japan using highly fit individuals. It consists of very-high-level cardiovascular work for 20 seconds, followed by 10 seconds of rest, repeated 8 times. The original research was done using athletes on stationary bicycles and reported very significant gains in VO_2 max. This protocol has since been applied to other forms of exercise but without the same research approach. There has also been some concern that high-intensity muscle workouts can result in **rhabdomyolysis,** the rapid destruction of skeletal muscle resulting in leakage of myoglobin (muscle protein) into the urine. Myoglobin clogs the kidneys and can result in kidney failure. Although this disorder is normally associated with muscle-crushing injuries and severe burns, there is evidence that extreme physical activity can also cause it. More research is needed on HIIT; in the meantime, remember that a workout should build you up, not tear you down; modify the intensity as needed.

If you decide to try one of these or another commercial program, be smart: use the exercise principles of progression and individuality, and make sure that you know how to perform the exercises properly (with hands-on instruction from a qualified instructor) so that you can prevent injury and maximize your outcome. Remember that the HIIT programs aim for a level of fitness that is well above that required for health.

WATER AEROBICS

Water aerobics (aqua aerobics) is a great way to get all the benefits of an aerobic workout with motivating music, a comfortable environment, and little or no impact stress (Figure 9.8). Anyone, of any age

Figure 9.8

and fitness level, can do it. The routines can be easily modified so that people of different abilities can exercise together. Unlike swimming, in water aerobics you do not have to get your hair wet—unless the weather is very hot, in which case wetting your hair will help keep you cool.

Water aerobics has a distinct advantage for people who are body conscious or who worry about being seen making mistakes; the water provides a certain degree of anonymity. It is also an excellent form of aerobic exercise for individuals who are overweight, have joint problems, or are recovering from an injury.

Two types of water aerobics have developed. Shallow-water aerobics are performed in standing-depth water. Deep-water aerobics uses flotation devices to suspend individuals in a vertical position in water over their heads. Deep-water aerobics is generally for swimmers, whereas shallow-water aerobics can be enjoyed by swimmers and nonswimmers alike. Both types of water aerobics classes are similar to other forms of aerobics in their class format. Class begins with a warm-up (which is usually done in the water but may be performed on the deck), an aerobic workout, an aerobic cool-down, a muscle-toning section, and finally, flexibility work. Water provides buoyancy; the deeper the water you work out in, the more buoyancy you experience. This buoyancy decreases the impact stress you experience as you push off the bottom of the pool. This means that the aerobics workout can be extended (for participants who want a longer workout) with less risk of injury. Working out in waist-deep water can lessen impact stress by about 50%, and as much as 90% in water at the shoulder/neck level. Most instructors prefer to have students exercise in water that reaches only to the chest- or armpits, because it is difficult for participants to control their movements in water that is deeper than this. Deep-water aerobics, in which a student does not use the bottom of the pool at all, is impact-free.

The benefits of water aerobics lie in the fact that water is 12 times more resistive than air. For example, because it is 12 times harder to walk through water than air, you burn more calories walking through water. Water aerobics programs also take advantage of the fact that both directions of a movement meet with resistance. There is no rest phase as there is in land-based resistance exercises. For example, on land, a leg lift to the side works the abductor muscles (outer thigh), whereas the same exercise in water provides resistance not only to the abductors but also to the opposing adductor muscles (inner thigh) as they draw the leg back to its starting position. Water aerobics, as a result, is an excellent medium for achieving a balanced muscle workout.

Monitoring exercise intensity with heart rate is not as straightforward for water-based activities, such as swimming and water aerobics, as it is for land-based activities, such as running, biking, and aerobic dance exercise. People who perform both land and water exercises often find that their heart rate is lower during water exercise even when the aerobic benefits are the same. Several theories are being tested about why heart rates vary in relation to oxygen consumption during water-based activities. Remember, heart rate is a good indicator of workout intensity only when it correlates with oxygen consumption. In water, this relationship seems to be affected by a number of factors, including water depth and temperature. Anything that reduces the workload of the circulatory system will result in a reduced exercise heart rate. Body heat generated through exercise is more easily dissipated in water. The cooler the water, the greater the cooling effect, and the lower the heart rate. The greater the percentage of the body submerged in cool water—the deeper the water—the more pronounced the effect. Water exercise performed in warmer water can produce heart rates similar to land-based exercise. Aerobic exercise in hot water is not recommended, because this prevents body cooling. Wearing a wet suit or a bathing cap in a warm environment can also interfere with body cooling and can drive the heart rate up. Heart rate changes due to temperature conditions are independent of the amount of oxygen being used during exercise.

Deep water offers more buoyancy. When gravity is affected this way, blood is more easily transported back to the heart. Water also acts to compress the blood vessels, which is believed to aid in venous return. This compression factor is also thought to help oxygen diffuse into the blood. The deeper the water, the greater the compression effect. Exercise in water lowers the demand on the heart, which results in lower exercise heart rates.

One important point should be stressed. Even though most people experience lower exercise heart rates in water than in land workouts, the benefits they receive from the exercise are usually the same. The question, then, is, How much lower a heart rate results in the same benefits? Research has documented reductions in water-based heart rates ranging from 10 to 20 bpm. The Cooper Institute for Aerobic Research recommends lowering the target heart-rate zone by 17 bpm. Others would argue for less of a reduction, and some claim that healthy participants can safely attain and benefit from the same heart rates during water exercise as they attain during land-based exercise. Recent large scale research studies by Dr. Luiz Fernando Martins Kruel's research group in Brazil suggest a way

to identify an individualized heart rate deduction. The individual takes a one-minute HR after standing out of the pool for 3 minutes and a one-minute HR after standing arm-pit deep in the pool for 3 minutes. The aquatic HR is subtracted from the land HR. This number is then subtracted from HRmax before calculating a percentage range. The Aquatic Exercise Association (AEA) recommends the use of the Kruel Aquatic HR deduction. Research also indicates that ratings of perceived exertion vary with the depth of water and speed of an individual's movements. Much depends on the environment, the individual's fitness and body composition, and program. If you decide to participate in water aerobics, work with your instructor to determine how best to monitor and adjust your intensity.

The principles of exercise presented earlier in this book apply to exercise in the water. And many of the exercises you are already familiar with can be used in the water. But, in addition to heart-rate monitoring, there are some significant differences between water- and land-based exercises, a few of which are described here.

1. If you are supplying the music, be sure your music box runs on batteries or that the electrical outlet you are using is above the deck and meets both state and local bathing codes. Burn fat, not the rest of you!

2. Music tempo is slower for water movements, usually between 124 and 136 bpm. When instructors use music with a tempo greater than 136 bpm, they use it at half time (that is, they use every other beat).

3. Optimum water temperature is between 83°F and 86°F. Cool water is good for people with multiple sclerosis, whereas warmer water is good for people with arthritis. Hot water would be good only for a class performing stretching movements.

4. Dehydration may occur more easily. Most classes are held outdoors in warm weather or indoors in a heated area. Because you are in water, you may not realize how much you are sweating. Drink water from a plastic container (glass is not allowed in pool areas) throughout class. Much of the body's heat is lost through the head, so be careful about wearing a swimming cap that traps heat because it may cause heat stress in warm weather. If you are in a pool that requires a cap (to help keep hair from clogging the pool filter) and you don't mind getting your hair wet, you can wear a Lycra cap and wet it periodically.

5. Pool attire might seem obvious, but here are a few tips to consider. If you get cold easily, wear tights and a bathing suit or leotard in the pool. Wash out clothing immediately after changing—chlorine is very hard on fabrics. Lycra blends tend to hold up better in pools. Women may prefer one-piece suits with a good built-in bra for support when jumping. Wearing a pair of aqua shoes can help prevent abrasions caused by pushing off the pool bottom, provide cushioning, and supply traction in and out of the pool.

6. A variety of movements and movement speeds results in a good overall workout. When speed is added to a movement, the water resistance increases, which means the workout is more intense. For example, it is much more difficult to run through water than walk through it. When speed is reduced, intensity decreases, but larger ranges of motion with more extended limbs can occur. For more discussion on methods of increasing and decreasing resistance in the water, see Chapter 11.

7. Special equipment is available for water aerobics. Webbed gloves and plastic or foam barbells can be used to increase resistance. For deep-water work, you can use flotation belts, jogging vests, kickboards, and other devices to support your body while you perform running-type exercises. Some devices are contoured better than others to fit comfortably under your arms.

Water aerobics is popular, and it has expanded into a variety of forms. Some classes resemble land aerobic dance exercise, some use a weighted step for aqua step aerobics, others have participants run in deep water, and some use circuit- and interval-training principles. As a side note, racehorses have been doing deep-water running in harnesses for years. Trainers know that they can train the horses longer and harder without risking stress fractures. So you see, you, your family, and your horse can all perform water aerobics together!

SUMMARY

There are many fun ways to get fit, and for those who like to do it with others, group fitness is a great way to do it. Camaraderie, motivating music, and sharing of achievements can make group fitness a very rewarding experience. Also, knowing that others expect you to be there helps you stay with the program. Many places create their own names for group fitness classes, so it is difficult to compare or describe them by name. Read the descriptions offered, and if that isn't enough, contact the instructor for a better description. When participating in a class, always keep the basic fitness principles in mind. Work at your own level, adjust the intensity as needed, and overload in small increments. You want to walk away energized and looking forward to the next class.

COMMONLY ASKED QUESTIONS

Can a beginner join any group fitness class?

It depends. Some classes are set up to handle a range of fitness levels; others cater to beginner, intermediate, or advanced participants. Check with the instructor to find out whether you need prior experience or some level of fitness to participate in the class.

Is one kind of group fitness better than another?

Different classes emphasize different things, so the one that matches your personal goals is the best. Some are more cardio oriented, while others are more muscular fitness oriented. Fusion classes offer cross training by offering two distinct kinds of activities within one class (i.e., spinning, Pilates), while most group fitness classes cross train by including a more generic variety of aerobic, resistance, and flexibility exercises. Follow your interests and goals.

KNOWLEDGE TIPS

1. Group fitness consists of an activity performed with small to large groups of people led by an instructor and usually, but not always, performed to music.

2. Group fitness can occur in many venues, including on cardio machines, in the water, in a gymnasium with a variety of equipment, or even outdoors.

3. All forms of group fitness use a warm-up, exercise, and cool-down format.

4. Indoor cycling provides an excellent cardiorespiratory workout and muscular workout for the legs. For all-around fitness, cycling should be supplemented with upper-body muscle work and additional work for the hamstrings to balance the considerable demands on the quadriceps.

5. Kickboxing for fitness can provide both an aerobic and muscle strengthening workout. This format involves kicking and punching air as opposed to sparring with a partner.

6. Functional training aims to improve fitness that supports daily movements. It involves a variety of exercises to gain strength and neuromuscular control, including exercises for balance, coordination, and stability.

7. Cross training uses two or more types of activities to achieve the same kind of fitness (i.e., running and swimming for aerobic fitness) *or* two or more types of activities to achieve total fitness (i.e., yoga and cycling for strength, flexibility, and aerobic fitness).

8. High-intensity training (HIT or HITT) consists of repeating cycles composed of short bursts of intense physical activity, followed by a rest or recovery interval.

9. Water aerobics provides an aerobic and muscle fitness workout in an impact-free environment, which is beneficial for all participants but is especially good for those who are overweight. Buoyancy and surface area equipment can add resistance challenge to the workout. Both shallow and deep water workouts are options.

THINK ABOUT IT

1. What kind of group exercise appeals to you? Why?

2. How can group fitness help you attain your fitness goals?

3. What types of group fitness classes are available to you?

4. What is cross training, and why might this be important to you?

5. Are there activities you like to do with a group and activities you like to do on your own?

6. Have you ever gotten hurt doing a daily activity? Can you think of a functional exercise you could do to strengthen yourself so that your body would be ready for that movement?

REFERENCES

Alkurdi, W., Paul, D.R., Sadowski, K., & Dolny, D. The effect of water depth on energy expenditure and perception of effort in female subjects while walking. *International Journal of Aquatic Research and Education*, 2010, 4, 49-60.

Aquatic Exercise Association. *Aquatic Fitness Professional Manual.* 6th ed. Champaign, IL: Human Kinetics, 2010

Bonelli, S. *Aquatic Exercise.* San Diego: American Council on Exercise, 2001.

Casten, C. *Aqua Aerobics Today.* Minneapolis/St. Paul: West Publishing Co., 1994.

Chewing, June M., Paula S. Krist & Paulo A. Poli de Figueiredo Monitoring Your Aquatic Heart Rate: Increasing Accuracy with the Kruel Acquatic Adaptation. Aquatic Exercise Research Committee Project May 2008-July 2009. www.aeawave.com/Portals/2/Research/Kruel_research.pdf

Kennedy-Armburster, C. & Yoke, M.M. (2009) *Methods of Group Fitness*, 2nd ed., Champaign, IL: Human Kinetics.

Knopf, K. *Make the pool your gym: no-impact water workouts for getting fit, building strength and rehabbing from injury.* Berkeley, CA: Ulysses Press, 2012

Kruel L.F.M., Peyré-Tartaruga LA, Alberton CL, Müller FG, & Petkowicz R. (2009). Effects of hydrostatic weight on heart rate during immersion. International Journal of Aquatic Research Education; 3:178-175.

Seabourne, T. *Complete Guide to Cardio Kickboxing.* Boston: YMAA Publication Center, 1999.

Sova, R. *The Complete Reference Guide for Aquatic Professionals.* Port Washington, WI: DSL Limited, 2000.

Spitzer, T-A., and W. W. K. Hoeger. *Water Aerobics for Fitness & Wellness.* 2nd ed. Englewood, CO: Morton Publishing, 1999.

Wilson, B. R., D. C. Nirwtsu, and J. M. Lindle. "Metabolic Responses to Three Water-Aerobic Exercises." *Research Quarterly for Exercise and Sport* 63 (March 1992 Supplement): A-30.

10

Muscular Fitness: Building Strength and Endurance

"Look well into thyself; there is a source of strength which will always spring up if thou wilt always look there."

MARCUS AURELIUS ANTONINUS

- Why do I need muscular strength and endurance?
- What kinds of exercises build muscular fitness?
- What is the difference between training for muscular endurance and for muscular strength?
- How many sets and repetitions should I do?
- What are the advantages of training with equipment?
- Are there special techniques and safety tips I should know about?

MUSCULAR fitness: What does that mean? It actually means a whole range of things, and it is time to move past the singular image of a super-muscled individual. Although a few people may aspire to large, developed muscles, the possibilities of toning, shaping, and firming muscles has a broader appeal that brings with it both health and appearance benefits. In this chapter, you will be introduced to exercise concepts underlying muscular fitness, and then you will learn more about ways to achieve it including the use of body weight, free weights, exercise bands, stability balls, and water.

Before diving into the specifics of muscular fitness development, let's take a brief look at the history behind it and define some terms that have been used to describe it. Prior to the aerobics movement, the main way to get "fit" was to perform calisthenics. The roots of this type of activity are found in the German and Swedish systems of gymnastics that emigrated to the United States with natives of those countries during the 19th century.

In the 1950s, body builder and fitness guru Jack LaLanne used television to popularize callisthenic-based workouts that included exercises like squats and push-ups to which he often added homemade weights such as soup cans. Typically, women performed "body-toning" exercises with the hope of eliminating the "jiggly stuff" on the backs of their arms and thighs, while men focused more on developing a muscular appearance, particularly with respect to their abdomens and chests. Although these appearance-oriented goals remain strong motivators for people starting an exercise regimen, people who sustain muscle fitness activity quickly discover the benefits of additional strength and endurance as well as improvements in appearance. It is also important to note that muscular fitness will alter body composition primarily by increasing muscle; aerobic exercise is still the best way to take off fat. Getting rid of the "jiggly stuff" or unwanted "belly" requires fat loss, but at the same time you can build up your muscles so that as the fat comes off nicely toned muscles are revealed.

The phrase "body toning" has historically been used to describe a series of muscle exercises performed predominantly by women. This term is still used occasionally today, but more current terms have taken its place. There has been a shift especially among women from the idea of "body toning" to the idea of muscular fitness (strength and endurance). Men who were not focused solely on muscle size have appreciated the increased opportunities provided by exercise programs intended to develop overall muscle fitness as well.

Body toning is more accurately expressed as "muscle toning," because it is the skeletal muscles that are firmed and shaped. When sufficient resistance is used, muscles not only become toned, but also increase in size, strength, and endurance. It is therefore more accurate to refer to them generally as "resistance exercises" or more specifically as "muscular strength" or "muscular endurance" exercises. These then, are the terms that will be used in this text. Another label you may hear is "floor exercises." This is what some fitness classes call the resistance exercises that are performed sitting or lying down on the floor. There are also trade names such as Vertifirm™ that refer to resistance exercises performed standing up.

Most hour-long aerobic fitness classes incorporate 10 to 20 minutes of muscle-developing exercises. If you want to devote more attention to muscle development, you can perform additional resistance exercises on your own or take a specialized course. You may find resistance training courses offered under titles such as weight training, body sculpting, body building, body shaping, and power lifting. How the muscles are worked, and whether the emphasis is on body contouring, hypertrophy (increasing muscle size), muscular strength, or muscular endurance, will differ among these programs. Some group fitness classes blend muscular fitness exercises with aerobic activity. These cross training and fusion-type classes are described more in Chapter 9.

Muscular strength and endurance have always been important in the sports world, but for a time they were overshadowed in the public eye by the health-conscious aerobic movement. The idea that you are more likely to die prematurely from a poorly conditioned cardiorespiratory system than from weak skeletal muscles was supported by research on lifestyle diseases. However, experts now agree that muscular strength and endurance play a vital role in physical health and wellness, and professionals have become more outspoken about incorporating exercises that develop muscle strength, recommending that individuals perform a series of resistance exercises at least twice a week (see the Benefits of Resistance Training box). Group fitness classes can be a wonderful package of both aerobic and total-body muscle conditioning. Depending on how much resistance training is done, the class may be more than an hour long. Some classes just use body weight to create the load, and others incorporate a variety of equipment. Aerobic activities often have a muscle endurance component built into them. Cycling and running, for example, are highly aerobic and also provide a really good muscle endurance workout for the legs. When an activity targets one part of the body, and not the whole body, a supplement of resistance exercises can be used to create a balanced workout. In this case, upper-body, core, and lateral moving lower body resistance exercises should be added.

BENEFITS OF RESISTANCE TRAINING

RESISTANCE TRAINING:

- increases your muscular strength and endurance
- enables you to do more work with less fatigue
- improves posture and trunk stability
- reduces your risk of injury, especially to the lower back
- helps increase or maintain bone density
- improves body composition
- can create a more aesthetic body build (shape)
- provides the muscular energy for recreational activities in addition to normal life demands
- improves your ability to perform physical skills such as skills needed for specific sports
- lowers risk of premature death and incidence of cardiovascular disease events
- lowers blood pressure for those with pre-hypertension or stage 1 hypertension
- increases insulin sensitivity

BENEFITS OF MUSCULAR STRENGTH AND ENDURANCE

Good strength and endurance are important for getting through the day without muscle fatigue. This also means having enough "muscle" to enjoy recreational activities and deal with any emergencies that might arise. If you find yourself sitting down because your legs and back are tired, or stopping something because your arms feel heavy, you are suffering from weak muscles. The more physically demanding your daily and recreational activities, the more strength and endurance you will need. Being in good muscular shape also helps prevent injuries and is especially helpful in preventing back pain. Another important reason to perform resistance exercises is to prevent osteoporosis, a disease characterized by a weakening of the bones. When bones are stressed, they get denser and stronger. Both the aerobic and muscle-building sections of a group fitness class will strengthen and/or maintain bones. Finally, if you enjoy sports activities, muscular strength and endurance play an important role in skill performance. For example, you can hit a softball farther with good strength, and you can keep up good footwork longer on the tennis court with good muscular endurance.

As muscle tissue is built, body composition, the ratio of lean body mass to fat, changes. Muscle is lean body mass, and even if fat is not lost, building more muscle improves the ratio of lean body mass to fat, which means that your percentage of fat decreases. When fat loss (through diet and exercise) accompanies muscle building, even greater body composition changes occur. Metabolic factors such as blood pressure, insulin sensitivity, and blood glucose levels have also been found to improve with regular resistance training. Mental health benefits may also be a benefit, but these have not been well documented at this time.

RESISTANCE EXERCISES: BEFORE, AFTER, OR DURING AEROBICS?

The question of when to do resistance exercises arises in group fitness classes that include separate sections focused on aerobics and on muscle fitness. Resistance exercises may be performed at the beginning of class following a good warm-up, or they can be done closer to the end of class following the aerobics and aerobic cool-down. Doing them early in the class may do the following:

- help lower the body's store of glycogen, thus encouraging more fat burning during the aerobic part of class.
- promote better resistance-exercise technique since the muscles are less fatigued.

- lessen the chance of a person experiencing postural hypotension, the disorientation or dizziness that occurs when you go from one position to another, such as sitting to standing. (Those who prefer to do resistance exercises after the aerobic section avoid postural hypotension by doing a thorough cool-down and starting with resistance exercises that don't drop the head.)

Performing resistance exercises after the aerobic cool-down may do the following:

- result in slightly more cardiorespiratory conditioning and calorie burning, because the heart rate remains higher for a longer period of time. This is most true if big-muscle endurance exercises are done first, such as a series of lunges.
- promote good technique during the aerobic portion of class, because the muscles are not fatigued from the resistance exercises.

At this time, there is no conclusive evidence that it is better to perform resistance exercises before or after aerobic conditioning. In fact, many instructors do both by incorporating standing muscle-toning exercises after the warm-up and performing additional exercises that require a sitting or lying position toward the end of class. There have been some attempts to add resistance such as small weights to step or low-impact aerobic routines, but research indicates minimal advantage in doing this and a greater risk of injury. Resistance training can be performed with the best technique, concentration, and safety during its own segment of class. If you have a personal preference and schedule flexibility, select an instructor who does it in the order you like.

Individuals who are less fit can also increase their muscular endurance (and strength to a lesser degree) during the aerobic phase of class. Arm movements and stepping patterns for 20 to 30 minutes develop muscle endurance. Even if you are highly fit in one way (for example, if you are a runner), you may find that you are less fit in another way (for example, in upper body strength) and will benefit from the full-body workout of the aerobic section.

ACHIEVING RESISTANCE

You can achieve resistance in a number of ways. Calisthenic exercises use the pull of gravity and the weight of body parts to achieve resistance. For example, doing a push-up means extending your arms and lifting up your torso against gravity. To achieve more resistance, you can add weights, the pull of an exercise band, the instability of an exercise ball, or the drag of water.

Exercises incorporating the use of weights, bands, and balls are discussed in Chapter 11. Sometimes you can also achieve more resistance by using a different body position both with and without a stability ball.

Here are some examples. The easiest push-up to do is one performed against a wall. Place your hands shoulder-height on the wall, and put your feet about 2 feet away from the base of the wall. Bend your arms. You can progressively increase resistance by doing a push-up (1) on your hands and knees, (2) on your hands and toes, (3) on your hands and toes with your toes up on a bleacher, step, or ball. You can make side leg lifts more difficult by beginning with a bent leg lift and progressing to a straight leg lift. Curl-ups are easiest when your arms are down at the sides of your body, harder when your arms are crossed over your chest, still harder with your hands up by your head, and most difficult when your arms are extended over your head. Curl-ups can also be made more difficult by putting your feet up on a step or ball or by performing them on a stability ball.

When an exercise is being performed in class, select the position and intensity that suits your personal needs. There are limits, however, to the amount of resistance you can achieve through body position. For more resistance and greater strength and endurance gains, you will have to use outside sources such as weights, weighted balls, exercise bands, or even a partner resisting your movements through a range of motion.

THE MUSCULAR STRENGTH–ENDURANCE CONTINUUM

To understand the relationship between strength and endurance, picture a continuum with strength at one end and endurance at the other. Exercises performed with heavy resistance (weight) exhaust muscles in just a few repetitions and build strength. Exercises with light to moderate resistance performed with many repetitions build muscular endurance.

STRENGTH ←——→ ENDURANCE
Heavy Resistance   Light-Moderate Resistance
Few Repetitions   Many Repetitions

Because there is no definitive point along the continuum where strength ends and endurance begins, the target zones for these two fitness components overlap. For health-related purposes, resistance training intensities that fall in the middle, where the two target zones overlap, are used to develop muscular strength and endurance, collectively referred to as muscular fitness.

THE FITT PRINCIPLE

As mentioned in Chapter 3, the FITT principle, incorporating Frequency, Intensity, Time, and Type of exercise (the variables used in locating and exercising within your target zones), can be used to create an optimal muscular fitness program to achieve your desired outcome. Time is represented in terms of volume of exercise, and the length of rest intervals is an additional key variable.

FREQUENCY

If you want to build muscular strength and endurance, you should incorporate resistance training (muscle toning, weight training) into your fitness program at least twice a week, and if possible, three times a week, on alternate days. You should not work the same muscle tissue twice in less than 48 hours because the tissue needs time to rest and rebuild. If you work out too frequently, your muscles will weaken over time. Serious weight trainers may work out more days of the week, but they use one set of muscles one day and a different set the next. This type of training is called a split-body program. A person might do chest, back, and abdominals one day and arms and legs the next; a 4-day-a-week schedule might consist of trunk on Monday and Thursday and limbs on Tuesday and Saturday.

INTENSITY

"Intensity," in the context of resistance training, is described by how much physical work you are able to do. The initial focus is on the amount of load (weight or resistance) you can move or hold. But there are other factors that influence intensity including the number of times (repetitions) you move the load, how fast you move, and how long you rest between movements. If you are holding the load rather than moving it, the intensity is affected by the position in which you hold it, how long you hold it, and how long you rest between the holds. The load can be created using body weight, a dumbbell or other free-weight equipment, or another form of resistance such as machines, bands, or water. For simplicity, the following discussion about intensity uses the word "weight" to refer to the load and "lift" to refer to movement of the load. Keep in mind that lifting a weight can involve pushing, pulling, or lifting.

The amount of weight you can lift only one time is called **one repetition maximum (1 RM)**. Muscular strength is emphasized when you lift a high percentage of 1RM, which you can do only a small number of times because the weight is so heavy. In comparison, muscular endurance is emphasized when you lift smaller percentages of 1RM; you can do more of these lifts because the weight is lighter. Robust gains in both hypertrophy and strength result from using a resistance equivalent to 60% to 80% of the individual's one repetition maximal (1RM) effort.[1] ACSM recommends that novice through intermediate strength trainers work out at an intensity equal to 60% to 70% of their 1RM (i.e., moderate to hard intensity), whereas experienced exercisers can work at above 80% of 1RM (i.e., hard to very hard intensity). These levels can be achieved by working out with a resistance that can be lifted 8 to 12 times, resulting in fatigue but not complete exhaustion. If muscular endurance is a person's focus, then the intensity is lowered to less than 50% of 1RM, and 15 to 25 repetitions are performed. Consecutive numbers of lifts such as those just described are called **repetitions**. One group of consecutive repetitions is called a **set**. The recommendation for strength building is 2 to 4 sets, with the understanding that just one set can have a positive training effect on beginners. Because endurance sets have higher numbers of repetitions, a limit of 2 sets is generally recommended. If you are older or very deconditioned, work with very light to light intensities for 10 to 20 repetitions. These ACSM recommendations are for general fitness.

It should be noted that you can also achieve strength and endurance through isometric (held) positions. These can include, for example, a wall sit and a variety of yoga positions that are held. Holding very difficult body positions for short periods of time emphasizes strength, whereas holding more moderate poses for extended times emphasizes muscle endurance.

Group fitness classes vary in how they approach muscular fitness, but most tend to emphasize muscular endurance or a level of exertion that is in the middle of the endurance-strength continuum. Select a resistance (weight) that allows you to do the repetitions without complete exhaustion. If you need to do fewer than the instructor, you can do one movement for every two of the instructor's and still be moving the whole time. It is also certainly acceptable to stop, take a rest, and then continue. You can also adjust your resistance midstream by adjusting your body position or switching up your equipment. For example, you might perform 5 push-ups on your toes and finish with 15 on your knees. Or, start with 5-lb dumbbells and finish with 3-lb dumbbells. Progressively overload your workout when the repetitions are starting to feel easy at the end of the set. For example, if your goal is

15 to 20 repetitions and you are challenged when you reach 15, then you are in your intensity target zone. But if you can go all the way to 20 without too much difficulty, it is time to increase the resistance by 5% to 10%. If you were lifting 5 lbs, this would mean no more than a 1-lb increase. Sometimes the equipment you are using won't allow so small an increase. So, you may need to start with a heavier resistance (8 lbs) for a few repetitions and then back off to a lighter resistance for the remainder—or keep training until you can handle the jump the equipment allows.

You may become curious about what your maximal lift ability is, or you may wish to know your 1RM so that you can calculate a percentage of it. Although it is possible for experienced lifters to directly test for 1RM, lifting a maximal load is not recommended for most individuals and especially not for those just getting started. Instead, if you are interested in your 1RM, it can be estimated from finding the weight you can lift 10 times and not an 11th. This is 10 repetitions max, or 10RM. Lifting to failure means that you cannot lift the weight another time OR that you cannot lift the weight another time with good form. Going to "failure" is different from going to a level of fatigue as previously recommended, and it is therefore even more important to maintain good form during this test. Once you know your 10RM, you can enter it into a max rep calculator such as the one found at the following site: www.exrx.net/Calculators/OneRepMax.html. This site will tell you not only 1RM, but also what weight represents 60%, 70%, etc., of 1RM.

Intensity can also be measured based on how hard it feels. The OMNI scale, introduced for aerobic work in Chapter 4, also has a scale for use with resistance training. Recall that the ACSM recommends that the novice through intermediate strength trainer work to an intensity equal to 60% to 70% of 1RM, which is described as moderate to hard intensity, and that experienced exercisers work to an intensity of 80% or higher of 1RM, which is described as hard to very hard scale (Figure 10.1).

Although intensity is measured as the load you lift, it is influenced by more than just load. The number of repetitions and the amount you rest between sets of repetitions also affect intensity and how your muscles will develop. (Rest intervals are discussed in a separate section.) Experts widely debate what combination of these variables creates the optimum stimulus for muscle development, especially when competitive levels of performance are desired. In general, those individuals seeking maximal strength use low reps (3 to 8), whereas those seeking health-related strength use a moderate number of reps (8 to 12), and those seeking endurance use high reps (15 to 25 or more).

---

[1]   Wernbom M, Augustsson J, Thomeé R. The influence of frequency, intensity, volume and mode of strength training on whole muscle cross-sectional area in humans. *Sports Med.* 2007;37(3):225–64.

Figure 10.1 The Omni Scale for resistance training

The number of sets can also range from 1 to 5, and the number of exercises increases as strength and definition are targeted.

TIME

No specific amount of time has been determined to be optimum for muscle fitness in terms of health benefits. It is much easier to make recommendations of time for aerobic exercise. Experts disagree on the numbers of repetitions and sets needed for strength, endurance, power, hypertrophy, etc., but it is the combination of these factors and the rest intervals between sets that will ultimately make up the amount of time (and the intensity) a workout requires. In resistance training, the volume (reps multiplied by sets) is often spoken of rather than minutes. High-end athletes spend hours in the weight room. Most of us are content with the results attained from just 20 to 30 minutes, which can easily be achieved through group exercise.

Research shows that performing two sets of each exercise is more effective in building strength than one set. Therefore, time permitting, it is recommended to build up to 2 sets. More can be accomplished with 3 to 4 sets, but of course this requires a greater time commitment. If you have the time, you can also add more exercises to your workout. For example, squats work the hamstrings, quadriceps, and gluteals. With additional time, each of these muscle groups can also be targeted separately or through additional single or combination exercises.

If you are interested in muscle endurance, a good question is, How many repetitions are enough?

It is impressive to be able to do 100 push-ups in a row, but does that make you healthier than when you could do 25? To answer this question, you must consider the amount of endurance you need for the things you like to do (recreational activities, job requirements, competitions, etc.), the psychological benefits of being able to perform a certain number, the wear and tear on your body, and the amount of time you have to train. Usually, it is more effective to increase resistance and do fewer repetitions than to do a really large number of repetitions. Moving closer to the strength end of the continuum also has a hidden benefit for endurance. Increases in strength actually increase muscle endurance. An example will best illustrate this. Imagine two people, one who can lift 50 pounds (lbs), and another who can lift 25 lbs. When they each lift 5 lbs repeatedly, the first person is lifting only 10% of his or her maximum, whereas the other person is lifting 20%. It is easier to keep lifting a smaller percentage of your maximum.

Group fitness classes tend to be oriented toward either muscular endurance or a combination of muscular endurance and strength, but when a simple exercise, such as push-ups, is being performed, two different people can get very different types of workouts if they are not careful to individualize the task. The person who can do 15 to 20 push-ups is working endurance, but the one who can do only three push-ups is working at the strength end of the continuum (heavy load, few repetitions). If both individuals are working with the same body weight (for example, 130 lbs), this illustrates the principle that the actual amount of weight or resistance is not what determines the training effect, but rather how hard it is for the individual to handle. The introduction of equipment like weights, bands, tubing, and weighted balls has allowed group exercise settings to better target the strength end of the continuum. Stability balls can challenge even advanced-level participants and can be combined with handheld weights. Barbells can also be loaded with increasing weight to challenge advanced participants. If you are interested in pursuing high levels of strength, you will want to seek out additional sources of free or machine weights and use a spotter when appropriate.

REST INTERVAL

When you work muscles more than one set, you generally rest between sets. This rest is critical to letting the muscle recuperate so that it can perform well on the next set. The length of the rest depends on the type of workout you are doing. Very heavy loads lifted only a few times require a much greater rest interval than lighter loads done more frequently. For general fitness, ACSM recommends 2 to 3 minutes of rest between sets. This type of workout falls in the middle of the endurance-strength continuum. You do not have to stop and sit around during this time. You can continue with other exercises, as long as they target different muscles; then, when enough time has elapsed, you can return to your previous exercise or move on to one that works the same muscles. For example, you can do squats, then let the legs rest while you do shoulder presses and abdominal curls, and then return to a leg exercise. The rest interval may change when you go beyond a general fitness program. For example, someone focused on muscle endurance may drop to a 30-second rest interval, whereas someone lifting very heavy loads may need to rest for 3 to 5 minutes. Individuals seeking strength and maximal size (a hypertrophy program) use about a 90-second rest interval.

Sometimes sets are done back to back, without any rest. This is an intermediate-level technique that provides the muscles with a different stimulus. Changing the exercise pattern after a while helps stimulate the muscles to keep improving. Supersets are two sets, done back to back with no rest, that use opposing muscles (e.g., biceps, triceps). Compound sets are similar but use two exercises that work the same muscles (e.g., push-ups and bench press).

TYPE: STATIC AND DYNAMIC TRAINING

There are two types of exercises for muscles: static and dynamic. Most people know static exercises as isometrics. During an **isometric contraction,** the muscle contracts, but it doesn't change in length. You perform isometrics by pushing against an immovable object (like a wall) or by holding a weight in one position. The weight can be the weight of your own limb, your whole body weight, or a weight you are holding. For example, you might hold yourself in a curl-up position for 10 seconds, or you might exert force by pressing one hand against the other. To increase strength, you would use short-duration holds of heavier weights or short-duration exertion using near-maximal force. To develop endurance, you would hold lighter weights or exert less force for longer durations. Isometrics can be very useful for strengthening a muscle in one position, which is particularly helpful for rehabilitating a weak point in a muscle's range of motion or strengthening postural muscles. One important word of caution: Isometric contractions can result in a rapid rise in blood pressure; therefore, people with high blood pressure and pregnant women should check with their physician before performing them.

In exercises that use **dynamic (isotonic) contractions** a force is applied through a range of motion. A curl-up is a good example of a dynamic exercise. Since most of our daily and recreational activities use a range of motion, dynamic exercises are usually the preferred way to train muscles. All of the resistance exercises in this chapter are dynamic in nature. However, there will be certain position-holding (stabilizing) muscles performing isometric holds. For example, during a regular push-up, the arms, chest, and shoulders perform dynamic contractions, but the abdominals, gluteals, and leg muscles perform isometric contractions. In more advanced weight training, you may find that isometric holds are incorporated within a dynamic movement to target specific parts of the range of movement.

You may also hear about **isokinetic contractions**. During these, the speed of movement is controlled, while the force exerted by the muscle can vary. These require special equipment that moves at a set rate and matches the force you apply with an equal resistance. Normally, if you push hard on a weight machine, the weights fly up. But this is not the case with isokinetic equipment. This type of exercise is especially good for rehabilitation, since you can push hard and receive high resistance during the healthy part of a movement and still push hard but apply less force and receive less resistance through the part of the motion where the muscle has been weakened by an injury.

ADDING RESISTANCE

Resistance training, now recognized as an important element of good fitness for everyone, has long suffered from myths and misunderstandings. Coaches once worried that an athlete who lifted weights would become muscle-bound and lose flexibility and coordination. Women worried that they would develop bulky, unseemly muscles. High-protein diets, including amino acid supplements, also have been touted to enhance muscle building. And at one time, circuit weight training was claimed to be a good aerobic workout. Today, we know that resistance training improves muscle performance, maintains and sometimes even improves flexibility, and does not cause women to develop bulky muscles (see Chapter 1). We also know that a high-protein diet is not needed to enhance muscle building; most resistance workouts require only a small increase in protein consumption in order to rebuild muscles and a lot of carbohydrate to fuel the exercise session. (See the discussion on protein in Chapter 13.) And although circuit weight training does increase heart rate into the training zone, it does not boost oxygen consumption to the same extent. Therefore, individuals who are less fit may improve aerobic fitness, but for the most part, resistance training benefits muscles and aerobic exercise strengthens the heart and lungs. Resistance training can, however, assist with some metabolic factors, such as blood pressure and insulin sensitivity.

More and more people have become aware of and are taking advantage of the benefits of resistance training. A basic program (moderate resistance for 12 sets of 8 to 12 repetitions) does not take long to complete, results in a firm physique, and develops a healthy combination of strength and endurance. Weights and bands used to be reserved for more advanced students, but in most cases, beginners can start with light weights, easy resistance bands, and movements in the water. Remember, too, that although some people are beginners at cardiorespiratory conditioning, they may not be beginners in strength and endurance. A person may also have more strength in some muscles and less strength in others. For example, many women have weaker upper body strength than lower body strength.

As a safety precaution, individuals with injuries, joint disease, or other medical conditions should discuss resistance training with a physician. You will also want to review the technique tips presented in Chapter 11. Technique becomes increasingly more important as you increase resistance. (Chapter 11 has many examples of how to add resistance to your exercises using body weight, free weights, bands, and stability balls.)

TYPES OF RESISTANCE

Things that create a resistance to muscles as they move can be used to increase the muscle's strength and endurance. Today, a variety of approaches and equipment can be used to achieve resistance, but that was not always true. Group exercise classes have changed a lot over the years. The weights that were first introduced in aerobic dance classes were handheld weights (many of which were not dumbbell shaped), elastic weights that slid onto a limb, and weights that wrapped around the limb with Velcro® attachments. These weights were limited to 1 to 3 lbs. As resistance training has grown in popularity among the general public and as more women have become involved in it, the equipment has shifted toward the use of dumbbells, barbells, and weighted balls. The amount of weight available is now greater, although workloads are usually still in the low to moderate range because the main focus is on muscle endurance. Another important reason to keep the resistance moderately low is that more challenging levels of **free weights** (dumbbells and weighted bars) should be performed only if a spotter is available. Group exercise classes do not usually involve paired activity with a spotter, although they can.

Resistance can be achieved in a number of ways, and each has its advantages. The simplest form of resistance is that of moving your body against gravity. When you want more resistance you can have a partner push or pull against you while you perform an exercise. To increase the resistance even more, you can use a variety of equipment. Resistance training machines are safe, usually do not require spotting, and can provide challenging loads without having to load weight plates. They do, however, restrict you to a certain motion, and they are designed for average-sized individuals. Newer machines allow for greater adjustments to accommodate body sizes. Unfortunately, they are not conducive to group exercise.

The use of free weights—equipment that you hold, such as dumbbells, bars, and weighted balls—allows you to recruit more muscle fibers than machine exercises because you must stabilize the weight in addition to pushing or pulling it. Free weights are also more versatile in that they allow motions to be performed in more directions, angles, and planes. Free weights also prevent one body part from lifting for another. For example, during a machine bench press, the right arm can push more than the left. In a free weight press—especially with dumbbells, but also with a bar—this imbalance will become obvious (if one arm is capable of more, the bar tilts) and can be corrected. Smaller barbells are becoming popular. Some bars themselves are weighted, whereas others are very light and allow you to load and clip into place weight plates ranging from 1 to 10 lbs. This arrangement works nicely with a step bench in a group setting for a variety of resistance exercises set to music.

If you chose to use free weights that wrap on to the body or are elastic and slip onto the wrist or ankles, be sure to reserve this equipment for the muscle-toning portion of class; do not wear it during the aerobic portion. This type of weight works well for people who do not like to, or cannot physically, grasp a dumbbell. You can also position the weight along the limb and adjust the difficulty of an exercise. For example, during a side leg lift, it is more difficult to lift a weight at the ankle than one placed above the knee.

Medicine balls and smaller weighted balls are also free weights, but they are softer and can be used in many ways. You certainly wouldn't want to throw and catch a dumbbell, but you can do so with a medicine ball. You can develop a specific kind of strength by moving a weighted ball through the motions you use in daily life, creative activities, sports, and recreation (Figure 10.2). Because they are weighted, they build strength in whatever range of motion you use them. You can use them on the go, such as tossing and catching while walking or jogging. You can balance on them with your feet or with your hands (i.e., push-up positions) for core strength, or turn and pass them to a partner to develop core stabilization during rotation (Figure 10.3). You can hold on to them and do many of the exercises described in Chapter 11 (lunges, squats, curl-ups, etc.), or if you are looking

Figure 10.3

for explosive strength, you can use them in "give-and-go" motions with a partner. The possibilities are endless and, unfortunately, beyond the scope of this book, but there are other books and professionals who can share this information with you.

There are two other forms of free weights not yet mentioned that add a unique aspect to a workout. One is the kettle bell. This is a round iron ball with a loop at the top that forms a handle. To use a kettle bell, you hold on to the handle and then swing the ball through the range of motion you wish to work. One of the most common exercises is the basic two-hand swing, where you swing the ball between the legs and then up to shoulder height using power from thrusting the hips, not from the arms. The technique involved requires skilled instruction, and because the weight is amplified by momentum, maintaining proper technique is critical. Mistakes with the kettle bell can cause serious injury, so beginners must work with very light weights until they master proper form. The value of kettle bells lies in the fact that they work multiple muscle groups at one time to build strength and stability in ranges of motion we use in everyday life. Kettle bells come from Eastern Europe, where they have a long history of use. If you are interested in kettle bells, it is best to find an instructor certified in their use.

A relative newcomer to fitness equipment is the SmartBell®, a brightly colored oval about 1-inch thick and 8 inches long with two handholds cut out. It arrived on the scene in 2000, looking something like a potato chip that won't lie flat because of its concave curve. Its two holes allow you to grip it with two hands

Figure 10.2

at once, or with one hand if desired, or to share one of the handholds with a partner. The SmartBell® was conceived, designed, and even initially made by Paul Widerman, a talented wrestler who, after suffering spinal compression injuries from traditional weight training, went in search of something better. Yoga changed his life, and after exploring dance, tai chi, and other martial arts, he sought to develop a piece of equipment that would complement the flowing, sweeping movements of these art forms. As he explains, the idea is to use circular movements that blend with gravity. This is in marked contrast to the unidirectional movements used with machines and most free weights. The curve to the SmartBell® allows it to wrap around the head or body, as well as to be used as an unstable platform for push-ups and other balance moves. Figure 10.4 shows an example of how it can be used together with a partner. It is a wonderfully versatile piece of equipment that, if used as intended, adds a whole other dimension to resistance training. You can purchase a SmartBell® and instructional DVD or look for a class that offers this unique program.

Exercise bands provide resistance in a somewhat different way than free weights do. They provide what is known as dynamic variable resistance, which means that as you stretch them, the resistance becomes greater. The disadvantage of this type of resistance is that at the end of a motion, the resistance may be more than you want, in which case you will have to use a less resistive band. But overall, they work very well. They are easily transported, easy to store, and inexpensive to buy. They also have the advantage of being able to stretch in many directions.

Two additional sources of resistance are stability balls and water. Stability balls take advantage of an unstable environment and body position to challenge the muscles. In addition to being fun, the balls are very

Figure 10.4 Partner work with SmartBells ©

versatile and easy to do at home. Pushing and pulling water can create resistance and offer the major advantage of being nonimpact; aqua or water aerobics is a very popular form of exercise for all ages.

FREE WEIGHTS

Weight should only be added to an exercise when the exercise is relatively easy to perform without weight, and you have established good technique. Start with light weights and work your way up in resistance. You will need to use lighter resistances with smaller muscles and heavier resistances with larger muscles. Fixed ends on dumbbells (as opposed to screw-on ends) are generally preferred because they cannot become loose and fall off accidentally. Dumbbells used in group exercise classes generally range in weight from 1 to 20 lbs. and bars weigh from 9 to 15 lbs.

Weighted limbs should always be moved with fluidity and control. When you add resistance to an exercise, it becomes even more important to maintain good alignment and control. When a weight is swung through the air, speed and momentum give it a force greater than its actual weight. The muscles, tendons, and ligaments around a joint have to stop the weight at the end of their range of motion. Too much weight, amplified by indiscriminate flinging of the arms or leg, can tear these tissues. (Think of the damage a wrecking ball can do when it is swung into a building.) An appropriate weight is one that you can move through a desired number of repetitions with the last few repetitions being difficult. If you find yourself recruiting extra muscles and losing your alignment for the last few repetitions, the weight is too heavy. Be sure to breathe comfortably throughout the exercises. With heavier resistance (difficult repetitions regardless of actual poundage), it is important to breathe out during the work phase and in during the recovery phase. This prevents a buildup of pressure in your chest.

RESISTANCE EXERCISES WITH FREE WEIGHTS

Exercise order and tempo are important components of a free weight workout. When performing a basic muscle workout, it is generally recommended to perform multi-joint and large muscle exercises first, followed by smaller muscle and single-joint exercises. Exercise order can also ensure that opposing muscle groups both achieve a workout and that the same muscle is not worked in back-to-back exercises, a technique reserved for more advanced workouts. For example, to complement the exercises of a standard workout, add the toe flexion exercise with a band shown in Figure 11.81 (on page 176). If more emphasis on the inner and outer thighs is desired, leg lifts with wrapped weights (or band) can also be added. The tempo generally recommended is 2 counts on the work phase and 4 counts on the recovery phase. However, in a group exercise setting, where only light to moderate weights are used and where an instructor is trying to use the rhythm of the music and/or the cadence of stepping up and down on a bench, it is common to see exercises counted with 2 (or 4) counts in both directions. When time is short, multi-joint exercise and exercises that provide the most balance for the aerobic workout and your personal weaknesses should be selected. Choreography or job-related or recreational activities can sometimes work one group of muscles more than its opposing group. Resistance exercises can restore balance.

Here are some additional important tips for working with dumbbells and barbells in a group fitness setting:

- Always *breathe out* during the *work* phase. On an arm curl, the work phase occurs when you are bringing the weight to your body. On a chest press, it occurs when you are pushing the weight away from the body. On a squat or lunge, it occurs when you are coming back up. An easy way to remember this is to *Exhale on Exertion*.
- Grip the equipment firmly, but not so tightly that it causes hand and wrist tension.
- There are several different ways to grip the equipment. In a closed pronated grip, the palm faces downward when you first pick up the equipment, and the thumb is wrapped around. When you change the position of the dumbbells or the barbell for some exercises (such as a shoulder press), the palms will end up facing forward even though you are still in a closed pronated grip. In a closed supinated grip, the palms face upward and the thumbs are wrapped.
- If you sweat a lot and the equipment feels slippery in your hands, wear weight-lifting gloves.
- Stick to light to moderate weights with which you can perform a higher number of repetitions rather than very heavy weights you can only lift a few times. *Never* perform heavy, demanding loads (weights) without a spotter. It is best to do these exercises outside a group fitness setting.
- Technique is critical to your success. If you feel yourself breaking form, stop, take a break, perhaps lighten the load, and then begin again if it is appropriate. Exercising to **failure** means to go until you can't do another repetition or until you break form. In a group fitness class, you want to challenge yourself but avoid working to failure. (In strength training with excellent form and with a spotter, working to failure can be a good challenge to the muscle.)
- If you are using a barbell with weight plates, be sure to clip the weights in place.
- When lifting a barbell, make sure to keep the bar level.
- When lifting with two dumbbells, move them both through the action simultaneously or alternate arms.
- If you have a history of joint problems such as arthritis, bursitis, ligament damage, or knee surgery, you should not use weights unless cleared to do so by a physician.

EXERCISE BANDS AND CABLES

Exercise bands, sometimes referred to as resistance bands or cables, are an inexpensive and versatile tool to increase the resistance during a muscle-toning exercise. They come in a variety of forms, including colorful flat sheets of rubber 5 to 6 inches wide resembling strips of inner tubes, cables with handles, and surgical tubing. The first are produced commercially for fitness classes and therapeutic clinics under several names such as Dyna-bands and Thera-bands®. They usually come in several colors; each color represents the amount of resistance, such as light, medium, or heavy.

Bands come in different widths and thicknesses. The wider or thicker the band, the more difficult it is to stretch. Some exercises require long bands that may be referred to as double bands. You can buy bands in different lengths and amounts of resistance. Most bands contain latex, but it is possible to purchase latex-free bands. Be sure to store latex-free bands in a separate bag.

If you choose to use a band, take off any jewelry that may cut into the band and always check the band for small cuts or tears before using it. (You can wear weight-lifting or bicycling gloves to take the pressure off your hands and to cover jewelry you do not want to remove.) Using the recommended range of 8 to 12 repetitions, you should change to a thicker or more resistant band when you can easily perform 12 repetitions and try a thinner or less resistant band if you can't do at least 8 repetitions. You may have to reduce band difficulty further if your goal is more endurance oriented and you intend to do more than

12 repetitions. For more resistance, you can use two bands at once and/or grasp the band farther from the end.

Bands and cables with handles can be interchanged in most exercises. If you are using a band, grasp or wrap the band. If you are using a cable, hold it by the handles. Many different cables are available in a variety of lengths and resistances, and some types of cables have loops built into them for inserting a hand or foot. If using a straight band, you can create a loop by tying the ends of the band together with a square knot.

If you have high blood pressure or have suffered a cumulative trauma disorder such as carpal tunnel syndrome, have a previous joint injury or chronic joint disease, check with a physician before using bands or cables. If you have knee problems, always work with the band above your knees. Bands may pull on leg hair, so socks, tights, or sweatpants are recommended. When pulling a band with your hand, be sure to keep the hand in line with the forearm. In other words, do not allow the wrist to "break" or "lay back."

Resistance Exercises With Bands

The band exercises in Chapter 11 are a representative sample of what can be done with bands. Note that each flexion exercise is presented with an opposing extension exercise and in some cases an additional lateral moving exercise. The large muscle, multi-joint exercises for a body area are presented before corresponding small muscle or single-joint exercises because this is usually the preferred order for performing them. In some cases, exercises for opposing muscles or muscle groups (for example, bench press and seated row exercises) are performed back to back with no rest period, a practice called **supersetting.** This method of training is more demanding and is therefore appropriate for more experienced and more fit individuals. The same order of exercises, but with a rest between exercises, is appropriate for all fitness levels. For more exercises and information on exercise bands, look for books written by qualified experts.

Stability Balls

Stability balls are large, heavy-duty inflatable balls that are used as exercise equipment in many fun and effective ways. They are a versatile tool for developing strength, balance, and flexibility. (Some instructors are even using them in aerobic routines.) Just sitting on one of these large exercise balls makes all kinds of muscles work to keep you balanced. The ball creates an unstable environment in which your muscles, especially your core (trunk) muscles, have to work to stabilize you. This not only strengthens the muscles, but it also enhances the communication between the nervous system and the muscles. The improved neuromuscular efficiency results in better overall coordination. Stability balls have many aliases, including **exercise ball, physioball,** fitness ball, and resistance ball, but the name **Swiss ball** has historical importance because the balls were first introduced in Switzerland as a rehabilitation tool. The term stability ball will be used here to reflect their use for developing body stabilizing strength.

Unlike traditional resistance training programs that target one muscle or muscle group, stability ball exercises work a combination of muscles in the body. This more closely imitates normal body movement. During each of the stability ball exercises presented in Chapter 11, one or more muscles will be performing dynamic full range-of-motion contractions, while others will be busy making small stabilizing adjustments to maintain the body's position on the ball. One of the nice things about stability ball exercises is that the difficulty of the exercise can be easily adjusted by changing your body position on the ball. A softer, less inflated ball is also easier to work on than a harder, more inflated ball. As a result, stability ball exercises can be equally effective for beginners working on developing functional (everyday and postural) strength and for college athletes trying to maximize their strength and performance.

The benefits of using a stability ball include the following:

- improves muscular strength and endurance and is especially effective for increasing abdominal and back strength
- improves flexibility, including healthy motion ranges of the spine
- enhances balance and coordination of the muscles that are used to stabilize the spine and control proper posture
- helps you learn and maintain a healthy (and injury-preventing) neutral spine position to use during exercise
- improves core muscle strength, which translates into greater control for athletic skills

Stability balls can be made of vinyl or plastic. When purchasing a ball, be sure you are getting heavy-duty vinyl that is burst-resistant and will not tear if punctured; if a ball is punctured, it deflates slowly to prevent injury. The balls are inflated using a hand or electric pump. Some balls come with what looks like an udder (three-pointed extensions) on which the ball can rest. When using the ball, the udder is rotated out to the side so that the ball can roll properly during exercises. The udder is strictly a means of keeping the ball from rolling around when not in use.

It is best not to wear sharp items (jewelry, belt buckles, etc.) when working on inflated balls. Also be aware that plastic balls can be damaged by heat or excessive sunlight. Supplies that are useful for maintaining stability balls include a variety of hand or electric pumps, stands to keep the ball from rolling away, plug removers, carrying straps, and storage accessories.

RESISTANCE EXERCISES WITH A STABILITY BALL

The following are key technique points to keep in mind when using a stability ball:

- Use a ball that is large or small enough to allow you to maintain a 90-degree (or slightly greater) angle at the knees when you sit on it. Your thighs will be parallel to the ground or will point down slightly. Smaller and larger balls also may be used for different exercises to achieve different angles, but for the exercises depicted in Chapter 11, the 90-degree rule is a good one. A 45-centimeter (cm) ball is generally used for individuals under 5 feet (ft) tall, a 55-cm ball for 5-ft to 6-ft tall individuals, and a 65-cm ball for those over 6 ft tall. A good-quality ball will hold up to 500 lbs.

- Always wear a shirt. A sweaty body can make you slide off the ball.

- Use progressions. When placing the lower body on the ball, the easiest position is to have the hips on the ball followed by the thighs and feet.

- Only perform exercises for which you have enough core strength to maintain a safe position. If you feel yourself losing alignment, select an easier version of the exercise or use one that doesn't involve the ball.

- Work with a neutral spine (natural curves) unless the exercise calls for spinal flexion or extension.

- Avoid scapular collapse (e.g., don't let your chest sag in a push-up position).

- The more external support you use, the less strengthening you will achieve, because the support stabilizes your position for you. One exception is presented in Figure 11.43 on page 160, where you will see that the student is using another student's feet to stabilize the side-lying position. This is done to keep the feet from sliding across the floor, not to control the person's position. On a nonslip floor this stabilization will not be needed.

You can make exercises more difficult by reducing the amount of your body that touches the ball surface, such as using only the lower legs instead of whole legs, or using one leg on the ball instead of two (advanced). Placing arms or legs farther apart on the ball makes holding positions easier, whereas placing them closer together results in a greater balance demand. (Ball exercises for posture control and flexibility have been included in Chapters 7 and 11.)

There are other types of balance and stability-challenging equipment available that are fun to use, such as foam rollers, Bosu balls, balance discs, and balancing boards. But because of the cost of these types of equipment, they are less often available for large groups.

WATER

To move your body through water, you have to move the water that is in your way. Pushing or pulling against the water provides a resistance that can be used for strength and endurance conditioning. Out of the pool, the air resistance you encounter during muscle toning is minimal, but the effect of having to work against gravity is significant. On the other hand, you are more buoyant in the pool (which lessens the effect of gravity), but the water offers 12 times more resistance to movement than does air.

You can increase water resistance using the following methods:

- Move the broadest body surface possible through the water. For example, moving a flat palm through the water creates more resistance than moving the edge of the hand through water. Moving a webbed glove or plastic barbell (Figure 10.5) through the water similarly increases the amount of surface and therefore the amount of resistance.

Figure 10.5

- Increase the length of the resistance arm of a lever. The arms and legs of the body act like levers. When the arm or leg is extended, it meets more resistance going through the water than when it is bent.
- Exert more force against the water. Moving a body part through the water quickly (with more force) is harder than moving it slowly through the water.
- Change the direction of moving water. Sweeping water in one direction and then reversing directions forces your muscles to work harder as they fight the current.
- Move as much water as possible. When you get a block of water moving, momentum will keep it moving and your limb will get to rest a little. Instead of continuing to push right behind the block of moving water, change the position of your arm up or down and pick up a new block of water. Circular and undulating movement patterns move more water than do straight-line movements.

Resistance exercises performed in water are similar to those on land, but aqua muscle toning has two distinct advantages. First, resistance is applied in both directions of an exercise. As the leg sweeps out to the side in a leg lift, the outer thigh muscles work against the water. As the working leg is brought back in, the inner thigh works against the water. As long as equal force is applied in each direction, muscle balance is achieved. (It takes two exercises, an outer and inner leg lift, to accomplish the same thing on land.) Second, people of all abilities can exercise together, because it's simple to adjust the intensity of the exercise. For example, participants can perform a lower-body exercise of jumping off the bottom of the pool by pushing off with a little or a lot of force. Grandparent and grandchild can do this together and both benefit! The intensity can also be adjusted in very small increments, unlike using weights or bands that require you to jump to the next available resistance level. For more resistance, webbed gloves, bands, Styrofoam dumbbells and noodles, kickboards, and pull buoys can all be added to the workout. Kickboards and pull buoys are more often used in a deep-water workout than a shallow-water one.

RESISTANCE EXERCISES IN WATER

Many of the resistance exercises you perform on land can be performed in the water. Some have to be adjusted to account for body position and stability requirements in the water, and some can be adapted to take advantage of the floating environment. Still others are unique to water aerobics. Described here are a handful of exercises to help you see how muscle toning is achieved in the water. If you like the idea of exercising this way, consider taking a course or purchasing a good water aerobics book.

You can perform exercises such as triceps extension, biceps curl, toe raise, and lateral arm raise in the pool just as you do on land. Flies, instead of being done lying down, are performed vertically and you can do them while walking backward to increase the resistance against the water. Leg exercises like squats and lunges have to be modified because of the buoyancy factor—you actively push off the bottom of the pool when performing these exercises. This jumping is not hard on the body, since the landing impact is cushioned by the water. You can do leg lifts while bracing the body against the side of the pool.

You can also use exercise bands in the pool. Again, you can perform many of the exercises that use bands the same way that you do them on land. Side stepping and walking forward and backward with bands around the ankles are good ways to work the legs during a shallow-water workout. For deep-water work, two bands can be tied together in the middle with loops tied into each end. A person floating in a waist belt can then insert a foot and a hand in the loops and perform various exercises like leg extensions and arm curls. Figure-eight bands (with loops at each end) are also commercially available.

Deep-water workouts borrow movements from swimming strokes, water polo, and synchronized swimming. For example, you can develop leg endurance by kicking laps with a kickboard, treading water with an eggbeater leg kick (used in water polo), or performing scissor kicks under or on the surface of the water (used in synchronized swimming). You can also use the pool edge (deck) or gutter edge to advantage.

Depending on the depth of the water and strength of the participant, triceps push-ups can be performed by gently pushing with the legs off the bottom or by kicking to assist the arms. You can work on abdominal muscles by placing your back against the pool wall and stretching your arms up on the deck, and then, in this position, draw your feet up to your chest. Or you can perform similar curl-ups in deep water while holding a noodle across your upper back and under the arms for support; or, to add upper-body work, do the abdominal curls while treading water. Finally, you will find that motions that are difficult to perform on land with resistance can be executed easily in water. For example, you can move your hands and arms in a figure-eight pattern or using a pattern that simulates a golf stroke. The possibilities are endless. Water aerobics can be a great stand-alone activity or an excellent way to cross-train.

SUMMARY

You can increase your muscular strength and endurance by progressively overloading. One way to achieve an overload is to increase the resistance against which the muscles work. You can increase resistance by adding weights or exercise bands to muscle-toning exercises, by performing the exercises in water, or by adjusting your body position. You can also use stability balls to add resistance or increase the number of muscles being used during an exercise.

COMMONLY ASKED QUESTIONS

Do I need muscular fitness, or is aerobic fitness enough?

They both do different things for you. Aerobic activity improves your cardiorespiratory fitness and gives you related benefits. Muscular fitness makes you strong, which can help you do activities that require "muscle," such as lifting and pulling things, or recreational activities, such as paddling a canoe. A balance of both makes for the healthiest and most able body.

Will weight training give women big muscles?

Not in the same way that men's muscles can get big. Women's muscles do hypertrophy (get bigger), but the fibers are smaller compared to those of men. For that reason, even when a woman's muscles grow, they still don't have the same "bulk." In addition, women do not have as much testosterone as men, and testosterone is needed to build large muscle fibers. Women who do hypertrophy more than average may have genetically higher levels of testosterone and growth hormones. In such cases, women can de-emphasize hypertrophy by working with light to moderate weight instead of heavier loads.

Will weight training decrease fat?

Any exercise that uses calories can help decrease fat storage. However, weight training does not use fat as a fuel the way aerobic activity does. Weight training that involves lower weight loads and more repetitions (muscle endurance) is going to burn more calories than strength-oriented programs with high loads and low numbers of repetitions.

Do I need a special diet for muscle building, such as adding more protein?

It depends on your goals and the program you use. For general fitness, you normally need just a well-balanced diet with enough calories to support both daily activity and the workout. In general, people tend to short their carbohydrates and overeat protein. In contrast, you need carbohydrates and only a small increase in protein to fuel the workout. (Chapter 13 discusses this in more detail.)

KNOWLEDGE TIPS

1. As resistance increases, so does the importance of body alignment and movement control.

2. Beginners should start with low levels of resistance and use progressive overloads to achieve higher levels of fitness.

3. Light to moderate resistance loads develop muscular endurance and are appropriate in group fitness classes. Heavier loads or working to failure must, for safety, be performed on a machine or with a spotter.

4. Individuals of all fitness levels should overload gradually by increasing the resistance or the number of repetitions (or sets) being performed.

5. Resistance training, which involves a minimum of 1 set (preferably 2–4 sets) of 8 to 12 repetitions for each of the major muscle groups, is recommended for most adults.

6. Individuals with joint injury, high blood pressure, heart disease, orthopedic problems, or other health concerns should discuss resistance training with their health care provider before beginning.

7. Resistance can be increased through the use of free weights, exercise bands, or stability balls, by performing exercises in the water, or by adjusting body position.

8. Stability balls add the element of instability, which results in increased strength, balance, and coordination. Body position on the ball can increase or decrease the difficulty of an exercise.

9. Water exercises can be made more difficult by presenting the broadest body surface to the water, extending a limb, moving through water with greater force, changing the direction of moving water, and moving more blocks of water.

THINK ABOUT IT

1. What are the benefits of having muscular fitness?

2. What is the difference between muscular endurance and muscular strength?

3. Explain the FITT Principles for muscular endurance and muscular strength.

4. Explain how increasing strength can help increase muscular endurance.

5. Resistance can be created using machines, body weight, free weights (dumbbells, barbells, medicine balls), stability balls, exercise bands, and water. Explain the key advantages to each type.

6. Stability balls, Bosu balls, and core boards all create an unstable environment in which to exercise. Explain why an unstable environment can be an advantage.

REFERENCES

Aaberg, E. *Resistance Training Instruction.* 2nd ed. Champaign, IL: Human Kinetics, 2006.

American College of Sports Medicine. *ACSM's Guidelines for Exercise Testing and Exercise Prescription.* 8th ed. Media, PA: Lippincott Williams & Wilkins, 2010.

———. "The Recommended Quantity and Quality of Exercise for Developing and Maintaining Cardiorespiratory and Muscle Fitness in Healthy Adults." *Medicine and Science in Sports and Exercise* 30 (No. 6, 1998): 975–91.

Brooks, G. A., Fahey, T. D., and K. Baldwin. *Exercise Physiology: Human Bioenergetics and Its Applications.* 4th ed. New York: McGraw-Hill, 2004.

Cassidy, C. "Should You Add a Little Weight to Your Workout?" *Women's Sports and Fitness* 8 (March 1986): 38–9, 47.

Delavier, F. *Strength Training Anatomy.* 3rd ed. Champaign, IL: Human Kinetics, 2010.

Fardy, P. S. "Isometric Exercise and the Cardiovascular System." *The Physician and Sportsmedicine* 9 (No. 9, 1981): 42.

Fleck, S. J., and W. J. Kraemer. *Designing Resistance Training Programs.* 3rd ed. Champaign, IL: Human Kinetics, 2004.

Goldenberg, L., and P. Twist. *Strength Ball Training.* 2nd ed. Champaign, IL: Human Kinetics, 2007.

Hopson, J. L., R. J. Donatelle, and T. R. Littrell. *Get Fit, Stay Well!* 2nd ed. San Francisco: Benjamin Cummings, 2012.

Kirk, E. P., J. E. Donnelly, B. K. Smith, J. Honas, J. D. Lecheminant, B. W. Bailey, D. J. Jacobsen, and R. A. Washburn. "Minimal Resistance Training Improves Daily Energy Expenditure and Fat Oxidation." *Medicine and Science in Sports and Exercise* 41 (No. 5, 2009): 1122–9.

MacFarlane, P. A. "Out with the Sit-Up, In with the Curl-Up." *Journal of Physical Education, Recreation, and Dance* 64 (August 1993): 62–6.

National Association of Sports Medicine, M. A. Clark, S. C. Lucett, and R. J. Corn (editors). *NASM Essentials of Personal Fitness Training.* 3rd ed. Baltimore, MD: Lippincott, Williams & Wilkins.

National Strength and Conditioning Association, T. R. Baechle and R. W. Earle (editors). *Essentials of Strength Training and Conditioning.* 2nd ed. Champaign, IL: Human Kinetics, 2005.

___. *NCSA's Essentials of Personal Training.* 3rd ed. Champaign, IL: Human Kinetics, 2008.

Page, P., and T. Ellenbecker. *Strength Band Training.* 2nd ed. Champaign, IL: Human Kinetics, 2010.

Ricci, B., M. Marchetti, and F. Figura. "Biomechanics of Sit-up Exercises." *Medicine and Science in Sports and Exercise* 13 (No. 1, 1981): 54–9.

Rose, S. *exercise Ball.* Bath, UK: Parragon, 2005.

Santana, J. C. The Essence of Stability Ball Training Vol 1 & Vol 2 (1998) DVD.

Seibert, R. J. *Group Strength Training.* 2nd ed. San Diego: CA: American Council on Exercise, 2004.

Silvestri, L., and J. Oescher. "Use of Aerobic Dance and Light Weights in Improving Measures of Strength, Endurance, and Flexibility." *Perceptual and Motor Skills* 70 (April 1990): 595–600.

Thompson, C. W., and R. T. Floyd. *Manual of Structural Kinesiology.* 18th ed. St. Louis, MO: Mosby, 2011.

VanGalen, P. A. *Exercising with Dyna-band, Total Body Toner.* Hudson, OH: Thomas B. Gilliam Ent., 1987.

Veit, K. "Bodysculpt." *Women's Sports and Fitness* 14 (January – February 1992): 52.

Vincent, W. J., and S. D. Britten. "Evaluation of the Curl-up—A Substitute for the Bent Knee Sit-up." *Journal of Physical Education, Recreation, and Dance* 51 (1980): 74–5.

Webb, Tamilee. *Tamilee Webb's Original Rubber Band Workout.* New York: Workman Publishing, 1986.

Wellness Letter, University of California at Berkeley. *The New Wellness Encyclopedia.* Boston: Houghton Mifflin, 1995.

11

Resistance Exercises: Weight, Bands, and Balls

"The undertaking of a new action brings new strength."

EVENIUS

- Which exercises work which muscles?
- Is there more than one way to exercise the same muscle or muscle group?
- What is the proper technique for each of the exercises?
- How can I maximize muscular fitness and minimize injury and soreness?
- Does it matter the order in which I perform the exercises?
- How many repetitions and sets do I need to do?

READY to build, shape, and tone your muscles? This chapter is filled with resistance exercises you can use to develop muscular fitness. You can perform many of these exercises with body weight alone, or you can add more resistance using weights, stability balls, and exercise bands. The technique for each exercise is detailed and illustrated so that you can perform the exercise correctly. However, if you perform these exercises without a careful plan, you may experience less than optimal results and unnecessary muscle soreness or injury. Therefore, it is important to team these exercises with the technique tips section of this chapter on page 140 and the information presented in Chapter 10. Muscle balance, for example, is important for appearance and to prevent injury. Someone not aware of this concept might select an array of exercises in this chapter that do not represent a well-balanced workout. Your instructor and/or courses specifically for muscular fitness are also excellent resources for putting together a muscular workout beyond the scope of the class in which you are presently enrolled.

The exercises in this chapter are organized by body part, starting with the upper body, then trunk and core exercises, then lower body. Each of these sections presents the multi-joint exercises first, followed by single-joint exercises. There are two reasons for performing

combination (multi-joint) exercises before single-joint exercises. The first involves making the best use possible of your available exercise time—if you have limited time, you can get the most out of your workout by doing combination exercises that hit all the major joints and muscles with the fewest number of exercises. The second has to do with preserving the strength of specific, often smaller, muscles so that they don't limit combination exercises. For example, if you perform triceps kickbacks that isolate the triceps muscle, and then try to bench press or do push-ups, the fatigued triceps will give out before the larger pectoral (chest) muscles have been fully worked. You will have pre-exhausted the smaller muscle in the single-joint exercise and limited your ability to work the chest and shoulders adequately. Here are two more examples: (1) perform squats before doing leg extensions or leg curls and (2) do shoulder presses before lateral arm raises.

Following multi-joint exercises, you can choose to add single-joint exercises to further strengthen individual muscles. (Purposefully pre-exhausting specific muscles is a technique used in advanced training but is beyond the scope of this text.) So begin your workout with combination and large muscle exercises and then, time permitting, follow those with single-joint and small muscle exercises. Another important pairing consideration involves back exercises and abdominal

muscle balance

exercises. Although both sets of exercises are multi-joint, you should do the back exercises first so that the abdominals are not too fatigued to help support the back during the back exercises.

Within body part sections (i.e., the upper body, core, and lower body), some exercises are grouped to show you how to work the same muscle(s) using different forms of resistance including body weight, dumbbells, barbells, exercise bands, and stability balls. Variety is good for muscle development, so when you are comfortable with one method, you may want to try another form of resistance. Switching up your exercise routine also keeps workouts mentally fresh.

The exercises in this chapter are not all inclusive; there are many variations and methods of training. The selected exercises provide a balanced muscle workout and are those commonly performed in group exercise classes. Many of the exercises require that you work first one side of the body and then the other. To save space, the exercise descriptions give the action for only one side (the side shown in the photograph, if provided), but be sure to work both sides equally. Because you need to include exercises that work opposing muscle groups, this chapter provides flexion exercises and extension exercises, abduction (away from the center of the body) and adduction (toward the center of the body) exercises, and pushing and pulling exercises. The names of the muscles being exercised and the function of the muscles are labeled for each type of exercise. When variations work slightly different muscles, this is indicated as well. To help you focus on where major muscles are located, there are icons accompanying many of the exercises that show the basic position of the muscles being worked by each exercise. In addition, you can refer to the more detailed diagram of the muscles in Appendix 1.

Finally, as you perform these exercises, do not confuse muscle toning with spot reduction. The idea that a toning exercise will remove fat from a specific body part is false. Toning and strengthening exercises work the muscle so that when good body composition is achieved (fat burned through aerobic exercise and energy balance achieved through good diet), toned muscles that were hiding under the fat will appear. And don't forget that developing muscular fitness has many benefits other than appearance!

Can't spot reduce

TECHNIQUE TIPS FOR RESISTANCE EXERCISES

Look over the following technique tips before you try any of the exercises in this chapter, because your technique is important in performing the exercises safely and effectively. These tips are even more important to remember when performing exercises with added resistance.

- Warm up thoroughly before beginning your workout.
- Perform multi-joint and large-muscle exercises before single-joint and small-muscle exercises (i.e., squats before hamstring curls; push-ups before triceps extensions).
- Isolate the muscle(s) you want to work. Some additional muscles will be used to stabilize your position; the rest should remain relaxed. It is very easy, but not advantageous, to recruit extra muscles to help do the work. For example, you can lift more weight in an arm-curl by leaning back, but the targeted biceps muscle doesn't receive any additional benefit, and your back may become sore.
- Maintain good body alignment throughout the exercise. When correct alignment and body position cannot be maintained, stop.
- Perform resistance exercises at a moderate pace. Fast movements mostly strengthen muscles in the positions in which a change of direction occurs. Momentum does most of the work between the turnaround points. Fast ballistic movements are required in certain power lifts, but they are not used for any of the basic resistance exercises presented in this text.
- Use fluid, controlled movements. Do not swing your limbs indiscriminately, especially if you are using weights.
- Use a full range of motion. This promotes flexibility and improves strength and endurance through the complete range of motion. Only use a range of motion in which you can maintain good technique. For example, less flexible individuals will have to use smaller ranges of motion until flexibility is improved.
- Avoid locking your joints. When a joint is locked, the potential for injury is greater.
- Breathe! Breathe during resistance exercises. Breathe naturally during repetitions with lighter resistance. With heavier resistance, breathe out during the work phase and in during the recovery phase. For example, breathe in as you bend your knees in a squat, and breathe out as you straighten your legs. Breathe out in an arm-curl when you draw your arms up, and breathe in as you lower your arms. Never hold your breath, since this can create dangerous pressure in the chest, especially when heavier resistance is used.
- Rest muscle groups for 30 seconds to 3 minutes before exercising them again. Shorter rest

breaks promote muscle endurance. Longer rest intervals are needed for recovery between heavy resistance strength exercises. While the muscle(s) are resting, you can exercise the opposing muscle(s) or perform a series of exercises repeating the series, starting with the first exercise.

- Exercise opposing muscle(s) to prevent soreness and maintain a balance between agonists and antagonists. (Examples of opposing muscles include biceps/triceps, hamstrings/quadriceps, pectorals/latissimus dorsi, and abdominals/ erector spinae.)
- Stop if you feel pain at any time. Pain is your body's way of telling you that you have imposed too much of an overload. If pain persists, see a health care practitioner.
- Stretch the muscles following a resistance workout.

EXERCISES FOR THE UPPER BODY

The exercises in this section target your arms, shoulders, and upper back. Most women (and some men) lack upper body strength. If you are weak in this area, it is important to begin with light resistance and build up to more resistance. A stronger upper body can be empowering and protective. You are less apt to recruit low back muscles when your upper body and abdominals are strong. You will also experience less fatigue in a number of daily activities as well as in recreational and sport activities. You will be able to swing harder, push harder, and pull yourself up (i.e., out of a pool) more easily. Working the upper back also acts to balance the forward posture used in keyboarding.

Upper Body Multi-Joint Exercises
Shoulder Press

Muscles worked: deltoid, triceps brachii

Deltoids

Triceps brachii

POSITION—BANDS

Sit on the floor with your legs crossed (or with your legs extended and knees bent), or sit straddling a step bench. Place the center of the band under your buttocks or under the step. Grasp the ends of the bands with your palms facing forward, elbows bent, and hands up by your shoulders. Sit up tall so that your back maintains a neutral posture (natural curvature of the spine). The band should have a little tension on it; if not, adjust the length of the band.

ACTION Extend your arms up over your head (Figure 11.1). Make sure your wrists stay firm and in line with your forearms and your palms stay facing front. Do not lean forward or arch the back. Slowly return your arms to the shoulder position.

VARIATION You can also do this exercise with just the weight of the arms.

Scan to view video ▲

Figure 11.1

POSITION—WEIGHTS

DUMBBELLS Sit on the floor with your legs crossed (or sit on a step bench). Sit up tall so that your back is in good alignment. Hold the dumbbells with a closed pronated grip to the outside of the shoulders. (Palms will be facing forward, thumbs wrapped.) Keep your wrists in line with your forearms. (You can also do this exercise while standing.)

BARBELL Stand with your feet shoulder width apart, knees slightly flexed. Hold the bar with your hands slightly wider than shoulder width, with a closed pronated grip (palms down, thumbs wrapped). Balance the bar on your collar bones and across the front of your shoulders (deltoids). At this point your palms should be facing forward. Keep your wrists firm and inline with your forearms. (This exercise can also be done seated.)

ACTION Press the weight overhead (Figure 11.2), extending your arms fully but without locking your elbows. Keep your wrists firm with palms facing front. Do not lean forward or arch the back. Slowly lower the weight.

Scan to view video ▲

Figure 11.2

Push-up

Muscles worked: pectoralis major, deltoid, triceps brachii

Muscle action: elbow (arm) extension, shoulder horizontal flexion

---

Pectoralis major

Deltoids (anterior)

Triceps brachii

Scan to view video ▶

Scan to view video ▶

Figure 11.3a

POSITION

Assume the push-up position with your hands on the floor, a little more than shoulder width apart. Extend your legs to the back. Beginners can rest their weight on their knees (Figure 11.3a). If you are more advanced, rest your weight on your toes (Figure 11.3b). In either case, your body should be straight with just a slight lift of the gluteals (buttocks).

Figure 11.3b

ACTION Bend your elbows to approximately 90 degrees. Then straighten elbows and return to starting position.

VARIATIONS

1. Place your hands farther than shoulder width apart.
2. Place your hands very close together.
3. Place your hands (easier) or feet (harder) on a step (Figure 11.4).

POSITION—BALL

Lie prone on the ball with your hips on top of the ball (beginner) or the lower legs (more advanced) on the ball. Place your hands shoulder width apart on the floor in front of the ball.

ACTION Bend your arms until your elbows are at a 90-degree bend (Figure 11.5). Keep your body straight (neutral spine) or slightly piked at the hips throughout the exercise.

VARIATION For more difficulty, place the toes on top of the ball. For even more difficulty, raise one leg off the ball.

Figure 11.4

Figure 11.5

Chest Press

Muscles worked: pectorals, deltoids, triceps brachii

Muscle action: shoulder horizontal flexion, elbow extension

Pectoralis major

Deltoids (anterior)

Triceps brachii

POSITION—BAND

Stand with your knees slightly flexed. Hold one end of the band in each hand with the band running across your shoulder blades and under your arms.

ACTION Extend both arms forward (Figure 11.6a). Slowly flex (relax) your arms.

ACTION Perform the same exercise lying down on a bench with the band or cable running under the bench. Keep your knees bent and your back in a neutral position (Figure 11.6b).

Figure 11.6a

POSITION—WEIGHTS

DUMBBELLS Lie on your back on the floor (or on a bench) with your knees bent and feet flat on the floor (or bench). Hold the weights in your hands, palms facing your knees. Start with your arms fully extended with the dumbbells held directly above the shoulders (Figure 11.7a, back figure). Keep your elbows slightly flexed to prevent locking. Keep the dumbbells parallel to each other.

BARBELL Lie on your back on the step bench in a stable position, with your feet flat on the floor and knees bent. Grasp the bar with a closed pronated grip (palms down, thumb wrapped) slightly more than shoulder width apart. Hold the bar directly over your shoulders with slightly flexed arms (to prevent locking the joint). Wrists should be in line with your forearms (not laid back).

ACTION Lower your arms toward your chest (Figures 11.7a and 11.7b) until your elbows reach a 90-degree angle. The dumbbells will finish near your armpits and

Scan to view video ▶

Figure 11.6b

should be lowered in unison. The barbell will come close to your chest and should cross your body at the nipple line. Press the weight back up.

Scan to view video ▶

Figure 11.7a

Figure 11.7b

Flies

Muscles worked: pectoralis major, anterior deltoid

Muscle action: shoulder horizontal adduction (horizontal flexion)

POSITION—BAND

Stand with your knees slightly bent. Hold your arms out to the side, with your arms parallel to the floor and with the elbows slightly bent. Hold the ends of the band, letting the band run across the top of your back.

ACTION Bring your arms forward until your hands meet in front of your chest (Figure 11.8). Return arms out to the side.

Pectoralis major

Deltoids (anterior)

POSITION—DUMBBELLS

Lie on the floor (or on a bench) with your knees bent and feet flat on the floor. Hold the weights in your hands with palms facing each other and arms extended above your chest. Keep a slight bend in your elbows.

ACTION Slowly open your arms out to the sides, drawing an arc (Figure 11.9) and lowering your hands until they are even with your shoulders or chest. Keep your wrists in line with your forearms. Maintain a little flexion (bend) in the elbows. Weights should move in unison. Return them to the above-the-chest position.

Scan to view video ▶

Figure 11.8

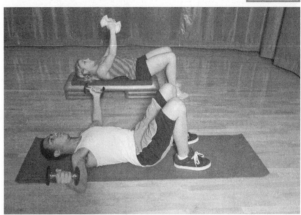

Figure 11.9

Row

POSITION—STANDING

Muscles worked: trapezius, posterior deltoid, rhomboids, latissimus dorsi, biceps group

Muscle action: scapular retraction, shoulder extension, elbow flexion

Trapezius

Deltoids

Rhomboids

Latissimus dorsi

Biceps brachii

Stand with your arms in front of your body parallel to the floor.

Figure 11.10a

ACTION Draw your elbows back, keeping your arms parallel to the floor (Figure 11.10a). Initiate the movement with the muscles in your back. Try to pinch your shoulder blades together (Figure 11.10b). Relax your shoulders and arms.

Figure 11.10b

POSITION—SEATED WITH BAND

There are two similar rowing exercises that can be done in a seated position; each targets the back but with a different emphasis on the muscles used. The seated low row (Figure 11.11a) uses more of the lattisimus dorsi and the teres major (located under the rhomboids), whereas the seated high row (Figure 11.11b) targets the middle trapezius muscle and rhomboids. Look carefully at the position of the elbows in these two pictures. The starting position for both is seated, with the legs extended forward and the knees slightly bent. The bend of the knees helps you sit up tall so that the spine can be in neutral alignment throughout the exercise. Shoulders are down and back. The band for low seated row runs across the bottom of the shoes and then straight up to the hands, which grasp the band with the palms facing each other (thumbs up). The band for high seated row passes across the bottom of the shoes and then crosses over the knees before being grasped with the palms facing down.

Figure 11.11a Seated low row

Figure 11.11b Seated high row

ACTION Seated low row: Initiate the movement by pulling the shoulder blades together. Then pull the elbows straight back (row) while keeping the arms close to the body. The hands will finish just below breastbone height (Figure 11.11a). Keep the hips and back still and shoulders down throughout the movement. Wrists should stay in line with the forearms. Slowly extend the arms to return to the starting position.

ACTION Seated high row: Initiate the movement by pulling the shoulder blades together. Then pull up and back with the elbows while lifting the arms away from the body and keeping them parallel to the floor. Finish with the upper arms extending to the sides at shoulder height, the elbows bent to 90 degrees and the forearms extending forward parallel to the floor (Figure 11.11b). Keep the wrists in line and the hips and back still throughout the movement. Slowly extend the arms to return to the starting position.

POSITION—UPRIGHT ROW WITH WEIGHTS

Muscles worked: middle deltoid, upper trapezius, biceps brachii

Muscle action: shoulder elevation

Scan to view video ▶

Trapezius
Deltoids

Biceps brachii

DUMBBELLS Stand with your feet shoulder width apart, knees slightly bent. Hold the weights with your arms extended down in front of your body, with your palms facing your legs.

BARBELL Stand with your feet shoulder width apart and your knees slightly flexed. Hold the bar in front of your body with a closed pronated grip (palms down, thumbs wrapped) and your hands slightly narrower than shoulder width. Rest the bar on your thighs. Your elbows should be extended.

ACTION Draw your hands up your torso (Figures 11.12a and 11.12b) toward your chin. Your elbows should point outward and slightly upward at the end of the movement. Slowly extend your arms to return to the starting position.

POSITION—BENT-OVER WITH WEIGHTS

Muscles worked: rhomboids, latissimus dorsi, middle trapezius, posterior deltoid, biceps brachii

Muscle action: scapular retraction (adduction)

Rhomboids
Latissimus
dorsi

Trapezius
Deltoids

Biceps brachii

Dumbbells—One Arm Stand in a forward lunge position, bend forward, and place your left hand on your left thigh for support. The fingers of your left hand should face inward. Extend your right arm down toward the ground and slightly forward (near the opposite knee). Hold the weight in your right hand with your palm facing in (Figure 11.13a). With a step bench, your front foot can be placed on the bench, or you can place one knee and your support hand on the bench.

BARBELL Stand with your feet shoulder width apart. Using a squatting motion, pick up the bar with a closed pronated grip (palms down, thumbs wrapped), with your hands more than shoulder width apart.

Scan to view
video ▲

Figure 11.12a

Figure 11.12b

Extend your arms and rest the bar on your thighs. Bend forward at your waist with a straight back until the bar is just above parallel, while simultaneously bending your knees and sitting back with your buttocks. Allow the bar to hang in front of your legs with straight arms. Focus a short distance in front of your

Scan to view
video ▲

Figure 11.13a

Figure 11.13b

feet. This position is more advanced; there is no support, and the bent position must be well controlled throughout.

ACTION Using only your shoulder and back muscles, pull your elbow(s) up and back (Figures 11.13a and

11.13b). Make sure your elbow(s) stay close to the side of your body. Maintain the forward body position until all the repetitions are completed. Bring the dumbbells/bar up to your chest, keeping your elbows pointed up. Slowly lower the weight.

Shoulder Shrug

Muscles worked: trapezius

Muscle action: shoulder elevation

POSITION—WEIGHTS

Stand with good posture.

ACTION Hold the dumbbells at your sides with palms facing inward. Shrug the shoulders up (Figure 11.14), hold for 3 to 5 seconds, and then relax down.

POSITION—BAND

Stand on the middle of the band with your feet shoulder width apart. Grasp far enough down the band with each hand so that tension is in the band when you stand up with good posture.

ACTION Shrug the shoulders up without bending the elbows. Hold for 2 seconds and then relax down.

Trapezius

Scan to view
video ▲

Scan to view
video ▲

Figure 11.14

Kneeling Back Extension (Back Hypers)

Muscles worked: erector spinae, latissimus dorsi

Muscle action: back extension

Erector spinae   Latissimus dorsi

Scan to view video ▶

Figure 11.15

POSITION—BALL

Kneel in front of the ball with your trunk on the ball. Rest your hands lightly on the small of your back (beginner), or place your hands up by your ears (advanced).

ACTION
Lift your torso off the ball until the back is straight (neutral spine). Do not hyperextend (Figure 11.15).

VARIATION
To add difficulty, move from your knees to your toes. This will allow your torso to be farther over the top of the ball. You can also place your arms above your head, with a right-angle bend in your elbows.

Lat Pull-Down

Muscles worked: latissimus dorsi, biceps brachii, deltoids

Muscle action: arm adduction

Latissimus dorsi   Biceps brachii   Deltoids

Scan to view video ▲

Figure 11.16 Increasing elbow bend will work the biceps.

POSITION—BAND

Stand with your knees slightly bent. Hold the band overhead in both hands, palms forward, with the anchor hand (left) directly above the shoulder and with the elbow slightly bent.

ACTION
Pull the band down and to the side by drawing the working elbow (right) down toward your waist (Figure 11.16).

Slowly relax the working arm and allow it to return to its original position. The band should be pulled down in front of your head.

UPPER BODY SINGLE-JOINT EXERCISES

Arm-Curl (Flexion)

Muscles worked: biceps brachii, brachialis, brachioradialis

Muscle action: elbow flexion

Biceps brachii

POSITION—BAND/CABLE

Stand with your foot on one end of the band. Grasp or wrap the band around your hand on the same side as the foot you are using to anchor the band (Figure 11.17). Start with your arm in an extended, relaxed position. Anchor your elbow at your waist. Cables or long bands allow you to work both arms simultaneously. Stand on the middle of the band or place it under a step bench.

ACTION Flex your arm(s), bringing your palm(s) toward your shoulder (Figure 11.17). Slowly lower your hand(s).

Figure 11.17

Figure 11.18a

Figure 11.18b

POSITION—WEIGHTS

DUMBBELLS Stand with your feet shoulder width apart and knees slightly flexed. Hold the weights firmly in your hands, with your arms down at your sides and palms facing forward or inward (Figure 11.18a). If the inward position is maintained, this is called a hammer curl.

BARBELL Stand with your feet shoulder width apart and knees slightly flexed. Grasp the bar with a closed supinated grip (palms up, thumbs wrapped) with your hands shoulder width apart. Extend your arms and let the bar rest on your thighs.

ACTION Keeping your wrists in line with your forearms, curl the weight up toward your torso until your hands are within 4 to 6 inches of your shoulders (Figures 11.18a and 11.18b). Do not allow any swaying or movement in your torso. Slowly lower the weight until your arms are straight but the elbow joint is not locked. A combination of hammer and regular curl can be performed by rotating the palms upward during the curl.

Arm Extension

Muscles worked: triceps brachii

Muscle action: elbow extension

Triceps brachii

POSITION—OVERHEAD PRESS: DUMBBELL

Stand with your knees slightly bent. Extend your arms straight up overhead. Your elbows right by your ears, flex your arms, allowing your clasped hands to fall behind your head (Figure 11.19).

ACTION Extend your arms until they are straight overhead. Relax and return to the flexed position. This exercise is sometimes called the French curl.

POSITION—DIPS

Assume the crab position, on all fours with your abdomen to the ceiling. You may place your hands on the floor or on a step (Figure 11.20). (If your arms are weak, place your hands and buttocks on the floor.)

ACTION Bend your arms to a 90-degree angle. Extend your arms and then return to starting position.

POSITION—BAND

Stand with your knees slightly bent. Grasp the middle of the band with one hand and hold it against your

Figure 11.20

Scan to view video ▶

Figure 11.21

chest next to the opposite shoulder. Grasp one or both of the ends of the band with your other hand. The lower hand should be directly below the upper hand.

ACTION Pull down with the bottom hand until your arm is extended (Figure 11.21). Keep your elbow by the body throughout the motion. (You may have to grasp higher on the band with the lower hand to get a full range of motion.) Slowly flex (relax) your arm.

POSITION—DUMBBELL KICKBACKS (STANDING)

Stand in a forward lunge position, with your elbow drawn up and back, and your left hand and arm in a support position on your thigh.

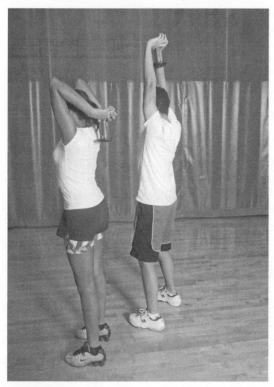

Figure 11.19

ACTION Holding your elbow in position, extend your right arm (Figure 11.22). Slowly bend your arm at the elbow and return to the starting position. This exercise may be combined with the bent-over row (page 147).

POSITION—BARBELL LYING ARM EXTENSION "SKULL CRUSHERS"

Lie on your back on the step bench in a stable position with your legs bent and feet flat on the floor. Hold the bar over your chest with a closed pronated grip (palms down, thumbs wrapped), hands shoulder width apart. Position the bar directly above your shoulders and extend your arms with a slight elbow bend to prevent locking the joint. Point your elbows toward your knees. Do not allow them to go out to the sides. (**Note:** This exercise can also be done holding the middle of a dumbbell with both hands turned so that it is on end.)

ACTION Slowly lower the bar (Figure 11.23) until it is just above your forehead. Maintain your upper arm position throughout—arms parallel, wrists in line with your forearms, and elbows pointing away from your face. Raise the bar back up.

Figure 11.22

Scan to view video ◄

Figure 11.23

Lateral Arm Raise

Muscles worked: deltoids

Muscle action: arm abduction

POSITION—BAND

This exercise can be performed with one arm at a time or both arms simultaneously. To perform it with one arm, stand on one end of the band and grasp the other end. Stand with your feet shoulder width apart and with good back alignment. Your knees should be slightly bent. Extend your arm down alongside your leg with your palm facing your leg. There should be a little tension on the band. Move your hand up or down the band to adjust the tension. To perform it with two hands, place the center of the band under your feet.

Deltoids

Grasp the ends of the band with your hands, and adjust the tension by sliding your hands up or down the band as needed.

POSITION—DUMBBELL

Stand with feet shoulder width apart, knees slightly bent, and spine in neutral alignment. Hold a dumbbell with each hand, with a closed grip (thumb wrapped) at the sides of the body with extended arms. Palms face into the respective legs. The elbows should be a little bent. Keep the shoulders down, chest up, and core engaged.

ACTION (BAND OR DUMBBELL) One or both arms can be moved at a time. Raise the arm(s) outward and upward (Figure 11.24a) until parallel with the ground (shoulder height). Maintain good shoulder rotation by keeping the little finger a little higher than the thumb as the arms come up.

Scan to view
video ▲

Figure 11.24a

VARIATIONS

Arms raises can also be performed to the front or diagonally across the body (Figure 11.24b). Start in the same position, and raise the arms in the direction you wish to strengthen.

Figure 11.24b

External Shoulder Rotation

Muscles worked: infraspinatus, teres minor

Muscle action: external shoulder rotation

Infraspinatus   Teres minor

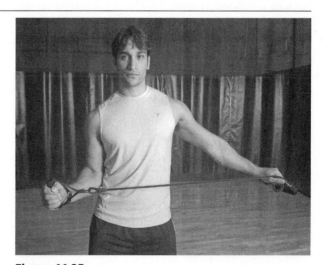

Figure 11.25a

POSITION—STANDING WITH BAND

Stand with feet shoulder width apart, knees slightly bent, and with a neutral spine. Wrap the band around the anchor hand and place it against your body at hip height. Grasp the other end of the band (cable handle)

Figure 11.25b

with the hand of the working arm, and anchor this arm with the elbow against the body. The hand will be in a fist, with the thumb facing the ceiling. The forearm is held parallel to the floor. When the forearm is extended in front of the body, have some tension on the band (Figure 11.25a). "A partner can also assist by holding the band for you and a towel can be placed under the arm for comfort (Figure 11.25b).

ACTION Swing the forearm outward, leading with the back of the hand (Figure 11.25a, 11.25b). Keep the

Figure 11.26

wrist in line and the arm parallel to the floor. The forearm acts like a door swinging on the hinge created by the upper arm against the body. Breathe out as you rotate the arm outward.

POSITION—LYING DOWN WITH DUMBBELL

Lie down on your side with the working arm on top. Anchor the upper arm against the body. Bend your elbow 90 degrees, and place your forearm across your abdomen. Hold a dumbbell in your hand with a closed grip (thumb wrapped) and with the palm facing your torso.

ACTION Rotate the forearm upward, raising the dumbbell on an arc (Figure 11.26). Be sure to keep the upper arm anchored and to maintain the 90-degree elbow bend. Breathe out as you raise the weight.

EXERCISES FOR THE CORE

The core is composed of the muscles between the hips and shoulders. Some people define the core as only the abdominal and deep spinal muscles, and others also include the buttocks, chest, and shoulder girdle. Strengthening the core, or center, of your body is crucial because it is used in either a stabilizing or an active role in most movements. The core plays a major part in postural alignment (stabilizing and supporting the spine) and in allowing you to optimize sport movements. Some core training exercises are dynamic, such as the curl-up (page 156), whereas others are static, such as the plank (page 161).

These exercises are organized by those that focus on the abdominals, the trunk, and then the hips. Although some core exercises tap a large number of muscles, only the major ones will be identified in the exercises that follow. When you perform core

exercises, body position is very important; improper technique can easily lead to an unhealthy load on your back. As you strengthen your core, enjoy the new sense of power and alignment you will feel during both daily and recreational activity. For more discussion about the core, please refer back to pages 60–62 in Chapter 6.

ABDOMINAL EXERCISES

A general understanding of the abdominal muscles and their function will help you select specific exercises for your program. The rectus abdominis is a long muscle that attaches to the pubic bone at one end and the ribs at the other. The full length of the muscle will contract during any abdominal exercise. The oblique muscles run from the ribs to the pelvic girdle on an angle. When they contract, they twist (or rotate) the trunk with respect to the pelvic girdle. The transversus abdominis is the deepest of the abdominal muscles. It lies underneath both the rectus abdominis and the obliques. It is often referred to as the transverse abdominal muscle because the fibers run across the body. (Other common names include transversalis and TvA.) Its primary function is postural; practicing good posture by keeping your abdomen lifted and pulled in is one way to keep this muscle toned. It is very important to make sure this muscle is engaged during core exercises because it helps to support the lower spine. If this and other abdominal muscles can't maintain good spinal positioning during exercise, then the exercise is too difficult.

For many years, people have done sit-ups to develop abdominal strength. Sit-ups used to be performed with a relatively straight back and with the hands behind the head. Today, curl-ups are the exercise of choice because they are much easier on the lower back, and they are as or more effective than sit-ups. In a curl-up, your head and shoulders follow a natural curl as you lift. (At one time, people were taught to lift the chin straight up; this is incorrect.) You roll up, initiating the role with your abdominal muscles and engaging the transverse and then the rectus abdominis, until your shoulder blades come off the floor. If you sit all the way up, your abdominals are resting for the last one-half to one-third of the exercise because the pull of gravity lessens in this range. Your hip flexor muscles also come into action in this range, taking work away from the abdominals.

Arm placement can make curl-ups progressively more difficult. With your arms at the sides of your body, your abdominal muscles are lifting only the weight of your trunk and head. When your arms are placed across the chest, the abdominals must lift the weight of your arms, trunk, and head. When you move your arms up

toward the head, they represent even more weight. Figure 11.27 demonstrates these three positions.

Placing your hands behind your head can be stressful to the neck; for this reason, many exercise leaders do not use this position. Too often individuals use their arms to pull their body forward, which presses the chin to the chest and stresses the neck. In properly executed curl-ups, the arms remain passive, and the abdominal muscles do all of the pulling.

The position with the arms near or behind the head is included for two reasons. First, some individuals can clearly maintain good technique and handle the weight of the arms in this position. Second, a few individuals experience neck fatigue prior to abdominal fatigue and like to rest their head in their arms to relieve the neck muscles. However, the majority of individuals will achieve the best results by placing their arms alongside their body or across their chest. Weights can also be held against the chest to make curl-ups more difficult.

To concentrate on the oblique muscles, you have to twist before lifting the torso. (A common error is to lift and then twist.) One way to ensure good twisting action when the hands are behind the head is to leave one elbow flat on the floor while the other lifts across the body.

Eighty percent of all people have back pain sometime during their lives—pain that is often caused by a lack of abdominal strength and leg flexibility. Some exercises that seem as though they should increase abdominal strength end up being the cause of lower back pain. See Figures 11.28, 11.29, and 11.30. Double leg lifts are one such culprit. A double leg lift requires the abdominal muscles to stabilize the spine while about one-half the body's weight is lifted through hip

Figure 11.27

AVOID

Figure 11.28 Straight-leg sit-ups place stress on the lower back and emphasize hip flexor strengthening, not abdominal strengthening. Placing your hands behind your head and pulling forward puts stress on the cervical vertebrae.

AVOID

Figure 11.29 The weight of both legs is often more than the abdominals can handle. The result is stress on the lower back area.

CAUTION

Figure 11.30 The V-seat position is another form of a double leg lift. This may also stress the lower back.

flexion. If the abdominal muscles are too weak, the pelvis is pulled forward by the hip flexors and strain is placed on the low back. The iliopsoas muscle, for example, attaches to the spine in the lower back area. When it contracts, it pulls against the lower spine. If the abdominals are able to stabilize the spine and pelvis, both legs can be lifted without incident. However, when the abdominals are unable to stabilize the body, the iliopsoas pulls the lower back up off the floor. The result is stress to the low back and hip flexors instead of giving the abdominals a workout.

Only individuals who can keep the back in a neutral position and maintain the natural curves of the spine should lift both legs. Many exercises fall into the "double leg lift" category: straddling the legs 6 inches off the floor, sitting and pushing both legs out, scissoring at a low angle, and others. Exercises that are better for the majority of the population are single leg lifts, bicycling the legs, or reverse curls. Strengthening the abdominals will help support the spine and decrease susceptibility to back pain.

Curl-Up

Muscle worked: rectus abdominis (obliques and transversus abdominis stabilize)

Muscle action: trunk flexion

POSITION

Assume the curl-up position—lie flat on the back with your knees bent, feet flat on the floor and shoulder width apart. Hands may be at your sides, across your chest, or by your head.

Rectus abdominis

ACTION Lift your upper body up off the floor while pressing your lower back into the floor. Be sure to lift up and "curl" naturally with your body and neck (see Figure 11.27). Roll back down to the floor. Beginners can relax between curl-ups; more advanced participants should curl down until their shoulder blades touch and then curl up again.

VARIATION

1. Lift your feet off the floor, ankles crossed or uncrossed and knees bent. Curl up (Figure 11.31). Roll back down to floor.

2. Bend your left leg and place your left foot on the floor. Place your right ankle on your left knee. Perform curl-ups (Figure 11.32). Curl down to floor.

3. Reach for your toes with your legs extended up in the air (Figure 11.33). Reach with one hand and place the other hand behind your head if you experience neck fatigue. You can also bend your legs during the relaxation phase and extend them during the reaching phase. Curl down to floor.

4. If the abdominals are weak and you need assistance curling up, you can place your hands

Figure 11.31

Figure 11.32

Figure 11.33

Figure 11.34

Figure 11.35

behind your thighs and gently assist with your arms. If you can't reach with your arms, use a towel or band looped behind the thighs. Lower down slowly as this will also build abdominal strength.

POSITION—WEIGHTS

Lie on your back with your knees bent and feet flat on the floor. Hold the weights in your hands and cross your arms flat over your chest.

ACTION Curl up until your shoulder blades come off the floor (Figure 11.34). Slowly lower down.

POSITION—BALL

After taking a seat on top of the ball, roll down the ball until the small of your back is against it. Lean back until your back is in a relatively straight line. Place your hands across your chest (beginner) or up by your ears (more advanced). Sitting further back on the ball so that the trunk extends off more will make this exercise harder.

ACTION Curl up approximately 30 to 45 degrees (Figure 11.35).

VARIATION

1. Curls may also be performed lying on the floor with the feet up on the ball.

2. Twisting or oblique curls can be performed sitting on the ball and twisting the torso to one side before curling up. It is easier to perform these with the hips rolled down a little on the front of the ball so more of the back is supported in the starting position.

Reverse Curl-Up

Muscles worked: rectus abdominis (obliques and transversus abdominis stabilize)

Rectus abdominis

Muscle action: trunk flexion

POSITION 1

Lie flat on your back with your legs bent so that your knees are near your chest but your feet are extended upward.

ACTION Try to lift your hips toward the ceiling while moving your knees toward your chest (Figure 11.36). (Try not to roll or use momentum—make the lower portion of the abdominals work.) Relax hips to floor. This exercise is often called a reverse curl.

POSITION 2

Sit on the floor with your legs extended to the front. Lean back on your elbows. Roll your pelvis under so that your lower back is stabilized. (Some people are more comfortable lying flat and supporting the hips with the hands.)

ACTION Bicycle your legs (Figure 11.37). If fatigue causes you to arch your lower back, bicycle with just one leg. (This exercise works a static hold on the abdominals while using the leg and hip muscles to cycle.)

POSITION—BALL

Lie flat on your back with your knees bent and feet flat on the floor. Hold the stability ball firmly between your lower legs. Rest the arms on the floor alongside your body.

ACTION While holding the ball between your lower legs, curl the lower half of your body toward your chest, bringing the ball with you (Figure 11.38).

Figure 11.37

Scan to view video ◄

Figure 11.36 Reverse curl.

Figure 11.38

Twisting Curl-Up

Muscles worked: obliques, rectus abdominis (transversus abdominis stabilizes)

Muscle action: trunk flexion and rotation

Obliques   Rectus
             abdominis

Scan to view
video ▶

Figure 11.39a

POSITION

Assume curl-up position.

ACTION Twist your torso to one side before curling up (Figure 11.39a). If your hands are by your head in a more advanced position, leave one elbow on or near the floor while twisting and lifting with the opposite side of your body (Figure 11.39b). Curl-ups may be performed in a series to one side or alternating sides.

VARIATIONS

1. Alternately extend one leg out and hold it off the floor as you bend your other leg into your chest. As the legs change position, twist and curl, bringing your left elbow to your right leg or your right elbow to your left leg. (Figure 11.40 shows this with an advanced arm position.)

2. Lay your knees over to one side, placing your body in a twisted position. Curl up. (Figure 11.41 shows an advanced arm position.)

Figure 11.39b Advanced arm position.

Figure 11.40 Advanced arm position.

Figure 11.41 Advanced arm position.

Hip and Trunk Curl (Flexion)

Muscles worked: rectus abdominis

Muscle action: hip and trunk flexion

POSITION

Lie on your back, with your knees bent toward your chest. Tie the band around your legs just above your knees. Place your hands inside the band loop, with palms facing your feet.

Rectus abdominis

ACTION Curl your knees toward your chest while simultaneously holding the band in position or pushing it away. Your upper body can also be curled toward your knees (Figure 11.42). Slowly uncurl your legs and upper body.

VARIATION You can perform this exercise without the band; curl your shoulders and knees toward each other.

Figure 11.42

(**Note:** This exercise is a curl-up and reverse curl at the same time.)

Lateral Trunk Raise with Ball

Muscles worked: erector spinae, quadratus lumborem (abdominals stabilizing)

Muscle action: lateral lumbar flexion

Erector spinae   Quadratus lumborem

Scan to view video ▶

POSITION

Lie on your side on the ball. Extend your feet in a forward/backward stride position with the top leg forward. You can place your arms on the ball for balance

Figure 11.43 A partner is supplying stabilization at the feet. This would not be necessary on a nonslip floor and with practice.

purposes or bend your arms with your hands near your ears (advanced).

ACTION Bend at your waist, lifting the trunk up off the ball while maintaining a sideways orientation to the floor (Figure 11.43).

TRUNK EXERCISES

Prone Bridge (Plank)

Muscles worked: abdominals (rectus abdominis, obliques, transversus abdominis), pectorals, triceps, deltoid

Rectus abdominis

Latissimus dorsi

Transversus abdominis

Pectoralis major

Triceps brachii

Deltoids

POSITION

From a modified push-up position, drop down onto your forearms. Create a straight line from the knees to the top of your head, with just a slight break (lift) at your hips. Breathe normally. The variations provided make this exercise progressively more difficult.

ACTION Hold the position. Be sure to breathe normally throughout. If you start to shake, take a short break and then resume the position you started with, or if on toes, drop to the kneeling position. Start with short durations (10 to 20 seconds) and build up to longer durations (1 to 2 minutes).

VARIATIONS

1. Curl your toes under and lift your knees off the floor. Create a straight line from your heels to the top of your head, with a slight break (lift) at your hips (Figure 11.44, female).

2. Move up off your forearms to a standard push-up position. Keep the slight lift in your hips and flex your arms slightly to prevent locking the elbow joint.

3. From the standard push-up position described above, lift one leg straight out behind you. Lead with your heel. Do not allow your back to arch or your hip to rotate. After holding the position with one leg up, change legs (Figure 11.44, male).

Figure 11.44

Scan to view video ▶   Scan to view video ▶

Lateral Bridge (Side Plank)

Muscles worked: abdominals (rectus abdominus, obliques, transversus abdominus), latissimus dorsi, deltoid, triceps

Obliques

Rectus abdominis

Transversus abdominis

Latissimus dorsi

Deltoids

Triceps brachii

Scan to view video ▲

Scan to view video ▲

Scan to view video ▲

Figure 11.45

POSITION

Sit on the floor on your right hip with your knees bent. Place your right forearm on the floor directly under your right shoulder. Lift your hips off the floor. Create a straight line from your knees through your hips, back, shoulders, and head. Your left arm should lie alongside your torso. Make sure your hips are vertical, one on top of the other (Figure 11.45, female).

ACTION Hold the position described above. Be sure to breathe normally throughout. If you start to shake, take a short break and then resume the position you started with, or if on toes, drop to the kneeling position. Start with short durations (10 to 20 seconds) and build up to longer durations (1 to 2 minutes).

VARIATION To make this exercise more difficult, extend your legs so that your knees are no longer touching the ground. The top foot can be placed on the floor in front of the bottom foot for more stability. The straight line now runs from your feet to the top of your head (Figure 11.45, male).

Overhead Stabilization

Muscles worked: whole body with emphasis on core muscles

POSITION—BAND (WITH PARTNER)

Stand with your feet slightly wider than shoulder width apart and your knees slightly flexed (not locked), or take an athletic stance with one foot in front of the other. If using the latter position, switch the front foot periodically. Hold the band in the middle with both hands (or grasp the handle of a cable band). Extend your arms up overhead. Your partner will stand behind you and take hold of the ends of the band (or the other cable handle). Make sure you are maintaining excellent standing posture.

ACTION Your partner will pull down on the ends of the bands in various directions while you try to remain steadfast in your posture (Figure 11.46). Your

Figure 11.46

partner should begin gently and increase intensity (pull harder) only when you request it. Partners should use smooth (never jerky) pulling motions. Your partner can pull the band downward toward center and also downward and off to the sides. Partners must be attentive and trustworthy, or else injury can occur.

VARIATION Hold a stability ball overhead, and have your partner push on it from various sides.

HIP EXERCISES

Hip and Shoulder Extension (Prone Swim)

Muscles worked: deltoid, gluteus maximus, hamstrings (with assisted abdominal and erector spinae stabilization)

Muscle action: hip extension, shoulder flexion

Deltoids

Gluteus maximus
Hamstrings

Scan to view video ▶

Figure 11.47

ACTION Raise one arm and the opposite leg simultaneously. Keep both your arm and your leg straight. Hold for 5 to 10 seconds and then relax (Figure 11.47). If you experience any pain, discontinue this exercise.

VARIATION Kneel on all fours and raise a leg, an arm, or opposite arm and leg simultaneously. This is often called the quadruped.

POSITION

Lie prone with both arms extended overhead along the floor.

Elbow Roll Out with Ball

Muscles worked: rectus abdominis, erector spinae, latissimus dorsi

Muscle action: hip extension

Rectus abdominis

Erector spinae

Latissimus dorsi

POSITION—BALL

Kneel in front of the ball. Place your forearms on the near side of the ball with your elbows apart and hands near each other.

ACTION Roll the ball forward using your forearms until your lower body forms a straight line from your knees to your shoulders (Figure 11.48).

Figure 11.48

Scan to view video ▶

Prone Body Tuck with Ball

Muscles worked: quadriceps (rectus femoris), iliopsoas, tensor fasciae latae

Muscle action: hip flexion

Quadriceps

Iliopsoas

Tensor fasciae latae

Scan to view video ▲

Figure 11.49

POSITION—BALL

Lie prone (face down) on the ball. Position the ball under your hips (beginner) or thighs or lower legs (more advanced). Place your hands shoulder width apart on the floor in front of the ball. Your head and back should maintain a straight line (neutral spine) throughout.

ACTION Bend at your hips, and pull your thighs to your chest. To increase the difficulty, place your legs closer to each other on the ball (Figure 11.49).

VARIATION Perform a knee-tuck press by doing a push-up action when the hips are flexed. This approximates a military press or handstand push-up, which will engage the triceps, deltoids, and trapezious.

Pelvic Tilts with Ball

Muscles worked: quadratus lumborem, transversus abdominis, rectus abdominis

Muscle action: lumbar spine flexion and extension (hyperextension)

Quadratus lumborem

Transversus abdominis

Rectus abdominis

ACTION Tuck your pelvis under by contracting the abdominals and rolling the ball forward. Then roll the ball backward, tilting your pelvis forward and placing your back into slight hyperextension (Figure 11.50).

POSITION—BALL

Sit on the ball with your feet on the floor shoulder width apart. Place your hands on the ball near your hips or on your thighs. Sit up with your spine in a neutral position.

Figure 11.50

Lateral Hip Tilts with Ball

Muscles worked: quadratus lumborem, obliques

Muscle action: lateral hip and trunk flexion

Quadratus
lumborem

Obliques

Figure 11.51

POSITION—BALL

Sit on the ball with your feet on the floor shoulder width apart. Place your hands on the ball near your hips or on your thighs. Sit with your spine in a neutral position.

ACTION Using the muscles on the side of the trunk, roll the ball first to one side and then the other (Figure 11.51).

VARIATION Perform hip circles.

EXERCISES FOR THE LOWER BODY

Two basic positions used in leg exercises require special comment. When working on all fours, you can be on your hands and knees (Figure 11.52) or on your forearms and knees (Figure 11.53). In most cases, the latter position is recommended because it allows you to lift your leg higher without causing your back to arch. If you are more comfortable in the first position, lift your leg only until it is parallel with the floor. During exercises in these positions, it is important to use the trunk muscles to stabilize the body.

When you are performing exercises lying on your side, your arm and trunk can be flat along the floor

(Figure 11.54), or you can be resting on your forearm (Figure 11.55). Both positions are fine. If you use the latter position, resist the temptation to slouch into your shoulder. Stay pulled up and again concentrate on using the core muscles to maintain good positioning throughout the exercises. Lying flat has the advantage of eliminating undesirable spinal curvature during the exercise.

Figure 11.52

Figure 11.53

Figure 11.54

Figure 11.55

LOWER BODY MULTI-JOINT EXERCISES

Squat

Muscles worked: gluteals, hamstrings, quadriceps

Muscle action: hip and leg (knee) extension

Gluteus
maximus
Hamstrings

Quadriceps

Figure 11.56a

POSITION

Assume the squat position—feet slightly wider than shoulder width apart, heels down, knees bent, trunk on a forward angle. Some back arching is required to maintain balance, but avoid excessive curvature.

ACTION Bend your knees to about 90 degrees. Be sure to retain muscular control throughout the movement (Figure 11.56a). You should sit backward (as though you are sitting on a chair) and keep your head and eyes forward and slightly raised. Straighten legs and relax. Do not perform a full deep knee bend (Figure 11.56b), because this places stress on the knee ligaments.

POSITION—BAND

In a standing position, place the center of the band underneath your feet. Grasp the ends of the band with your hands. When you are standing straight with feet shoulder width apart and arms extended by your sides, the band should have some tension. Move your hands up or down the band (or wrap/unwrap the

Figure 11.56b Deep knee bends place stress on knee ligaments.

Figure 11.57

Scan to view
video ▶

Figure 11.58a

Scan to view
video ▶

Figure 11.58b

Scan to view
video ▶

band around your hand) to adjust the tension. Toes should be pointed slightly outward. Focus is forward and slightly upward. Chest up and out.

Action Bend your knees (Figure 11.57) to about 90 degrees while sitting backward as if sitting down in a chair. Be sure to retain muscular control throughout the movement. Keep your head and eyes forward and slightly raised. Straighten your legs slowly against the resistance of the band. Sit down only as far as you can while maintaining control and good back position-ing (natural curve), aiming to get your thighs paral-lel to the ground. The trunk leans forward and arches slightly as you squat. Flexibility may limit the range of motion.

POSITION—WEIGHTS

DUMBBELLS Stand with your feet slightly wider than shoulder width apart, heels down, toes forward or an-gled slightly outward, knees bent, trunk on a slightly forward angle. Hold the weights in your hands just above your shoulders (near your ears), palms forward, elbows out.

BARBELL Stand with your feet slightly wider than shoulder width apart, heels down, toes pointing for-ward or slightly angled outward, knees bent, trunk on a slightly forward angle. Hold the bar with your hands slightly wider than shoulder-width, with a closed pro-nated grip (palms down, thumbs wrapped). Balance the bar on your upper back, just above the scapula. Arms should be fully flexed (bent).

Action Bend your knees (Figures 11.58a and 11.58b) to about 90 degrees while sitting backward as if sitting down in a chair. Be sure to retain muscular control throughout the movement. Keep your head and eyes forward and slightly raised, chest up and out, shoul-der blades down and back. Keep good back alignment, natural curve; avoid excessive arching or rounding of the back. Straighten your legs slowly.

POSITION—BALL (WALL-SLIDE, DOUBLE-LEG)

Place the ball between a flat wall and your back at belt height. Place your feet shoulder width apart and about 12 to 14 inches from the wall (beginner) or place your feet under your hips (more advanced). Place your hands on your hips or extend them in front of your body parallel to the floor.

ACTION While maintaining pressure against the ball, bend your knees until they reach a 90-degree angle (Figure 11.59). Make sure your back stays upright (perpendicular), your hips stay under your shoulders, and your feet stay flat on the floor. Return to a standing position. As you improve, you can narrow your stance, which increases the balance requirement. Your knees should not extend over your toes.

Scan to view video ▶

Figure 11.59 This exercise should be performed against a flat wall. A pillar is used here to allow the reader to see both positions simultaneously.

Lunge

Muscles worked: lead leg—gluteus maximus, hamstrings, quadriceps

Muscle action: hip and knee extension

Gluteus maximus   Quadriceps   Hamstrings

POSITION—WEIGHTS

BODY WEIGHT Stand with your feet shoulder width apart, hips square to the front and hands on your hips.

DUMBBELLS Stand with your feet shoulder width apart and arms extended down by your sides (or up by your shoulders). Hold the weights in your hands with your palms facing in.

BARBELL Stand with your feet parallel and shoulder width apart, with your knees slightly bent. Hold the bar with a closed pronated grip (palms down, thumbs wrapped), hands slightly more than shoulder width apart. Place the bar on the base of your neck so that it is balanced by the upper back and shoulder muscles. Lift your elbows to help stabilize the bar. Lift your chest up and out. Look slightly upward. Pull your shoulder blades down and back.

ACTION Take a large step forward or backward with one foot, into a lunge position. Keep the knee of your front leg behind the instep of your front foot. Keep your hips square. Lower your hips (Figures 11.60a, 11.60b, and 11.60c) until the thigh of your front leg is

Figure 11.60a

Scan to view
video ▲

Scan to view
video ▲

Figure 11.60b

Figure 11.60c

Figure 11.61

parallel to the floor. The heel of your back foot should raise off the floor. Return to the starting position by pushing off the floor with your front leg. (Do not perform this exercise if it causes knee pain.) Flexibility may limit your ability to reach 90-degree flexion.

Note: Stepping backward prevents knee soreness for some individuals.

POSITION—BAND

Stand in a front lunge position with the center of the band under your front foot. Hold the ends of the bands in your hands with your arms extended down by your

sides. Move your hands down the bands or wrap the band around your hands until there is some tension on the band when your torso is upright. Keep your front knee over your ankle and your hips square. The heel of your back foot should be raised.

ACTION Lower your hips directly down (Figure 11.61) until the thigh of your front leg is parallel to the floor. Raise your hips against the resistance of the band. Repeat 8 to 12 times before switching legs. Make sure the front knee does not move forward; it should stay over the ankle.

Double-Leg Curls

Muscles worked: hamstrings, quadriceps (rectus femoris)

Muscle action: knee and hip flexion

Hamstrings   Quadriceps

POSITION—BALL

Lie on your back on the floor with your ankles and lower legs resting on the ball. Lift your buttocks up until your body forms a straight line between your shoulders and ankles. Arms remain on the floor.

ACTION Roll the ball toward you by pulling your heels toward you until your knees are flexed to a right angle (Figure 11.62). To increase the difficulty, place your feet closer together on the ball. If you keep your body straight, bending only your knees, this works primarily hamstrings. If you bend at the hips the quadriceps also become involved. The abdominals maintain an isometric contraction.

Figure 11.62

LOWER BODY SINGLE-JOINT EXERCISES

LEG CURL (FLEXION)

Muscles worked: hamstrings

Muscle action: knee flexion

POSITION

Lie prone on the floor. Fold your arms, turn your head to one side, and rest it down on your arms. Place your left ankle over your right ankle.

Hamstrings

ACTION
Flex your right leg (leg curl) while pushing downward with your left (Figure 11.63). Your left leg should provide enough resistance so that your right leg can only be brought up slowly. Stop when the right leg reaches a 90-degree angle. Be sure that the leg being curled stays in alignment. Do not allow the lower part of your leg to be pushed to the side.

Note: The leg creating the resistance also gets a workout. The quadriceps muscle is slowly lengthening against the push of the curling leg. This creates what is called an eccentric (lengthening) contraction.

Figure 11.63

POSITION—BAND

Lie prone. Tie the band around both ankles; leave about an inch between the ankles. Hands can be under your chin or under your hips.

ACTION
Bend one leg up toward the buttocks while holding the other leg down (Figure 11.64a). Slowly lower your leg.

VARIATION
For a more advanced exercise, stand and bend one leg up toward the buttocks (Figure 11.64b). Slowly lower your leg. The band can be wrapped around the foot to keep it from sliding.

Figure 11.64a

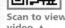

Scan to view
video ▲

Figure 11.64b

HIP EXTENSION

Muscles worked: gluteus maximus (with hamstring and abdominal stabilization)

Muscle action: hip extension

Note: Hip extension can be performed lying prone on the floor, kneeling, or standing. It can be done in isolation (just hip action) or combined with shoulder action. Two exercises which combine hip and shoulder movement were presented as core

Gluteus
maximus

exercises earlier in the chapter (see pages 154–165); Figure 11.47 shows you how to lie prone and lift one arm and one leg, and a variation explains how to perform a similar exercise in a kneeling position. The two exercises presented here isolate the hip extension action; using the band adds resistance.

POSITION

Assume an all-fours position. Lift the working leg up off the floor. Flex this leg 90 degrees. Keep your hips flat. Flex your foot (Figure 11.65a).

Figure 11.65a

Figure 11.66

Figure 11.65b

ACTION Keeping your hips flat, lift your leg upward. It probably won't lift very high if you are in a correct position (Figure 11.65b). Lower your leg.

POSITION—BAND

Tie the band around both ankles; leave about an inch between the ankles. Lie prone.

ACTION Keeping your legs straight, lift up one leg with the heel leading. Keep both hips in contact with the floor (Figure 11.66). Slowly lower your leg.

VARIATION A standing hip extension exercise (not shown here) is really an upright version of the prone exercise. Stand on one leg and extend the other straight back with or without a band. Lead with the heel, and maintain your back position.

POSITION—PELVIC TILT

Lie on the back with knees bent and feet on the floor about shoulder width apart.

ACTION Press your lower back into the floor by tilting your pelvis. Continue to roll your pelvis under while tightening your buttocks and lift your hips off the floor (Figure 11.67a) until your body creates a straight line. Lifting too high will arch your back. Roll down and release the pelvic tilt or lower your pelvis without touching your buttocks to the floor; repeat the lift. Rolling in and out of the position involves the abdominal muscles to a greater degree.

VARIATIONS

1. Vary the distance between the feet. (Some people feel knee discomfort when the feet are close together. If you feel knee discomfort, don't do this variation.)

2. Cross one leg over the other knee and lift as before (Figure 11.67b), or extend one leg upward and lift as before (Figure 11.67c). When one leg is off the floor, this becomes an advanced exercise, since it requires greater body stabilization.

3. Perform the exercise with the legs resting on a stability ball.

POSITION—WITH LEG FLEXION

Assume the all-fours position (on hands and knees). Lower your shoulders by taking the weight off your hands and putting it onto your forearms. Extend the working leg out to the back. Flex the foot with the heel facing directly up to the ceiling, toes touching the ground (Figure 11.68a).

Figure 11.67a

Figure 11.68a

Figure 11.67b Advanced.

Figure 11.68b

Figure 11.67c Advanced.

Figure 11.69

ACTION 1 Keeping a straight leg, lift the working leg until it is aligned with your back (Figure 11.68b). Lower and touch your toes to the ground. The gluteals and hamstrings are both active during this exercise.

ACTION 2 Lift the working leg until it is aligned with your back (Figure 11.68b). Maintain the knee position,

flex your leg, and bring your heel toward your buttocks (Figure 11.69). Then straighten your leg. In this exercise, the hamstrings are targeted while the gluteals act as stabilizers (along with the trunk and arm muscles).

Note: Muscle action 2 for this position includes both hip extension (Action 1) and leg flexion if the leg is brought down and up between curls of the leg.

LEG EXTENSION

Muscles worked: quadriceps

Muscle action: knee extension

Quadriceps

POSITION—BAND

Tie the band around both ankles; leave about an inch between the ankles. Sit with your knees bent and your feet flat on the floor. Lean back on your forearms. This exercise can also be performed sitting on a step or a stability ball.

ACTION Extend one leg forward (Figure 11.70). Slowly lower the leg.

Figure 11.70

POSITION—BALL

Sit on the ball with your feet on the floor shoulder width apart. Place your hands on the ball near your hips or on your thighs. Sit with your spine in a neutral position.

ACTION Extend one leg forward and parallel to the floor while maintaining good sitting alignment (Figure 11.71).

Figure 11.71

OUTER THIGH LEG LIFT

Muscles worked: gluteus medius, gluteus minimus, tensor fasciae latae

Muscle action: hip abduction

Gluteus medius and minimus

Tensor fasciae latae

POSITION—STRAIGHT LEG

Lie on your right side with your left hip directly above your right hip. Keep your upper body flat along the ground or support raised shoulders with your right

forearm flat on the floor. The bottom leg may be bent for balance.

ACTION Lift the top leg straight up, and then lower it down (Figure 11.72). Keep your knee facing directly toward the front. (If the knee rotates to the ceiling, the

Figure 11.72

muscles on the front of the leg, instead of the outer thigh muscles, do the work.)

VARIATIONS

1. Alternately point and flex your toe.

2. Raise the leg only halfway up, and then lower it down (smaller range of motion).

3. Raise the leg all the way up, and then lower it only halfway down. It is good to do this variation in combination with #2 so that the whole range is worked.

POSITION—BENT LEG (ACCORDIANS)

Lie on your right side with your upper body positioned as described in the straight leg lift. Bend both knees 90 degrees and flex slightly at your hips for comfort. Adjust the bottom leg for balance.

ACTION Raise the top leg, and then lower it. Keep your knee facing forward and the lower leg parallel to the ground (Figure 11.73). (If the knee points toward the ceiling, the muscles on the front of the thigh will work instead of the outer thigh muscles.) By bending your knees, you will lift less weight than when you keep your legs straight.

Note: This is a modified position, generally less difficult than the straight leg lift.

POSITION—ALL FOURS (HYDRANTS)

Support your body on all fours. Keep your weight centered. Your elbows should be straight but not locked.

Figure 11.73

Figure 11.74

Your head should be in line with your back. Turn your body sideways to the instructor so that your head can be turned (rather than lifted) to view the instructor. Place your hands shoulder width apart with fingers facing forward. Pull in your abdomen.

ACTION Keeping your weight centered and leg bent, lift your left leg to the side and then lower it (Figure 11.74). Lift until you feel resistance. Do not lift the working hip. If a yardstick was placed on your back, the yardstick should remain parallel to the floor throughout the exercise. Another test to see if your weight is centered is to raise your right arm when your left leg is working. (If your hip is allowed to rise, some of the back muscles are doing the work.) This exercise requires more core stabilization than the exercises performed lying down.

POSITION—SIDE STEP WITH BAND

Stand with your feet together and knees slightly flexed. Tie and place the band above your knees (beginner), or below your knees (intermediate), or around your ankles (advanced).

ACTION Step to one side, maintaining a slight knee bend. Slowly slide in the opposite foot, bringing your feet back together (Figure 11.75a). The outer thigh can also be worked using a side-lying leg lift (Figure 11.75b).

Figure 11.75a

Figure 11.75b

INNER THIGH LEG LIFT

Muscles worked: adductors (adductor magnus, adductor longus, adductor brevis, pectineus, gracilis)

Muscle action: hip adduction

Adductors

POSITION—STRAIGHT LEG

Lie on your right side. Bend your left leg, and allow the knee and lower leg to rest on the floor in front of your body (Figure 11.76). Keep your left hip directly above your right hip.

Figure 11.76

Figure 11.77

ACTION With your inner thigh facing the ceiling, raise and lower your right leg.

VARIATIONS

1. Lift your right leg up and slightly back.

2. Flex and point the toe of your right leg while holding the leg up off the ground. (This involves a static hold of the adductor muscles, while flexing the ankles uses the gastrocnemius and soleus muscles.)

3. Circle your right leg forward and then back.

4. Hold your right leg off the ground while bending and straightening your knee (Figure 11.77). (This involves a static hold of the adductor muscles, while flexing the knee uses the hamstring muscles.)

POSITION—STRADDLE

Lie on your back. Extend your legs straight up in the air. Straddle your legs, and place your hands or forearms on the inside of your thighs. (Lack of flexibility may make this uncomfortable for some, since it requires the hip flexors and abdominal muscles to hold the legs vertical.)

ACTION Bring your legs together while resisting with your hands (Figure 11.78), then relax. Start with easy resistance and build up. (Arm and shoulder muscles also work in this exercise.) This exercise can also be done with a partner providing resistance.

Figure 11.78

POSITION—SEATED (ADVANCED)

This is for people at an advanced fitness level only—it may cause lower back strain. Sit up tall with your legs extended forward along the floor. Place your hands on the floor behind your buttocks. Bend the nonworking leg so that your knee is close to your buttocks. Take the working leg to the side and rotate it at the hip so that your inner thigh is facing the ceiling.

ACTION   Raise your leg and then lower it (Figure 11.79).

VARIATION   Raise your leg and then lower it as you move it to the front and then back out to the side. (Hip rotator muscles are also worked in this exercise.)

POSITION—BAND

Tie the band around both ankles with about an inch between the ankles. Lie on one side with your top leg bent and the knee placed on the floor in front of the body.

Figure 11.79 Advanced.

ACTION   Lift your bottom leg up toward the ceiling (Figure 11.80). Slowly lower the leg to the floor. This exercise can also be performed in a standing position by pulling the working leg diagonally across the front of your body. You can make this exercise easier by placing the band closer to your knees. Wear socks to keep leg hair from being pulled.

Figure 11.80

LOWER LEG

ANKLE FLEXION

Muscle worked: tibialis anterior

Muscle action: ankle dorsi flexion

POSITION—BAND

Sit on the floor with your knees bent in front of your body and your hands supporting behind your buttocks. The band, tied snugly around both feet, should run across the top of the arch of your right foot and under the sole of your left foot.

Tibialis anterior

Figure 11.81

ACTION   Flex your right foot—that is, draw your toes toward your shin (Figure 11.81). Slowly point (relax) your foot.

ANKLE EXTENSION

Muscles worked: gastrocnemius, soleus

Muscle action: ankle extension, point toe

Gastrocnemius Soleus

POSITION—BAND

Sit on the floor with your legs extended out in front. Hold one end of the band in each hand with the band running across the ball of one or both of your feet. Your foot should be in a flexed position.

ACTION Extend your foot by pointing your toes (Figure 11.82). **Caution:** Do not let the band slide off the foot. Slowly flex (relax) your foot.

Figure 11.82

POSITION—WEIGHTS

Stand tall with good posture. Hold the weights in your hands down at your sides, palms facing inward.

ACTION Raise up onto the balls of your feet (Figure 11.83). Slowly lower back down until your heels touch. This exercise can be added to the end of a squat to save time.

VARIATION This exercise can also be performed with the balls of your feet on a bench so that your heels can drop below the level of the bench, thus effectively increasing the range of motion in which strength is developed.

Scan to view video ▲

Figure 11.83

SUMMARY

Working muscles correctly will increase your rate of improvement. Be sure to isolate the muscle or muscle group you are trying to train. If your muscles begin to cramp during an exercise, stop and stretch them out.

If the instructor and class are doing more of an exercise than you can do, perform one exercise for every two they do. To gain fitness, overload by working until you feel mild discomfort, but never perform an exercise that causes pain. Finally, don't be afraid to modify exercises to make them safer and more comfortable for you.

Don't overload more than 10%

KNOWLEDGE TIPS

1. Perform large-muscle, multi-joint exercises before smaller-muscle or single-joint exercises.

2. To progressively overload, increase resistance or perform more sets.

3. You can make an exercise more difficult (intense) by changing position or by adding resistance in the form of weights, bands, balls, or water.

4. Move at a moderate pace and maintain body control throughout resistance exercises.

5. Exercise both muscles of a muscle pair.

6. Use a curling motion during sit-up–type exercises.

7. Avoid exercises that strain the lower back.

8. Protect the lower back during exercises by contracting core muscles and maintaining a neutral spine.

9. If muscle cramping occurs, stop and stretch.

10. Breathe out during the work phase of an exercise and breathe in during the relaxation phase.

THINK ABOUT IT

1. Explain how increasing strength can help increase muscular endurance.

2. Resistance can be created using machines, body weight, free weights (dumbbells, barbells, medicine balls), stability balls, exercise bands, and water. Explain the key advantages to each type of resistance, or identify the resistance equipment you would use and why.

3. Identify pairs of exercises that work opposing muscles or muscle groups.

4. Put together a workout with 8 to 10 exercises using the major muscles of the body.

5. As you perform an exercise, try to identify three to five technique points you would use to teach the exercise to a friend. Include body position and proper use of equipment.

6. Stability balls create an unstable environment in which to exercise. Explain why an unstable environment can be an advantage.

7. Explain what proper breathing technique is when using resistance training.

Esmeralda

The Mind-Body Connection

"Where does the body end and the mind begin?
Where does the mind end and the spirit begin?
They cannot be divided as they are interrelated
and but different aspects of the same all-pervading
divine consciousness."

B. K. S. IYENGAR

* What does a mind-body connection mean?
* How do I develop a mind-body connection?
* How can I get myself to relax? Feel more connected? Less stressed?
* What is the difference between Pilates and yoga?

WHO among us has not said, "How I wish I could get some balance in my life! I want something more. I want to stop rushing and enjoy life more fully." Today many of us juggle a variety of demands, such as coursework, jobs, social events, and family responsibilities. All the while, the little voice in our head (the inner voice) is reminding us of our obligations and our to-do list and maybe chastising us for not being better at what we are doing. Sometimes the inner voice is helpful, talking through a problem, reminding us of important things, but sometimes it is just talking, talking, talking . . . and getting in the way. Seldom is the inner voice quieted and thought allowed to shift inward. Those who take the time to tune out the demands of the outer world and focus on the inner one often find an enhanced connection with their bodies and feel physically and mentally renewed. For this reason, over recent years there has been a growing interest in activities such as yoga, pilates, the martial arts, and meditation—activities that encourage a mind-body connection and promote healthy lifestyles.

Before discussing some of the specific methods of achieving a mind-body connection, let's look more closely at what it means to connect the mind and body. Stress, both good (eutress) and bad (distress) and the immune system are at the heart of this idea. That mental stress affects our bodies is pretty intuitive, but how

it does so and to what extent is not as obvious. Hans Selye, an astute observer of behavior, recognized in the 1940s that regardless of the type of stress, good or bad, the stress response was similar. For example, the physical stress response of nervousness, sweating, and a pounding heart can occur right before you ask someone out on a date or just before an exam. And a yes for the date provides an adrenaline rush, whereas a failing grade on an exam registers in the pit of our stomach. Interestingly, the stress response will occur whether the cause of the stress is real or perceived. In other words, if you think you are in danger, your body will react the same way as when you are in danger. Furthermore, people's perceptions of the same situation can be quite different. For example, for some people speaking in front of a crowd is frightening, and thus elicits a stress response, whereas others find it enjoyable.

Whatever the cause of stress, once the alarm has been raised you will experience physical reactions that are often described as the "fight-or-flight" response. One of the problems with modern living is that too often we confront stressful situations but do not have the opportunity to vent them physically. The hunter/gatherer who was surprised by a wild animal would run. Today, when presented with an unrealistic deadline, the college student whose blood pressure spikes doesn't usually run—although this might be a very healthy idea—at least initially! As we have become

179

more sedentary, we have lost our physical outlets for stress, and chronic stress with no relief is harmful to our health. Providing a physical outlet can be very positive both physically and mentally. This is when the body can help the mind, and by calming the mind, we help the body.

A Harvard study in the 1970s found physical evidence of the effects of our mental outlook on our immune system. Immune cells were discovered to have receptors for chemicals called neuropeptides. These chemicals are produced by the brain and vary with emotions. In other words, how you are feeling sends out chemicals to your immune system. Negative factors, such as academic difficulties, pessimism, loneliness, and chronic stress, lower the immune system and make us more susceptible to disease, whereas positive factors such as aerobic exercise, social support, laughter, and satisfying relationships, boost the immune system. The study of how our psyche (brain) influences our immune system is called **psychoneuroimmunology.** Negative thoughts, worry, anxiety, nervousness, and panic all work to bring our physical body down. Positive thinking, viewing life as a fun challenge, feeling in control, and good self-esteem can help us stay healthy.

Remember, some stress is good—it pushes us to new heights, allows us to take on challenges, and keeps us engaged in life. The trick is not to eliminate it, but rather to manage it. Blow steam in healthy ways, keep things in perspective, manage time well, and put a good spin on life. This leads to a healthier immune system and better quality of life. Here are a few ways to manage stress. All of the ideas presented here can be found in much more depth in stress management texts, courses, and resources. For more information, contact the psychology department or health center of your institution.

- Engage in physical activity. It can help clear your mind and give you a chance to regroup when you are feeling overwhelmed. Breakthrough thinking often happens during a walk, jog, golf game, dance, or exercise class. It is almost as though taking your mind off a problem allows your mind to solve it. In a grander sense, meditation or yoga can help you reconnect with what is centrally important so that you refocus your energies to what really matters to you.
- Develop supportive relationships. Share your feelings and accept support from those who truly understand your situation.
- Say no to activities and jobs that will put you over your limits. If you feel the need to help, rather than take on the job yourself, help find someone who can.

- Break the "big job" down into smaller, more manageable pieces and then schedule when you will get these done.
- Expect things to change, and allow yourself to adapt. Life seldom stays the same, and people who continue to hang onto what "was" have difficulty enjoying or coping with what "is."
- Take the time to get organized, physically and mentally. Set your priorities and then manage your time so that these things get done first.
- Spend time with positive people. Their attitude wears off on others! There is good evidence that laughter *is* one of the best medicines.
- Eat good foods and get enough rest. Life is much easier to cope with when we take care of our basic needs. You can get a lot more done when you've eaten energizing foods rather than junk foods that make you feel sluggish.
- Do something for someone else. Giving a gift or doing a kind act always makes you feel better.
- Take control of the stressors you can. Identify them and then work to eliminate them. One person who had difficulty getting the equipment she needed asked to be in charge of equipment. Another who hated traffic rearranged his morning routine so he could leave earlier and avoid it.
- Accept your limitations. You can't do it all, and the "I shoulds" will kill you. Maybe this isn't the semester you are going to organize your closets or fix up the car.
- Change your attitude toward stressors you can't change. We can't control everything, but we can control how we react to things. Try reframing. Here is an example. A term paper is due the next day and you cannot possibly finish in time. You can't change the due date. Rather than continue to worry and be unproductive, you can reframe the situation, accept that you will lose a letter grade for being late, take the extra day, and do it well so that even with the penalty you have a good grade.
- Put a positive spin on things. If you're stuck in traffic with children in the car, you have a choice: fret and swear, or spend some quality time with the kids.
- Learn to relax. Try some of the techniques presented in this chapter and create your own way of finding time for yourself.

You can help yourself achieve a more balanced life can be greatly assisted by participating in activities that forge a mind-body connection. The remainder of this chapter is dedicated to activities and techniques that do just that. Included are Pilates, yoga, progressive relaxation, mental imagery, and autogenic training.

PILATES NOT CARDIO IT'S STRE.

Pilates is a method of mental and physical conditioning that aims to develop strength balanced with flexibility. To fully appreciate the method and the choices available, here is a little background.

Pilates is the life work of German-born Joseph Pilates. After suffering from rickets, asthma, and rheumatic fever as a boy, Joseph focused his life on finding and honing a method of exercise that promotes strength and good health. He became strong through his dedicated study of exercise, and by age 14 he was modeling for anatomical drawings. By age 32 he had moved to England where he performed in the circus and became a self-defense trainer for English detectives. At the outbreak of World War I, Joseph was interned in England with other German nationals. During this time, he worked in an infirmary and developed a method of exercise he called "contrology," which he taught to others interned with him. He gained recognition when none of his "students" died during the influenza epidemic of 1918. In 1926, Joseph immigrated to the United States. With his wife Clara, he opened a small studio in New York City called Pilates Studio, Inc., to teach his method of exercise. Pilates caught the attention of the dance community, including influential choreographers George Balanchine and Martha Graham, who referred a number of dancers to them. Joseph lived a long, healthy life. When he died in 1967 at the age of 87, his wife continued to operate the studio with the help of one of Balanchine's former dancers, Romana Kryzanowska, who had studied with Joseph many years prior. Romana continues to teach and train instructors today in the original Pilates method, while many other students of Pilates Studio have set up their own classes. Some of them have also trained instructors who, in turn, have gone on to teach contemporized versions of the Pilates method. Although this is discouraged by those who prefer to teach the original method, others recognize the value of embracing more recent research. For example, Moira Stott-Merrithew, the founder of Stotts Pilates, teaches use of a neutral spine position rather than a flat back, because the neutral spine allows for the normal curvatures of the spine and is the position of greatest mechanical advantage.

Instructors who teach contemporized versions of Joseph Pilates' method had to refer to their classes as "like Pilates" or something similar, until the year 2000, when a court decision declared "pilates" a generic term (like yoga and karate) and rescinded the trademarks previously held by Pilates Studio, Inc. This means that now all who teach this type of exercise can use the name and advertise their classes as pilates classes, even if they do not teach the original method.

Joseph Pilates developed more than 500 exercises, most of which are performed lying down. Some are performed using special equipment he designed, and some are done on a mat (hence the pilates term "mat class" for a common type of instruction using no equipment). The equipment, which uses cables and springs to create resistance, adjusts for body size and needs. The most popular pieces of equipment include the reformer, Cadillac or trapeze table, chair, and different sized barrels. Multiple exercises can be performed on each piece of equipment. To see examples of pilates equipment, go online to www.pilates.com.

The Pilates method of body conditioning has six original principles.[1]

1. **Concentration:** One must pay attention to how the body moves and how each part of the body is interconnected with the rest of the body. The mind must be engaged during every move—the mind and body work as a team.
2. **Control:** All physical movement must be controlled by the mind.
3. **Centering:** One's center is the "powerhouse," which consists of the muscles of the abdomen, lower back, and buttocks. These muscles support the spine and internal organs and are important in maintaining good posture. All movement begins at the center and flows out from there.
4. **Flowing movement:** All movements are to be done smoothly and evenly, not in a rushed or jerky manner.
5. **Precision:** Control must be used to ensure that all movements are performed correctly each time.
6. **Breathing:** The bloodstream is purified (oxygenated and eliminated of noxious gases) with proper breathing technique. Breathe in to prepare for a movement, and breathe out as you execute it.

The "core," or basic, exercises of the Pilates method work the core muscles described in Chapter 2. The result is a flatter abdomen, strong lean muscles, and better control and coordination of movements involving the limbs. Pilates also:

- improves core strength and stability (balance)
- balances strength and flexibility (longer, leaner muscles)
- is a nonimpact exercise that is easy on the joints
- improves coordination
- improves circulation
- improves posture
- heightens body awareness (mind-body connection)

---

[1] S. P. Gallagher and R. Kryzanoska. *The Pilates Method of Body Conditioning.* Philadelphia: Bainbridgebooks, 1999.

Figure 12.1 The pilates roll-up exercise.

- helps prevent injuries and relieve low-back pain
- improves sports performance
- enhances functional fitness (ability to do daily activities)

Basic exercises include the roll-up, the hundred, the single and double leg stretches, and single leg circles. It is extremely important that these exercises be performed with proper technique and control of the spine. This is achieved by recruiting the deep postural muscles in addition to the more surface abdominal muscles. The roll-up (Figure 12.1) is similar to a straight leg sit-up, which due to the potential for low-back strain is contraindicated for many individuals. However, under proper supervision and with controlled precise rolling of the spine, this can be a safe and effective exercise. The hundred is another

example of an exercise in which the back position must be monitored carefully and a progression of positions employed based on the individual's core strength. It is critical that the back remain pressed into the floor (mat) throughout the exercise. (Some instructors refer to this as imprinting the back on the floor.) The easiest body position is lying on the back with the knees bent and feet on the floor. The next position in the progression is with the feet up (Figure 12.2a); shins can be parallel to the floor or higher depending on comfort and strength. The most difficult leg position (Figure 12.2b) is with the legs extended and lowered as far as the individual can go without shaking. This advanced position is, in essence, a double leg lift, which is normally considered an exercise to avoid. It comes off the avoid list when the individual has enough strength to maintain good spinal positioning. The arms extend toward the feet and are held just a few inches off the floor. The upper spine is curled upward lifting the shoulder blades off the floor. To begin the exercise, extend the legs to the desired position while simultaneously curling the upper body. While holding this position, the arms are pumped up and down (a few inches) in coordination with short breaths. The breathing is done in cycles. Each cycle is five short in-breaths and then five short out-breaths. The name of the exercise, the hundred, represents the goal of performing 100 arm pumps with coordinated breathing (10 cycles). The shoulders and neck should remain relaxed throughout. A modification, which leaves the head and shoulders on the floor, can be used as needed. All of the pilates exercises are to be initiated by the center of the body (the powerhouse). To be successful, participants must focus on the deep stabilizing muscles, clearing their minds of everything else.

Figure 12.2a Beginner's position for the pilates hundred. This can also be performed with the feet on the floor.

Figure 12.2b Advanced position for the hundred. When the legs are extended, it is critical that the low back remain in contact with the floor or mat.

Figure 12.3 An instructor's touch can help a pilates student focus on the right muscles and technique.

There are many excellent pilates classes being taught in both traditional and contemporary forms. Unfortunately, there are also classes being taught by instructors who have minimal training in pilates. Certification programs range from 600 hours of internship to weekend workshops. It is important to select an instructor with both training and experience. Mat classes are the most popular form of pilates because they can be taught in many locations and involve only mats for equipment. They are also more conducive for group instruction. Smaller groups are best because the instructor can better watch and assist participants. An instructor's touch can help a participant mentally and physically locate and focus on muscles and proper technique (Figure 12.3).

Joseph Pilates felt strongly that thought and movement have to emanate from the inside out. He believed that the stabilizing benefits of beginning all movement from the center, accompanied by focused mental practice, will carry over into daily life. He felt that the discipline of focus and the greater body awareness forge a mind-body connection that changes not only how a person moves but also how he or she approaches life. And he is not alone. Pilates exercise is now enjoyed by dancers, theatre groups, professional athletes, rehabilitation clients, and fitness enthusiasts around the world.

YOGA

At the end of the day, you sit down, tired, and a friend reaches over and massages your shoulders. You remark how good it feels and admit that you didn't even realize how tight you were. This is a small example of how becoming aware of your body and providing it

with what it needs can affect your outlook. Going a step further is to become aware of what caused you to be tight in the first place. Was it some physical work? A keyboard at the wrong height? Mental stress manifested through a tightening of the neck and shoulders? Becoming aware by tuning into your body allows you to make changes that keep the tightness from occurring, and you feel better. Once you feel calmer on the inside, it is easier to turn outward and show qualities such as generosity and compassion to others, which ultimately helps you develop a more peaceful existence.

To the observer, yoga is a series of poses that develop strength, flexibility, and balance. But to stop there is like describing "home" as a house made of wood, bricks, and glass without including the family relationships and emotional ties that make up the place we call "home." So too, yoga goes beyond the bricks and mortar of exercises and the development of the physical body to a state of awareness that unites the mind, body, and spirit in a way that fundamentally changes and guides how you live.

Yoga brings you to a state of mindfulness that asks you to be in the present, acutely aware of your physical self, and to use breathing and postures to renew and strengthen and bring balance and harmony into your life. Researchers have studied yoga and can give us "proof" of some of its benefits but the real proof is very individual and can be known only through the regular experience of yoga. The following discussion of yoga will provide you with some of its history, philosophy, postures, and vocabulary, but it is not meant as a tutorial on yoga. Rather, this information may encourage you to join a class and experience it first-hand.

BACKGROUND

Yoga is an ancient Eastern Indian philosophical tradition dating back 5,000 years that is practiced all over the world today. It has been growing in popularity in Western countries for a variety of reasons. Some people see it as a way to increase strength, stamina, and flexibility; some use it to reduce stress; others more fully embrace its philosophy and begin the "path to enlightenment."

Yoga embraces the ideas of living in harmony and achieving an inner peace, and its ultimate goal is a journey to *samadhi*, or self-realization. Yoga is accepted by, and influenced by, the Hindu religion. Yet, most people outside the Hindu faith find they can embrace the yoga philosophy along with their own religious beliefs. In yoga, there is no distinction between where the mind leaves off and the body begins. The practice of yoga is directed toward realizing this connection between the mind and the body.

Yoga is often described as a tree with deep tangled roots, a big stem, large branches, and many secondary branches. There are six major branches in yoga: hatha yoga, raja yoga, karma yoga, bhakti yoga, jnana yoga, and tantra yoga. (Some sources list just four pathways, with hatha subsumed under raja.) **Hatha yoga is the physical aspect of yoga and is what most Americans refer to when they speak simply of yoga.**

Hatha yoga is practiced through the use of various poses called *asanas*, through breathing techniques called *pranayama*, and through meditation. The goal of hatha yoga is to transcend the mind-body connection and fuse the mind, body, and soul into one.

GETTING STARTED

It is very easy to begin a class. You will want to wear clothing that is comfortable to move in and stays put when you move, that is form-fitting but not too tight. Form-fitting clothing will also allow the instructor to see whether your body is in alignment. The material should breathe well. You will also want to bring a water bottle and possibly a towel. A yoga mat is often supplied but check ahead of time to determine whether you need to bring your own mat.

You will be asked to remove your shoes and leave them either outside the room or just when you enter. Most people participate barefoot but if you prefer socks you may want to buy some yoga socks with nonslip bottoms. If the class uses equipment such as blocks, straps, or blankets, they are usually supplied, but if they are not you will need to bring your own.

It is a good idea to arrive well hydrated and to avoid eating a heavy meal for several hours prior to the class. A lighter meal is usually fine. If your blood sugar is too low you may feel light-headed during class—see how you feel, and adjust your eating pattern accordingly.

When beginning yoga, remember to be patient with yourself. Recognize that your body has limits and that it takes time to develop muscular strength, endurance, balance, and flexibility. Don't push too hard in the beginning. Also remember that the physical training is only part of the equation and that the mind and spirit connection with the body also takes time to develop. After a yoga class it is normal to feel all of the following: tired, stiff and sore, energized, and as though your joints and heart are more "open." Over time the tired feeling will be replaced with feelings of renewal and energy. And as your body becomes used to the postures and your alignment and modifications to suit your body are refined, the soreness will disappear. You will not be able to fully appreciate yoga's impact on how you think and move and feel unless you perform it regularly for a number of weeks.

ASANAS

The practice of the yoga postures and the postures themselves both bear the same name, *asana*. The asanas develop muscular strength, endurance, and flexibility, but also work at a deeper level to achieve health and spiritual contentment. Depending on the style of yoga being practiced, the number and manner in which asanas are performed varies. They may be held for extended periods of time to build strength and endurance; performed at a fast pace flowing from one to the next, resulting in strength and power; or in slower, more gentle manner to promote flexibility and relaxation.

Asanas are grouped according to the action or position in which they are performed: standing, seated, backward bending, forward bending, twisting, inverted, and lying down (prone and supine). Their names, translated from Sanskrit, bring to mind an image for the pose—everything from the Awkward Pose to animal names such as the Fish and Cobra Poses, to positional names such as the Revolving Lateral Angle Pose, to human names such as the Warrior Pose or Child Pose, and to places or things such as the Mountain or Tree Pose. Examples of several basic postures are described in this chapter so that you can appreciate the very specific awareness cues and imagery used to bring a participant into the right position.

Asanas are designed to allow for a progression of difficulty and to be modified to work with different body types and fitness levels. Basic poses like the Mountain Pose (Figure 12.4), standing correctly on

Figure 12.4 Mountain Pose

two feet, must be established first before a person can move on to more challenging poses such as the one leg stand called the Tree Pose (Figure 12.5). Notice that the person on the left performing the Tree Pose has placed her leg well above the knee (more advanced) whereas the person on the right has hers further down the leg (easier). They are also using one another to

establish balance and will eventually progress to standing by themselves. The series of Triangle Poses offers another good example of how an asana can be modified for different levels of ability. The beginner can use a block to bring the ground to the hand and can use a forward facing gaze (Figure 12.6a); at the next level, the hand slides down to the ankle (Figure 12.6b) or even more advanced, all the way to the floor and the gaze is turned upward looking at the extended arm. A third posture can be achieved by twisting the body to form the Reverse Triangle Pose (Figure 12.6c). When seated it is important to maintain good back posture. Sitting on a block can make it easier for less flexible individuals to achieve this while more advanced individuals can sit directly on the mat. The leg position can progress from a simple crossing of each other, Cobbler Pose, to the Lotus position (Figure 12.7). In Child Pose an individual can choose to extend the arms for an additional shoulder and back stretch or fold the arms back into the fetal position (Figure 12.8). What is of the highest importance in yoga is that individuals seek postures that are the right fit for their physical and mental state and to recognize that this can vary from day to day or even hour to hour.

Four asanas will now be described in detail. The Mountain Pose is an example of a standing pose that develops good posture. Downward Facing Dog is a forward bending pose and part of many basic sequences.

Figure 12.5 Tree Pose.

Figure 12.6a Triangle Pose with block

Figure 12.6b Triangle Pose with hand on leg and upward gaze

Figure 12.6c Reverse Triangle Pose

Figure 12.7 Cobbler Pose

Figure 12.8 Child Pose

The Warrior II Pose is an example of a strength pose. (Warrior I, not pictured, is a forward-facing lunge and considered more difficult.) Finally, the Corpse Pose is an example of a lying down asana. The Corpse is used to close most sessions by providing deep relaxation and an opportunity to let the body and mind integrate all that went on before it.

MOUNTAIN POSE – TADASANA (FIGURE 12.4)

(Standing)

- Stand with the feet parallel to one another and no more than hip-width apart. The inner side of the feet can be touching if this position is comfortable.
- Lift up the toes, fan them out, and as you place them, root them into the ground.
- Balance the weight evenly between the feet.
- Distribute the weight in each foot evenly around the foot – centered rather than leaning forward on the toes or back on the heels.
- Relax the shoulders and let the arms hang at the side.
- Feel the grounding of the body through the legs and feet.
- Engage the thigh muscles so that the kneecaps lift upward.
- Position the hips over the knees over the ankles.
- Pull up on the back of the legs to help tuck the pelvis a little to release and lengthen the low back.
- Pull in the abdomen gently.
- Rotate shoulders down and back while letting the shoulders feel relaxed and broad.
- Lift the chest slightly.

- Lengthen the whole spine as though the crown of your head were reaching for the sky.
- Feel the neck lengthen as the shoulders press downward and the head reaches upward.
- Look straight ahead while softening the eyes and the jaw.
- Lengthen as you breathe in; relax and lower the shoulders as you exhale.
- Quiet the mind, and let your body be strong and still like a mountain.

BEGINNER MODIFICATIONS: Stand with the back against the wall.

ARM VARIATIONS: The arms can be extended overhead with fingers interlaced and index fingers pointing upward or palms held together in front of the heart.

DOWNWARD FACING DOG – ADHO MUKHA SVANASANA (FIGURE 12.9)

(Forward Bending)

- Take a position on the hands and knees.
- Place the hands slightly forward of the shoulders.
- Spread the fingers, with the middle fingers facing forward and parallel to one another.
- Align the hips over the knees.
- Tuck the toes under.
- Look at the hands.
- Draw the hips back toward the feet and then lift upward (with the "sit" bones toward the ceiling).
- Straighten the knees while lengthening the back and maintaining the natural curves of the spine, especially in the low back.

Figure 12.9 Downward Facing Dog Pose.

- Modification: Keep knees bent if needed to maintain back alignment.
- Lower the heels to the floor.
  - Modification: Lower heels only as far as you can without losing the natural curve of the lower spine.
- Engage the thigh muscles (quadriceps) to take pressure off the arms.
- Rotate the thighs inward and pull them backward to take pressure off the arms.
- Lower front ribs toward the front of the thighs.
- Rotate the upper arms toward the center to spread the shoulder blades. (Rotate the bottom of the shoulder blades away from one another.)
- Maintain a straight line from the hips to the wrists.
- Push the mat away with the hands and arms – feeling the arms and hands as grounded.
- Relax the neck and jaw.
- To return to a stand, inhale, bend the knees, and drop the hips downward.
- Follow with Child Pose to provide a rest.

BEGINNERS:

- Place the toes or hands against a wall. Rotate the hands outward so that the thumb and index finger are against the wall.
- Place a pillow or blanket under the head.

ADVANCED:

- If you are very flexible, resist the inclination to sink the chest too far. Maintain the back alignment.

WARRIOR II POSE – VIRABHADRASANA II (FIG 12.10)
(Standing Pose)

- Start in Mountain Pose.
- Step (or jump) the feet apart while raising the arms to the sides, with the palms facing downward. The arms will be parallel to the floor.
- Turn the right foot out to point directly to the side. Turn the left foot in about 15 degrees.
- As you inhale, bend the right knee (90 degrees) until the thigh is parallel to the floor.
- Keep the knee directly over the ankle (not to one side or too far forward or back).
- Center the body; the trunk extends directly up (no lean).
- Press your weight down through the back of the left foot.
- Feel the openness in the left hip, which is rotated to the left.
- Feel the energy coursing through the arms and shooting out the fingertips.
- Turn the head, and look along the right arm.
- Inhale, lengthening the spine; exhale and sink into the lunge. Maintain a strong connection into the floor.
- Repeat on the left side.

Notes:

- The hips, shoulders, and arms all fall in the same plane, so much so that if this pose were performed in a very narrow hall, nothing would touch the walls.
- If the shoulders rise, try turning the palms up to help lower the shoulders. Then turn the palms back down while maintaining the improved shoulder position.
- Avoid the tendency to lean toward the side of the lunged knee.

CORPSE POSE – SAVASANA (FIG 12.11)
(Lying down – resting pose)

- Place a folded towel or pillow at the head of the mat (if desired). Only the head, not the shoulders, will rest on this.

Figure 12.10 Warrior II Pose

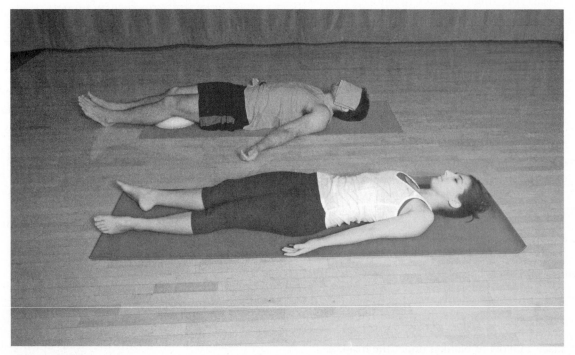

Figure 12.11 Corpse Pose

- Sit in the center of the mat with the knees bent and feet flat on the mat.
- Gently lean back until you are lying down.
- Push through the feet enough to raise the pelvis, and tuck it under slightly, helping to extend and relax the low back. Do not try to flatten the back into the floor – leave the natural curve.
- While inhaling, extend one leg straight along the floor. Repeat for the other.
- Relax both legs, especially the inner thigh area, letting the legs and feet rotate outwards.
- Check that both legs are the same in relation to the middle of the body (one not angled out more than the other, etc.) As a guide, you can place the feet near the edges of the width of the mat.
- Using the hands, lift the head, lengthen the neck, and replace the head to the ground.
- Extend the arms up over the chest, and, while exhaling, lower them to the ground alongside but not touching the sides of the body. Arms may be angled away as much as 45 degrees. Find the position that is comfortable.
- Turn the palms upward, evenly touching the knuckles of the fingers to the floor (not thumb).
- Relax the shoulders, trying to broaden across both the shoulder blades and the collarbones.
- Release tension in the face including the tongue, nose, eyes, and forehead. Think of letting the eyes and the brain sink to the back of the skull.
- Mentally "let go," surrendering yourself.
- Use abdominal breathing, allowing the body to sink into the floor (feeling heavy) on exhalation.
- Remain in this position for 5 to 10 minutes.
- When you are ready to get up, first wiggle the toes and hands. Then draw the knees to the chest, and roll over onto the right side into a sitting pose or Child Pose.

MODIFICATIONS: Place a folded towel, pillow, or bolster under the knees to assist the low back.

Place a mask over the eyes to help block out light.

Make sure interruptions will not occur for 5 to 10 minutes (cell phones on silent, etc.)

CAUTION: Try not to fall asleep. Concentrate on your breathing to avoid this. Practice also helps.

PRANAYAMA

The practice of *pranayama* unites the breath with the mind. It is not deep breathing, but rather the gentle, full inhalation and full slow exhalation during which the *prana*, which means "energy" or "life force", is absorbed by the mind and the body. A variety of breathing techniques are used – some to invoke relaxation, others to energize. Some are relatively easy to learn and others require the help of an experienced teacher.

Equal breathing (Sama Vritti Pranayama) is practiced by inhaling for the same length of time as exhaling. We don't normally breathe in this regular pattern—we typically speed up, slow down, and pause. So, regulating the breath brings a measure of control and order to the body, which is passed on to the brain. Sit or lie down in a relaxed position, and try mentally counting the length of your inhalation and exhalation. Try different counts, for example, 2 counts in and out, and then 3 counts in and out. Take a moment to see how this makes you feel.

A second type of breathing is called the three-part breath (Dirga Pranayama). In a relaxed pose, place one hand on your chest and one hand on your abdomen. Start by inhaling and trying to fill the abdomen and then exhaling. After doing this about 5 times, try filling the abdomen and then breathe in a little more, trying to fill the ribcage. Exhale first from the ribcage and second from the abdomen. After practicing this about 5 times, try adding the third part, which is the area of the chest around the heart. Breathe in and fill the abdomen, then fill the rib cage, and then fill the upper part of the chest around the heart. Exhale in reverse order—heart area, rib cage, abdomen. (This order may be reversed as well.) There are additional ways in which to control the breath; some are for calming, some aid in finding a balance, and others are vigorous and stimulating. Breath control takes time to develop, so patience is needed. Some types of breathing can lead to dizziness and hyperventilation if not learned properly.

Pranayama and asana can be studied and practiced separately. Some yoga programs insist that the breath be incorporated in the asanas immediately, but others encourage students to breathe as they normally do until the asanas are established, and only then add more breathing techniques.

STYLES OF YOGA

There are a number of styles of hatha yoga, ranging from meditative to highly vigorous. The different styles emphasize different aspects: the release of energy, relaxation, therapy, postural alignment, inner focus, detoxification, strength, balance, or flexibility.

In addition, yoga can be challenging or more relaxing, depending on how it is performed. Some styles challenge you by having you hold poses, whereas other styles have you link together poses in a single flow, which can be very physically demanding and result in cardiorespiratory benefits. Ashtanga yoga, Birkram's "Hot" yoga, Iyengar yoga, and Power yoga (based on Ashtanga) are some of the more physically challenging styles. Other types of yoga include Integral, Ananda (more gentle), Kripalu, Kundalini, Sivananda, and Viniyoga. These types of yoga all share a common lineage back to *Patanjali's Yoga Sutras*, an ancient text that outlines the basic philosophy and practices of classical yoga. For an informative description of the many styles of yoga, refer to the Yoga Styles Guide available on www.pearsonhighered.com/bishopaerobics.

Selecting a yoga class and instructor that meet your needs is very important. The styles are quite different, and hybrid styles are continually emerging. The class should feel comfortable and rewarding (not an obligation), and you can and should modify the movements to meet your energy and abilities. Many instructors teach an eclectic style using methods from more than one traditional approach. In recent years, some yoga teachers have adapted their classes for health club settings (e.g., Yogafit) in a way that brings more of a focus on the fitness aspects. Yoga may be offered as part of a fusion class that partners an activity such as spinning (cycling) with yoga or a combination of yoga and pilates (i.e. Yogalates). The name given to a class may not specifically tell you the style of yoga but a conversation with the instructor or observing the class will. Yoga studios are more apt to describe their classes in reference to a formal style. It takes considerable training and maturity to be a good yoga instructor. Look for someone with experience, and watch or take a trial class. Some instructors train for 3 to 5 years to become yoga teachers, whereas other instructors only take weekend workshops and then incorporate yoga into their classes. There are also programs that offer specialty classes for individuals who are pregnant, living with chronic pain or a debilitating disease, or are young. Yoga may also be part of a therapeutic program that aims for physical rehabilitation and restoring balance, a positive outlook, and vitality to one's life. Yoga offers us health-related fitness and much more.

PROGRESSIVE RELAXATION, MENTAL IMAGERY, AND AUTOGENIC TRAINING

PROGRESSIVE RELAXATION

Progressive relaxation is a technique that systematically relaxes your skeletal muscles. Edmond Jacobson developed the technique of progressive relaxation based on his beliefs that relaxing skeletal muscles will also relax nearby organs and involuntary muscles, and that a person cannot be nervous or tense in any body part where muscles are relaxed. The program of progressive relaxation consists of alternately tensing and relaxing muscles in a predetermined order. Purposefully creating tension in your muscles will help you recognize when your body is becoming tense at other times and consciously learn to relax it.

BENEFITS OF YOGA

Regular yoga practice can lead to a number of benefits. Yoga has been said to:

- Calm/relax and stimulate the body and mind
- Promote self-understanding, mental clarity, and inner peace
- Stimulate organs and glands
- Remove toxins
- Counteract stress and disease
- Produce fitness: muscular strength, endurance, flexibility, some cardiorespiratory
- Strengthen bones and correct posture

- Improve breathing (respiration)
- Increase energy
- Alleviate pain (or help tolerate pain) and promote healing
- Have a positive effect on hypertension (for some people)
- Have a positive effect on asthma (yoga is not a replacement for medication but may increase awareness of triggers and allow for calmer state during an event)
- Help control some aspects of epilepsy (not to replace prescribed medications)

Jacobson's full training procedure takes months, with whole sessions dedicated to relaxing a single muscle group. However, it is possible to achieve significant relaxation benefits in less time. A session should begin with muscle tensing, but most of the session should be devoted to achieving full relaxation. In the beginning, it may take a while to achieve muscle relaxation. But with practice (usually several months), you will be able to elicit the relaxation response quickly and counteract stress-induced tension. An example of this classic progressive relaxation technique developed by Jacobson is found in the Progressive Relaxation Exercise box.

MENTAL IMAGERY

Progressive relaxation, a physiological (physical) technique, is often combined with **mental imagery,** a cognitive (thought-based) technique. During mental imagery, you imagine yourself doing something special—often performing a task or athletic move that you want to perfect. You may use external imagery, in which you see yourself going through the movement, or you may use internal imagery, in which you feel yourself going through the movement. Research studies show improved performance when

mental imagery is used in conjunction with physical practice.

AUTOGENIC TRAINING

Autogenic training was developed by Johannes H. Schultz as a way to relax the body. It is a psychophysiological technique, which means it is a physiological technique that uses the relationship between physiological processes and thoughts, emotions, and behavior. It uses visual metaphors, such as imagining warmth and heaviness to relax. A variety of mental images can be used, such as imagining your body glowing warm like the sun and sinking into the deepest, downiest cloud to achieve even greater relaxation. To relax a tense muscle, a person might picture the aching muscle as red and then try to mentally change the color to a cool blue, or imagine the tension as a liquid and let it run out like water. The technique involved is very similar to Jacobson's progressive relaxation method and often begins with muscle-tensing and muscle-relaxing exercises. The full program, a series of six psychophysiological exercises, takes about four months to learn. Audio and video formats and workbooks are available commercially, in addition to course offerings with trained professionals.

PROGRESSIVE RELAXATION EXERCISE

 To begin progressive relaxation, take a comfortable position lying on your back on the floor with your knees straight or bent but not crossed and your arms by your side. Or sit relaxed in a comfortable chair. Spend a few minutes clearing your mind and concentrating on deep breathing. Begin to relax. Now clench your right fist; study the tension in your fist, hand, and forearm as you do so. Relax your fist. Feel the looseness in your hand and arm, and notice the contrast with the tension. Repeat this procedure with your right fist again; always notice as you relax that this is the opposite of tension—feel the difference. Repeat the entire procedure with your left fist, then both fists at once.

Continue this process of clenching and releasing as follows. Always repeat the exercise for each muscle at least once. Flex your biceps (one at a time, then both), scrunch your forehead, squeeze your eyelids closed, bite down with your jaw. Each time you

release, notice the sensation of looseness. Really appreciate the contrast between tension and relaxation. Press your tongue against the top of your mouth, purse your lips, press your head back against the floor or back of the chair, then press it forward against your chest, shrug and relax your shoulders.

As you release from each exercise, feel the comfort and heaviness increasing. Breathe in, filling your lungs completely, and hold your breath. Notice the tension. Exhale and let your chest become loose. Repeat several times; notice the tension draining from your body as you exhale. Continue relaxing and breathe freely and gently. Next, tighten your stomach and hold, then arch your back, while keeping the rest of your body as relaxed as possible. Move the clenching and releasing through the rest of your body, one body part at a time: buttocks, thighs, knees, calves, shins, feet, and toes. Feel the relaxation spread deeper and deeper as your focus moves down your body.

Let go more and more until you feel yourself completely relaxed.

SUMMARY

There is strong evidence that the mind and the body are inextricably connected. When either one is out of balance, it affects the other. The basis of pilates is that the focus of the mind helps control and train the body, and the fitness of the body then affects the way we act and think. In yoga, there is no distinction between where the body begins and the mind leaves off. Therefore, the physical training of the body necessarily trains the mind, and similarly the state and discipline of the mind influence the body. They are interrelated and cannot be considered separately. Progressive relaxation, mental imagery, and autogenic training use both the mind and body to help us leave our stressors behind and create a positive internal environment. The belief that the mind and the body are always connected allows us to use both in the healing process of either.

KNOWLEDGE TIPS

1. Many philosophies believe that there is a fundamental connection between the mind and body.

2. Techniques and philosophies such as those used by yoga, pilates, progressive relaxation, mental imagery, and autogenic training promote a mind-body connection and a healthy lifestyle.

3. Group fitness instructors sometimes incorporate aspects of mind-body techniques into their classes.

4. Pilates, a practice created by Joseph Pilates, is dedicated to developing a balance between strength and flexibility.

5. Yoga is an ancient Eastern Indian philosophical tradition dating back 5,000 years. It consists of physical, psychological, and spiritual aspects to realize the unity of the mind and body.

6. Hatha yoga is the physical aspect of yoga. It is practiced through poses called *asanas,* breathing techniques called *pranayama,* and meditation.

7. Pilates uses exercises on adjustable equipment as well as simple mat exercises to develop the powerhouse, or core muscles of the body: the abdomen, lower back, and buttocks.

8. The six original principles of the Pilates method are concentration, control, centering, flowing movement, precision, and breathing.

9. Progressive relaxation is a relaxation technique that systematically relaxes your skeletal muscles through tensing and releasing in a specific order.

10. Mental imagery is often used with progressive relaxation. During mental imagery, you imagine yourself doing something.

11. Autogenic training is a psychophysiological technique to induce relaxation through specific mental imagery and muscle-tensing and muscle-relaxing exercises.

THINK ABOUT IT

1. Explain how your mind can influence your body and vice versa. Give an example of a technique that uses the
   - body to influence the mind
   - mind to influence the body

2. If you feel yourself becoming distressed, what can you do to help return yourself to a healthy state of being?

3. What is the philosophical basis behind yoga?

4. What makes pilates different from other forms of strengthening and stretching?

5. Create a mental imagery scenario that will help you handle a stressful situation (i.e., a test).

REFERENCES

Bartholomew, J. B., and B. M. Miller. "Affective Responses to an Aerobic Dance Class: The Impact of Perceived Performance." *Research Quarterly for Exercise and Sport* 73 (No. 3, 2002): 301(9).

Bauman, A. "Is Yoga Enough to Keep You Fit?" *Yoga Journal* 158 (2002): 85–91.

Corliss, R. "The Power of Yoga." *Time,* April 23, 2001, pp. 54–56.

Feuerstein, G., and S. Bodian, with the staff of *Yoga Journal* (editors). *Living Yoga: A Comprehensive Guide for Daily Life.* New York: J. P. Tarcher/Perigee, 1993.

Freedman, F. B., B. Gibbs, D. Hall, E. Kelly, J. Monks, and J. Smith. *Yoga and Pilates for Everyone.* London: Hermes House, 2005.

Friedman, P., and Eisen, G. *The Pilates Method of Physical and Mental Conditioning.* Warner Books, 1982.

Iyengar, B. K. S. *Yoga: The Path to Holistic Health.* New York: Dorling Kindersley, 2001.

Kiecolt-Glaser, J. K., W. Garner, C. E. Speicher, G. Penn, and R. Vlaser. "Psychosocial Modifiers of Immunocompetence in Medical Students." *Psychosomatic Medicine* 46 (1984).

Reddy, P. R., and P. R. Kumar. "A Comparative Study of Yogasanas and Aerobic Dance and Their Effects on Selected Motor Fitness Components in Girl Students. *Research Bi-annual for Movement* 19 (No. 1, 2002): 30–37.

Silvananda Yoga Vedanta Center. *Learn Yoga in a Weekend.* New York: Alfred A. Knopf, 1998.

Stewart, K. *Pilates for Beginners.* Created and produced by Carroll & Brown Publishers, London. First published in the USA by Harper-Resource, an imprint of Harper-Collins Publishers, New York, 2001.

Stott-Merrithew, M. *Pilates Essential Matwork for Beginners: Stott Pilates with Master Instructor–Trainer Moira Stott-Merrithew.* 2nd ed. Merrithew Corporation, 2001. Videocassette.

Tran, H., J. Lashbrook, and E. A. Amsterdam. "Effects of Hatha Yoga on the Health-Related Aspects of Physical Fitness." *Preventive Cardiology* 4 (2001): 165–170.

13

Nutrition and Weight Control

"Life itself is the proper binge."

JULIA CHILD

- What is a balanced diet?
- What are the best foods to eat?
- Should I drink water or a sports drink?
- How can I best manage my weight?
- How do exercise and diet tie together?

PROPER nutrition and exercise are two of the most valuable tools for developing and maintaining a healthy body. Used together, they are more effective than either one alone. An exercise program without proper nutrition can leave you feeling run-down, depleted of energy, and without the building blocks for muscle and bone development. Similarly, a balanced diet without exercise doesn't result in muscle tone or aerobic efficiency. Put them together, and you not only get the positive effects of each one, you also experience combination benefits. When a weight-loss diet is combined with exercise, more of the weight lost is fat (as opposed to lean body mass) than when dieting is used alone. People are also more successful at maintaining a healthy weight (once they attain it) when exercise is part of the equation. This chapter starts with a review of basic nutritional information, then examines the combined effects of exercise and nutrition on weight control, and finally discredits some popular but false beliefs concerning dieting and weight management.

BASIC NUTRITIONAL INFORMATION

A car needs a variety of fluids to keep it running. You could say its nutritional requirements are gas for fuel; radiator fluid to keep the engine cool; and oil, transmission, and brake fluids to lubricate. If you fail to keep these fluids at appropriate levels, the car either runs poorly or doesn't run at all.

Your body, like a car, requires certain types and quantities of nutrients to function properly. The body's nutrients are chemicals that come from the digestion of food and drink. Your body needs about 50 different nutrients. Organized into six categories, they are referred to as the essential nutrients: carbohydrates, protein, fat, water, vitamins, and minerals.

Collectively, the six essential nutrients provide for the:

- production of energy
- construction and maintenance of cells
- regulation of body processes

Of these six, only three—carbohydrates, fat, and protein—provide energy for the body. When these nutrients are chemically broken down, energy is released. That energy is measured in kilocalories, which the general public calls **calories.** Fat provides almost twice as much energy (9 calories per gram, or g) as carbohydrates and protein (4 calories per g). Although no energy can be obtained from water, vitamins, or minerals, these nutrients play major roles in the many chemical processes of the body, including the processes that result in energy production.

How much of each nutrient do we need? This important question is continually being researched in this country and around the world. Every 5 years in the

United States, this information is reviewed and written into science-based advice (guidelines) on food and physical activity choices for health. The *2010 Dietary Guidelines for Americans* is available online at www. health.gov/dietary/guidelines or through the Government Printing Office. Some of the key recommendations are included in this chapter for easy reference.

In addition, the U.S. Food and Nutrition Board of the Institute of Medicine of the National Academies in collaboration with Health Canada released a report in 2005 to provide dietary reference values for the intake of nutrients for healthy Americans and Canadians. The report is titled "Dietary Reference Intakes (DRIs) for Energy, Carbohydrate, Fiber, Fat, Fatty Acids, Cholesterol, Protein and Amino Acids." A summary of some of the key points from this report follows. There will be more on these points in the chapter as the essential nutrients are discussed.

- Adults should get 45% to 65% of their calories from carbohydrates, 20% to 35% from fat, and 10% to 35% from protein.
- Added sugars should comprise not more than 25% of total calories consumed. Added sugars are sugars incorporated into foods and beverages during production, which usually provide insignificant amounts of vitamins, minerals, or other essential nutrients. Major sources include soft drinks, fruit drinks, pastries, candy, and other sweets.
- The recommended daily intake for total fiber for adults 50 years and younger is 38 grams for men and 25 grams for women.
- Using new data, the report reaffirms previously established recommended levels of protein intake, which is 0.8 grams per kilogram of body weight for adults; however, recommended levels for pregnancy are increased.
- The report doesn't set maximum levels for saturated fat, cholesterol, or *trans* fatty acids because increased risk exists at levels above zero; however, the recommendation is to eat as little as possible while consuming a diet adequate in important other essential nutrients.

You may have already noticed wider ranges on carbohydrates, fats, and proteins. These ranges were expanded to cover a broad spectrum of individual differences and with the goal of minimizing risk of chronic diseases and maximizing the intake of essential nutrients. The recommendations of other health organizations—50% to 60% carbohydrate, less than 30% fat, and 10% to 15% protein—fall within the range of the U.S.-Canada recommendations.

CARBOHYDRATES

Carbohydrates are the primary source of energy for the body and the only source of energy for the brain. They also play a role in the digestion of fat and protein, hence the expression that "fat is burned in a carbohydrate flame," and the concern that low levels of carbohydrates can result in an increased use of protein for energy rather than muscle-building and maintenance.

Carbohydrate foods (sugars and starches) are broken down into the simple sugar **glucose.** Glucose is absorbed into the blood and used by the cells. If it isn't used right away, glucose is stored in the muscles and liver as **glycogen** (long chains of glucose molecules). Glycogen is the preferred fuel for aerobic exercise. There are limits on how much glycogen can be stored. When these limits are reached, additional glucose is converted into fat and stored as adipose tissue.

There are two kinds of carbohydrates: simple and complex. The natural sugars found in fruits and milk and refined sugar are simple carbohydrates. Foods containing high amounts of refined sugars are easily digested and rapidly absorbed into the bloodstream. When enough refined sugar is eaten, it creates a surge in blood sugar. This triggers a release of insulin, which, in reaction to the high concentration of sugar in the blood, sweeps much of the sugar out of the blood. This, in turn, causes a sudden drop in blood sugar that leaves you feeling sluggish, tired, and often hungry. A sugary snack such as a candy bar is not a good way to get quick, lasting energy—that strategy generally backfires!

Foods that are composed of more complex sugars, such as whole-grain cereals and vegetables, are sources of complex carbohydrates. For the most part, these foods take longer to digest, so they are more slowly absorbed into the blood. This prevents quick rises and dips in the level of blood sugar. The resulting steady level of blood sugar helps you maintain your energy level and prevents you from feeling hungry between meals. At least half of all grains should be whole grains.

Foods can be categorized according to their glycemic index. Foods with a high glycemic index are easily digested and, if eaten alone, result in a surge of sugar in the bloodstream. It may surprise you to learn that some starches have a high glycemic index and can act on blood sugar like simple carbohydrates. These include pasta, white bread, white potatoes, and white rice. Good substitutes for these are brown rice and whole-grain breads and pasta.

Nutritionally speaking, it is better to eat complex carbohydrates and natural sugar foods (fruit, milk)

2010 DIETARY GUIDELINES FOR AMERICANS RECOMMENDATIONS

According to the *2010 Dietary Guidelines for Americans*, individuals should meet the following recommendations as part of a healthy eating pattern while staying within their calorie needs:

- Increase vegetable and fruit intake.
- Eat a variety of vegetables, especially dark-green and red and orange vegetables, and beans and peas.
- Consume at least half of all grains as whole grains. Replace refined grains with whole grains.
- Increase intake of fat-free or low-fat milk and milk products, such as milk, yogurt, cheese, or fortified soy beverages,
- Choose a variety of protein foods, which include seafood, lean meat and poultry, eggs, beans and peas, soy products, and unsalted nuts and seeds.

- Choose seafood in place of some meat and poultry.
- Replace protein foods that are higher in solid fats with choices that are lower in solid fats and calories and/or are sources of oils.
- Use oils to replace solid fats where possible.
- Choose foods that provide more potassium, dietary fiber, calcium, and vitamin D, which are of concern in American diets.

There are additional recommendations for specific population groups, including women capable of getting pregnant, women who are pregnant or breastfeeding, and individuals ages 50 years and older.

---

than refined sugars because the former contain vitamins, minerals, phytochemicals, and fiber, whereas refined sugars have no nutritional value. Of course, one can't deny that sweets made with those refined sugars have other benefits worth enjoying every now and then! The trick is to consume them in small amounts. As you reach for something sweet, consider also that when it comes to calories (and fat), some choices are better than others. For example, a piece of Chocolate Chip Paradise Pie from Chili's weighs in at 1290 calories, a typical piece of carrot cake with icing rings in at 540 calories but only 240 without the icing, pumpkin pie at about 240 calories, and chocolate pudding (4 oz.) or a brownie at about 150 calories. Of course, if you like to eat four brownies but would eat only one piece of cake, the point is moot.

Fiber (or roughage) is a general term for food substances that the body can't fully digest. Fiber is made up of complex chains of carbohydrates that the human digestive system lacks the enzymes to break. There are two types of dietary fiber: soluble and insoluble. Soluble fiber wraps around fats and promotes their excretion. Insoluble fiber combines with water and gives bulk to the stool. Bulk encourages waste products to move more quickly out of the body, thereby reducing the time that potential cancer-causing substances remain in the colon. Good food

sources of fiber include whole (not refined) grains, fruits, and vegetables. Animal foods do not contain fiber. A high-fiber diet:

- helps maintain regularity
- helps fill you up and keeps you from getting hungry so fast
- provides good nutrients because sources of fiber are nutrient dense
- helps prevent constipation, hemorrhoids, and diverticulitis
- reduces cancer risk, especially colon and rectal cancer
- lowers "bad" blood cholesterol (low-density lipoprotein, or LDL)

A coincidental benefit is that high-fiber diets tend to be low in saturated fats and thus help to reduce the risk of cardiovascular disease.

In general, the more a food is processed, the less fiber it contains. See the Fiber: Where It Is ... Where It Isn't ... box on page 197 for an example. Women need about 25 grams of fiber per day and men 38 grams—too much or too little can cause difficulties. Add fiber to your diet gradually, and drink plenty of fluids so that you don't experience gastrointestinal distress. Your body needs time to adjust.

PROTEIN

Your body needs **protein** to build and repair body tissues, to make hemoglobin (which carries oxygen), to form antibodies (which fight infection), to produce enzymes and hormones, and, when necessary, to supply energy. When protein foods are digested, they are broken down into amino acids. There are nine amino acids that the body cannot manufacture. These nine are called essential amino acids. Foods that contain all the essential amino acids are called complete proteins; those that contain only some of the essential amino acids are called incomplete proteins. Complete protein sources, such as meat, have all the essential amino acids. If, however, you are a vegetarian or eat very little meat, you need to eat a wide variety of grains, vegetables, and seeds to get all the essential amino acids. In the past, it was believed that two complementary incomplete proteins had to be eaten together at the same meal. Now it is known that as long as they are eaten on the same day, they will offer the benefits of a complete protein. Beans and rice, pasta and peas, and wheat bread and peanut butter are examples of good pairings of incomplete proteins.

It is not necessary to take amino acid pills; it is easy to get all the protein you need in a normal diet. In fact, most Americans eat too much protein. When too much protein is consumed, the extra amino acids are converted to fat and stored. The recommended protein intake for men and women over age 18 is 0.8 grams per kilogram of body weight per day. Research suggests that highly active individuals, such as endurance and strength-trained athletes require 1.2 to 1.7 grams per kilogram of body weight per day, and that this amount can generally be obtained through diet alone, without the use of protein supplements. However, even though they require more protein, they also need substantially more carbohydrate and overall calories; therefore, the recommended proportion of protein in the total diet doesn't change significantly. For the average American, protein consumption is about 15% of the diet, which falls in the recommended range. However, many Americans eat too many total calories, so 15% of that total can represent more protein than needed. As an example, 15% of 2,000 calories equals 350 calories, whereas 15% of a 3,000 calorie diet equals 450 calories.

To determine the protein requirement for a normal healthy adult, you must (1) convert pounds to kilograms, (2) multiply by the recommended amount of protein per kilogram of body weight, and (3) convert grams to calories by multiplying by 4, because protein contains 4 calories per gram. Here is an example using a 143-pound individual:

143 lb ÷ 2.2 = 60 kg (body weight)
60 kg × 0.8 = 48 g (protein required)
48 × 4 = 192 calories from protein

The 192 calories represents about 10% of a 2,000-calorie diet and is the equivalent of 6 ounces of steak. If you do not want to convert body weight to kilograms, a close approximation can be obtained (for the 0.8 g/kg) by multiplying body weight in pounds by 0.36.

Countries where meat is used more for flavoring and less as a primary food have lower incidents of cardiovascular disease. Although most experts recommend that we consume smaller portions of red meat, remember that it is a good dietary source of iron. Both animal and plant foods contain protein. Some good sources of protein include meat, poultry, eggs, milk products, legumes (beans and peas), whole grains, pastas, rice, and seeds.

FAT

Fat is an essential part of every cell in your body. No fat, no life. The absolute minimum for men is about 3% to 6% of body weight, for women about 8% to 12%. Fats, also known as lipids, have a bad reputation only because most Americans overconsume them. Fat is an excellent source of concentrated energy. It also acts as insulation from the cold and carries the fat-soluble vitamins A, D, E, and K. Fat helps provide energy for prolonged activities performed at low to moderate levels of intensity, but to do so, carbohydrate must also be present.

Dietary fat is 95% triglycerides. Tryglycerides are made up of three fatty acids and one glycerol. Fatty acids come in three varieties: saturated, polyunsaturated, and monounsaturated. Saturated fats in the diet are related to elevated blood cholesterol, stroke, and coronary heart disease. In addition, saturated fats are converted into cholesterol in the liver when the amount of dietary cholesterol is low. Therefore, eating a diet low in saturated fats is as important, if not more important, than eating a low-cholesterol diet. Saturated fats, which are generally but not always solids at room temperature, include animal fats, butter, cheese, chocolate, and coconut and palm oils. (Chocolate, however, does contain some healthful substances—especially dark chocolate.) Unsaturated fats are generally liquids or soft solids at room temperature. Polyunsaturated fats include most of the oils (corn, soybean, cottonseed, safflower, sesame, and sunflower), fish, some nuts (walnuts, pecans, flaxseed), and most margarines. Monounsaturated fats include peanut, olive, and canola oils; avocados; olives; and some nuts (peanuts and cashews).

FIBER: WHERE IT IS ... WHERE IT ISN'T ...

Fiber is in plant leaves, roots, seeds, and skins. The more plant foods are processed, the less fiber they will contain. Take, for example, an apple:

raw with peel	3.6 g
½ cup applesauce	2.1 g
apple juice	0.2 g

To make sure that you are getting whole grains, read the labels. Do not be fooled by labels with the following ingredients: wheat flour, enriched flour, or degerminated corn meal. Also be careful of 12-grain product labels. Check the ingredient list to see whether any of the 12 grains are whole.

There are many good high-fiber foods. This abbreviated list contains some that students on the go can obtain easily, carry with them, or keep handy in the car. And remember, these foods are excellent fuel sources rich in vitamins, phytochemicals, and minerals.

- salads containing lots of vegetables, tabouli salad
- sandwiches with vegetables: romaine lettuce, peppers, onions, etc.
- pizza with vegetables or fruit: broccoli, green pepper, pineapple, etc.
- apples, pears, and oranges
- pasta sauce with vegetables added
- whole-grain pastas
- whole-grain cereal (for breakfast or eat dry for snack; keeps well in the car)
- seeds or nuts, such as shelled almonds; these make handy "staying" snacks
- baked potato topped with vegetables, such as broccoli (choose instead of fries)
- soups containing whole grains, such as barley
- Whole-grain crackers

Fat consumption should be between 20% and 35% of energy intake. According to the *2010 Dietary Guidelines*, the average American intake of total fat and saturated fatty acids (SFA) has decreased significantly, to 33.6% and 11.4%, respectively—still higher than recommended, but certainly improved. Further, if a person eats too much food—even when the diet consists of the correct percentages of fat, carbohydrate, and protein—the extra calories are stored as fat. Twenty percent fat of a 2,000-calorie diet (400 calories) is different from 20% fat of a 3,000-calorie diet (600 calories). If you exceed what you need, your body will store it for future use. You don't have to work hard at getting your required fat, because fat is hidden in so many foods. Red meats, cheese, baked goods, and fried foods are all high in fat. One of the easiest ways to cut down on fat is to switch from whole milk to low-fat or fat-free milk. Nearly half of whole milk's 150 calories per serving come from fat. Reduced-fat milk (2%) derives 38% of its 120 calories from fat, while low-fat milk (1%) drops to 23% of its 100 calories. And the winner, fat-free milk (nonfat or skim), contains no fat in its 80 calories. As you look for the fat content of foods, be aware that many products are labeled by the percentage of *weight* that is fat rather than the percentage of *calories*. Using the milk example above, only 2% of the weight (or 5 g) of reduced-fat milk (2% milk) is fat, but notice that more than a third of its calories come from fat. Many people mistakenly think that only 2%, not 38%, of the *calories* are from fat. To convert grams of fat to calories, you simply multiply the grams by 9. Two-percent milk, for example, contains 5 g of fat, which translates into 45 calories from fat. So, depending on the type of milk you pour in your cup, you can consume as much as 72 or as few as no calories from fat.

Trans fatty acids, often referred to as **trans fats**, appear naturally in small amounts in beef, lamb, and full fat dairy products. But they can also be produced through a process called hydrogenation, which adds hydrogen to vegetable oil. The resulting *trans* fat doesn't spoil as easily, which means that foods containing it, especially baked goods, can have a longer shelf life. Unfortunately, *trans* fat also has the effect of lowering your "good" cholesterol (HDL) and raising your "bad" cholesterol (LDL), which increases your risk for heart disease.

Fast-food companies, under fire for using saturated fats to fry their foods, switched to *trans* fats and appeared to be making a healthier offering until research on *trans* fats showed it to be as bad or worse than saturated fats. In 2006, the U.S. Food and Drug Administration (FDA) required that *trans* fats be listed on nutrition labels under the saturated fats food line. If, however, a food contains less than 0.5 gram of *trans* fats, the content is allowed to be listed as zero. Even if you eat a food with a small amount of *trans* fats, eating several servings of it can add up. To see whether a food labeled as 0 *trans* fat does contain some, look under the ingredients list for the words "partially hydrogenated" vegetable oil. That is another term for *trans* fats. "Complete" or "fully hydrogenated" is fine; however, simply "hydrogenated" may indicate that the product contains *trans* fats. Especially check fried foods, baked goods, margarines, and shortenings for *trans* fats. As the public has demanded healthier foods, many manufacturers have produced products free of *trans* fats. Double-check these for their saturated fat content. And remember that restaurants may still be using *trans* fats.

The American Heart Association recommends that no more than 1% of your total daily calories be *trans* fat. That translates into just 20 calories, or 2 grams for a 2,000-calorie diet. Saturated fat should represent less than 10% of your fat intake. Another good area to check are snack foods—not all popcorns, crackers, etc., are equal when it comes to *trans* and saturated fats.

Fats that are health-enhancing include the polyunsaturated fats called omega-3. These are found in fish such as salmon, mackerel, herring, tuna, and sardines and can help reduce cholesterol and inhibit atherosclerosis in the coronary arteries. The American Heart Association recommends eating fish twice a week. Omega-3 fatty acids are also found in walnuts and flaxseeds. Consider little changes, such as adding walnuts to your whole-grain muffin for breakfast or making a tuna fish sandwich for lunch.

Cholesterol is a waxy fatlike substance found in the blood and in body tissues. The body naturally synthesizes it because it is essential in the formation of bile salts, which are used in fat digestion. It is also an essential component of all cell membranes; therefore, it is found in every cell of the body. It is transported through the blood by fat-protein particles called lipoproteins. Lipoproteins are named according to their density. The two major types of lipoproteins are **high-density lipoprotein (HDL)** and **low-density lipoprotein (LDL).** HDL picks up cholesterol from the cells and bloodstream and transports it to the liver, where it is used to make the bile salts. When the bile salts are used for fat digestion, some of them are excreted, thus eliminating cholesterol from the body. HDL is sometimes called the garbage collector of the blood, because it picks up cholesterol and dumps it in the liver. HDL is also referred to as "good cholesterol."

Cholesterol levels can be increased two ways: through our diet (eating cholesterol-rich foods) or through production of cholesterol in the liver. When the body has too much cholesterol, the LDL transporting cholesterol will give up some of its cholesterol to the walls of the arteries. As the fatty deposits (plaque) build up, the arteries become narrow and clogged. This condition, called atherosclerosis, is often accompanied by arteriosclerosis, a hardening of the arteries. Both of these can lead to **coronary heart disease**

CHANGES TO MAKE IN THE AMERICAN DIET

According to the *2010 Dietary Guidelines*, Americans should reduce the following foods and food components:

- Reduce daily sodium intake to less than 2,300 milligrams (mg). Persons who are 51 and older and those of any age who are African American or have hypertension, diabetes, or chronic kidney disease should further reduce their daily intake to 1,500 mg.
- Consume less than 10% of calories from saturated fatty acids by replacing them with monounsaturated and polyunsaturated fatty acids.

- Consume less than 300 mg per day of dietary cholesterol.
- Reduce intake of calories from solid fats and added sugars.
- Limit the consumption of foods that contain refined grains.
- If alcohol is consumed, it should be consumed in moderation—up to one drink per day for women and two drinks per day for men—and only by adults of legal drinking age.

(CHD), a degenerative heart condition caused by the thickening and hardening of the coronary arteries. To prevent these dangerous diseases, people must control their cholesterol level. This disease does not start only in middle age; plaque has been found in young adults and even in children.

Both the total amount of cholesterol in the blood and the amount of HDL in the blood are good indicators of heart disease risk. A desirable level for **total cholesterol** is below 200 milligrams per deciliter (mg/dl). A low level of HDL cholesterol, 35 mg/dl or lower, is considered a risk factor for coronary artery disease. A high level of HDL cholesterol, 60 mg/dl or higher, is considered protective. Another way to look at cholesterol is the ratio of total cholesterol (HDL + LDL) to HDL. According to the American Heart Association (AHA), you should keep your cholesterol ratio at or below 5:1. The ideal cholesterol ratio is about 3.5:1. For example, if total cholesterol is 200 and HDL is 50, the ratio is 4:1. If total cholesterol is 210 and HDL is 60, the ratio is 3.5. If you want to know your cholesterol levels, you can take a simple blood test. A combination of diet and exercise is the best way to control your cholesterol level. Aerobic exercise can increase the amount of HDL cholesterol, and a diet low in cholesterol and low in saturated and *trans* fats can decrease the amount of LDL cholesterol circulating in your bloodstream.

WATER *half-your body weight*

Water, which constitutes 70% of the body's weight, is the solvent for digestion and waste removal. Water is the major component of blood and of the lubricant found in and around joints and organs. It also acts as a coolant as long as sweat is evaporating. You should consume the equivalent of six to eight 8-ounce (oz.) glasses of fluid daily for normal activity. Most people in the United States do not have a problem staying hydrated. Fluid intake can come from both beverages and foods. Recent research indicates that even caffeinated beverages can assist in hydration.

However, warm environments and exercise can both increase fluid needs. Water losses as little as 2% to 3% of body weight can negatively affect physical performance. You can be this dehydrated and not even be thirsty. Furthermore, thirst can be quenched with small amounts of water, when, in fact, your body may need much more. Be sure to stay well hydrated, and don't trust your thirst as an indicator of dehydration. Water is the best thing to drink for exercise up to an hour. For exercise more than an hour, an electrolyte-replacing sports drink containing less than 8% carbohydrate may help boost energy and aid in endurance

activities. For the normal fitness exerciser, water is free, easy to digest, and great for rehydration. Be sure to start class hydrated, and drink again after class. If the environment is very warm, it is a good idea to have a drink in the middle of class. Some students like to keep a water bottle handy.

You want to drink the fluid that will leave your stomach the most quickly and get out to the body where it is needed. Cold drinks (40° to 50°F) leave the stomach more quickly than do warm drinks. They also help cool you off. Even ice-cold water won't hurt you, although you should drink it slowly. Sugars (glucose, fructose, sucrose) in drinks slow down the rate at which the fluid leaves the stomach. If you do use a sport drink and the carbohydrate percentage is higher than recommended (4% to 8%), you can dilute the drink. Soft drinks are not good sources of rapidly absorbed fluid. Fifteen minutes after drinking 12 oz. of a regular soft drink, 95% of it is still in your stomach. In addition, the carbonation can cause stomach bloating and upset. Fifteen minutes after drinking 12 oz. of water, only 30% of it is still in your stomach. Water, under normal conditions, is the most effective drink and also the least expensive.

Don't worry about replacing the electrolytes lost during a regular aerobics class. Sweat is really very diluted. The small amounts of minerals and electrolytes (including sodium [salt], potassium, and magnesium) that are lost through sweat can, under normal conditions, be replaced during your next regular meal. Avoid salt pills during exercise; they create a high salt concentration in the stomach that prevents rapid fluid absorption. They may also cause stomach irritation and nausea. Sports drinks with low levels of sodium are helpful during endurance exercise lasting over an hour.

VITAMINS

Vitamins are organic compounds that are essential for the process of releasing energy from food. As a result, they help to control the growth, maintenance, and repair of body tissues. Vitamins cannot be manufactured by the body and must therefore be obtained through a balanced diet. Research evidence suggests that the lack of vitamins impairs physical performance, but no evidence has proven that large doses enhance performance. Large doses of the fat-soluble vitamins (A, D, E, and K) can accumulate over time and cause serious toxic effects. Excess water-soluble vitamins (B, C, and others) generally wash out of the body daily. However, megadose levels of intake of these vitamins can also result in serious problems. A balanced diet will usually provide all the vitamins you need. Some exceptions include pregnant women, who are usually prescribed vitamins, strict vegetarians, and individuals on low-calorie diets. If you think that your diet is not sufficiently vitamin rich, you may want to do a diet analysis, consider a nutrition supplement or multivitamin, and consult a registered dietician or other qualified health care provider.

MINERALS

Minerals are inorganic compounds that perform a variety of functions in the body. Some minerals, such as calcium and phosphorus, supply strength and rigidity to body structures like bones and teeth. Adequate calcium intake is important to the prevention of osteoporosis (weakening of the bone). The mineral iron is critical to the formation of hemoglobin, which is the oxygen-carrying pigment in the red blood cell. Lack of iron can cause fatigue. Menstruating and physically active women require more iron than other women, and women in general need more iron than men. Other minerals play a role in the production of hormones, such as zinc with insulin, and still others are involved in the regulatory functions of the body such as muscle contraction, nerve transmission, and blood clotting. A balanced diet will normally provide adequate amounts of all the minerals, although in some cases individuals may benefit from supplementation. Most Americans, especially teenagers, women, and the elderly, do not consume adequate amounts of calcium and iron. Note that some vitamins and minerals, such as calcium and vitamin D, must be taken together to ensure proper absorption and use in the body. Others, such as selenium and vitamin C, should be taken separately. Selenium, which helps reduce the risk of some cancers, can interfere with vitamin absorption. Taking a vitamin C supplement an hour ahead of the selenium supplement solves this problem. Sodium also deserves special mention because many Americans greatly exceed the recommended 2,300 milligrams (mg) a day—the equivalent of one teaspoon of table salt. For sodium-sensitive individuals, high salt intake increases their risk for hypertension. Excess sodium also increases calcium loss through the urine which adds to the risk of losing bone density. See the box, Sodium and Potassium.

ANTIOXIDANTS AND PHYTOCHEMICALS

An **antioxidant** is an organic substance that can neutralize particles called free radicals without becoming a free radical itself. Reducing free radicals in the body is believed to prevent or reduce the risk of diseases like cancer, heart disease, and stroke. Vitamins C, E, and A (which is converted from beta-carotene), selenium (a mineral), and phytochemicals are antioxidants. **Phytochemicals** (meaning "plant chemicals") are food components that help ward off cancer, cardiovascular diseases, diabetes, and hypertension. They are found in a wide variety of foods, including colorful fruits and vegetables, grains, legumes, and seeds. Carotenoids (one type of phytochemical), the most common of which is beta-carotene, are the pigments that give many vegetables such as carrots and sweet potatoes their color. Other good sources are green tea, garlic, licorice, and soy.

Free radicals are naturally formed during chemical processes in the cells as well as through exposure to things like solar or cosmic radiation and cigarette smoke. The most damaging source of free radicals in humans comes from oxygen. During oxygen's role of producing energy from carbohydrates and fats, it is usually converted into water and carbon dioxide, but sometimes it loses an extra electron and becomes a free radical. This free radical then steals an electron from another source, which sets up a chain reaction that can result in damage to cell walls, other cellular structures, and the genetic information within the cell. If left unchecked, such damage can become irreversible and lead to disease. When an antioxidant meets and neutralizes a free radical, the chain reaction stops.

Antioxidants are being actively researched. To date, the research is very promising but not conclusive,

---

SODIUM AND POTASSIUM

KEY RECOMMENDATIONS

- Consume less than 2,300 mg (approximately 1 teaspoon of salt) of sodium per day.

- Choose and prepare foods with little salt. At the same time, consume potassium-rich foods, such as fruits and vegetables.

especially concerning antioxidant supplements. Most of the research has been done using antioxidant-rich foods, so the benefits being documented may be the result of something else in the food, or a combination of the antioxidant with something else in the diet. Furthermore, many studies have been carried out on populations with inadequate dietary intake of antioxidants, thus leaving open the possibility that supplements for individuals with healthy diets may not be necessary or beneficial. Some studies, however, suggest that benefits are derived from antioxidant levels above what can be obtained through diet. Before taking a supplement, consult with your health care provider. To make antioxidants part of your diet, consume lots of fruits, vegetables, and whole grains. Sweet potatoes, carrots, spinach, cantaloupe, and mangoes are all great sources of antioxidants. Research consistently shows that people with the highest fruit and vegetable intake are the healthiest.

MYPLATE

The U.S. Department of Agriculture (USDA) has given us a new way to picture a balanced diet. The previous MyPyramid food guidance system has been replaced with MyPlate, which shows a plate divided into five food groups (Figure 13.1)—fruits, vegetables, grains, protein, and dairy—each represented by a colored section. The goals of MyPlate are to make meal planning, proportionality, and healthy choices easy to visualize, which will, it is hoped, translate into healthier eating in the United States. Nutrition information, resources, recipes, tips, food label information, graphics, and more interactive content are available on the website for MyPlate: ChooseMyPlate.gov. The SuperTracker feature lets you enter the food you are eating and helps you plan, track, and analyze your diet and physical activity. It is a great way to come up with a nutrition goal. And remember to fill half your plate with fruits and vegetables!

Figure 13.1 MyPlate.

FOOD LABELS

After you know what kinds of foods are good for you and how much of each kind to eat, you need to become a savvy food label reader. The FDA requires food labeling on most packaged foods. Figure 13.2 shows an example of a food label and offers guidelines for interpreting the information contained on the label. Label information is based on serving sizes. What many people don't realize is how much serving sizes, in terms of actual helpings, have increased over the years. The label, however, uses standard sizes that may seem small compared to what is on your plate. To interpret the label correctly, you must know what the label considers a serving. Figure 13.3 on page 203 provides a visual guide to some serving sizes. If you are consuming food in greater quantities, you need to multiply the label information by the number of servings you are consuming. For example, the USDA describes a standard 2-ounce bagel as two servings from the grain group. Many bagels are 6 ounces. This is the equivalent of six servings. Similarly, the label on a single large muffin may state that the package consists of two servings. If the serving size is 250 calories and 10 grams of fat and you eat the whole thing, you have consumed 500 calories and 20 grams of fat. Instead of "biggie-sizing," we should consider "junior-sizing," especially when fats and sugars are involved. One way is to drink a big glass of water and a smaller cup of soda. Note the website under the food label for a wealth of online information.

WEIGHT CONTROL INFORMATION

To control one's weight at a "desirable" level is one of this nation's most passionate goals. Well-founded weight-loss programs and rip-off fad diets flourish side by side in a society seeking the "beautiful" body. Differentiating fact from fallacy can be difficult at times. But two things are clear: (1) excessive weight, especially fat, can be harmful to your health; and (2) there are no magical diets that take off fat quickly and keep it off. In fact, even gradual weight loss through good nutritional dieting can be difficult to maintain. But it can be done, and when exercise is part of the plan, keeping the weight off is easier.

The extra weight many people carry around is an even heavier burden because of its relationship to disease and quality of life. Overweight individuals have a higher incidence of hypertension, high blood cholesterol, heart disease, stroke, some cancers, diabetes, and arthritis. And this does not even address the psychological pain that overweight people endure

1 pound of fat is 3500 calories

Using the Food Label

The food label carries an easier to use nutrition information guide. It is required on almost all packaged foods (compared to about 60% of products until now). The label below is only an example.

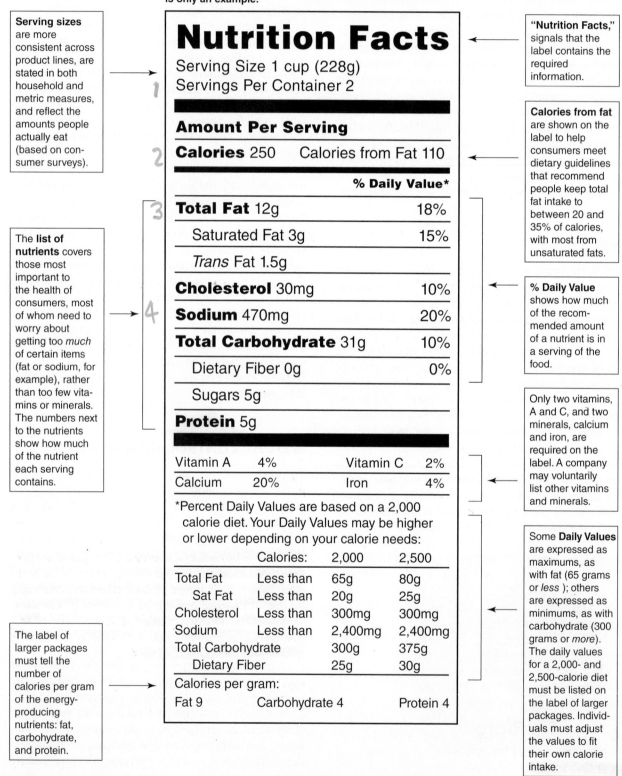

Serving sizes are more consistent across product lines, are stated in both household and metric measures, and reflect the amounts people actually eat (based on consumer surveys).

The list of nutrients covers those most important to the health of consumers, most of whom need to worry about getting too *much* of certain items (fat or sodium, for example), rather than too few vitamins or minerals. The numbers next to the nutrients show how much of the nutrient each serving contains.

The label of larger packages must tell the number of calories per gram of the energy-producing nutrients: fat, carbohydrate, and protein.

"Nutrition Facts," signals that the label contains the required information.

Calories from fat are shown on the label to help consumers meet dietary guidelines that recommend people keep total fat intake to between 20 and 35% of calories, with most from unsaturated fats.

% Daily Value shows how much of the recommended amount of a nutrient is in a serving of the food.

Only two vitamins, A and C, and two minerals, calcium and iron, are required on the label. A company may voluntarily list other vitamins and minerals.

Some **Daily Values** are expressed as maximums, as with fat (65 grams or *less*); others are expressed as minimums, as with carbohydrate (300 grams or *more*). The daily values for a 2,000- and 2,500-calorie diet must be listed on the label of larger packages. Individuals must adjust the values to fit their own calorie intake.

Figure 13.2 Nutrition label. For additional information, go to www.fda.gov/Food/ResourcesForYou/Consumers/NFLPM/usc274593.htm
Source: Food and Drug Administration, 2006.

1-2 a week
8 a month

SERVING SIZE CARD

Figure 13.3 Serving size card.

due to the unfeeling remarks and attitudes of others. Obese individuals can suffer from depression, poor self-image, poor self-esteem, and even job discrimination. Health risks grow with the percentage of over-weightness; therefore, those who are 10% to 15% over their desired weight have only a small additional risk, while the very overweight and obese carry the highest risk.

Body shape is also related to health risk. For reasons not completely understood, individuals with apple-shaped bodies (those who carry extra fat around the abdomen) have a higher incidence of heart disease than those who are pear-shaped (those who tend to store extra fat in the lower body). You can calculate a waist-to-hip ratio to determine if your shape puts you at more risk. Simply measure your waist at your navel, and then your hips at the greatest circumference around the buttocks. Using Worksheet 13.1 (provided at the back of the book and online at

www.pearsonhighered.com/bishopaerobics), divide the waist measurement by the hip measurement. A waist-to-hip ratio greater than 1.0 for men and 0.8 for women indicates an increased cardiac risk. Some experts believe that waist alone or waist, in conjunction with BMI, is a better predictor of risk than BMI alone. Women with a waist circumference greater than 35 inches and men with a circumference greater than 40 inches are considered as high risk regardless of their BMI (body mass index, discussed later in this chapter).

Weight control is a complex process involving a number of factors, including genetics, environment, race, gender, economic status, and psychological factors. Why one person stays thin and another doesn't is not as easily answered as one might think. For example, there is good evidence that obesity runs in families. But is this due to a genetic predisposition or to family eating habits and culturally driven food choices? One study using adopted children illustrates the complex, even contradictory evidence often facing weight control researchers. The adopted girls tended to "look" like their biological parents, especially their biological mothers, while the boys did not bear similarities to either biological parent.

The **set point theory** is a genetic-based theory that asserts that the body has a preset level of fat that it "believes" to be correct and that it will work to ensure. If a person tries to lose weight and drops below the set point, the body encourages weight gain and a return to the set point by conserving fats and increasing appetite. Even when obese individuals (in a controlled setting) are forced to gain weight, they quickly return to their previous weight when allowed to resume their normal eating habits. The biological mechanism at work in set point is still not fully understood. And there are some individuals for whom it doesn't seem to be true: lean people who can eat anything and not gain weight, and a small percentage of obese individuals who can lose weight and keep it off indefinitely. Encouragingly, there is some evidence that aerobic exercise can lower the set point. The fact, however, that so many people have become overweight in recent years lends doubt to this theory, but not to the idea that genetics plays a role. And remember, a genetic predisposition for something does not mean you will develop it. However, it does signal a need to develop good lifestyle habits in terms of eating well and exercising.

Environment plays the most obvious role in weight control. Environment includes everything from your schedule, to the availability of nutritious food, to cultural influences, to personal choices. It is awfully easy to succumb to high-fat foods when they are quick and convenient. And habits developed in childhood can be very difficult to change. The good news, however, is that personal behaviors, unlike genetics, can be changed. Nutrition awareness exercises can help identify environmental triggers, which can then be avoided or handled with good planning.

Overconsumption explains a lot of overweightness, especially when teamed with a sedentary lifestyle. But it does not account for the fact that many obese individuals eat the same, or less, food than individuals of normal weight and still don't lose weight. There is some evidence that obese individuals burn calories more efficiently and can therefore sustain the same activity level on fewer calories than can a person of normal weight. So again, the equation is not as simple as one would expect. Nor does simple consumption account for the thin person who can eat anything and not gain a pound. Some thin people just seem to "burn calories" sitting still—metabolism no doubt plays a role in this.

Psychological factors such as negative emotions also influence people's eating habits. When dealing with emotions such as rejection, anger, or depression, some people find comfort in eating. This can lead to overeating and/or unhealthy binge behaviors. Feeling "too fat" even though one isn't can also lead to unhealthy habits or eating disorders.

One has to wonder what socioeconomic and gender influences are at work when people under the poverty line are fatter than those at the top of the socioeconomic ladder, especially women. The research on weight control is many-faceted and is not always conclusive, but each study brings us a little closer to understanding the puzzle of weight control and management.

OVERWEIGHT, OVERFAT, OBESE

The word "overweight" comes from the idea that there is an ideal weight for each of us, and if you weigh more than that, you are overweight. In the past, if you wanted to see if you were overweight you checked a height/weight chart. One well-known chart was produced by Metropolitan Life, an insurance company that was interested in body weight as a predictor of life expectancy. One problem is that there are a number of charts with various weight ranges for the same height. Today, the phrase "ideal weight" has been replaced with "healthy weight," and in place of the traditional height/weight chart, many professionals recommend calculating **body mass index (BMI).** BMI is easy to calculate and provides a fairly good estimate of healthy weight when the more accurate methods of measuring body fat are not available. (See the section on body composition later in this chapter.) BMI is calculated by dividing your weight in kilograms by the square of your height in meters. The higher your BMI category, the greater your risk for health problems. To calculate your BMI and determine your weight category (healthy weight, overweight, or obese), turn to Worksheet 13.1 at the back of the book and online at www.pearsonhighered.com/bishopaerobics. For both a quick estimate of BMI and to see what category you are in at your height and weight, see Figure 13.4 on page 205. Healthy or normal weights, based on BMI, are believed to be protective. However, recent research suggests that a normal weight as determined by BMI may not be sufficient by itself to lower disease risk; it may be that normal weight must be coupled with cardiorespiratory fitness. This bolsters the argument that diet and exercise should happen together.

Only show height & weight

ARE YOU A HEALTHY WEIGHT?

BMI measures weight in relation to height. The BMI ranges shown above are for adults. They are not exact ranges of healthy and unhealthy weights. However, they show that health risk increases at higher levels of overweight and obesity. Even within the healthy BMI range, weight gains can carry health risks for adults.

Directions: Find your weight on the bottom of the graph. Go straight up from that point until you come to the line that matches your height. Then look to find your weight group.

Healthy Weight BMI from 18.5 up to 25 refers to healthy weight.

Overweight BMI from 25 up to 30 refers to overweight.

Obese BMI 30 or higher refers to obesity. Obese persons are also overweight.

Figure 13.4 Are you a healthy weight? BMI chart.
Source: Report of the Dietary Guidelines Advisory Committee on the Dietary Guidelines for Americans, 2000, page 3.

BMI is not without limitations. It may surprise you, for example, to learn that athletes and other highly muscular individuals weigh more than normal and may be incorrectly categorized as overweight. And BMI doesn't take into account where extra fat is stored. Remember that abdominal fat is associated with a higher risk of disease than fat stored in the lower body. Nor can BMI tell you how many of your pounds are fat rather than lean body mass (muscle, water, organs, etc.). In fact, no distinction can be made between a round, soft person and a lean, muscular person as long as they are the same height, weight, and gender. Using a waist circumference measure together with BMI does help establish risk level.

If instead of thinking in terms of being **overweight,** you think in terms of being overfat, the distinction can be made. **Overfat** is a condition in which the percentage of body weight that is fat weight is too high. A person can be a little or very much overfat. Using fatness as the measure, the muscular "overweight" person can be differentiated from the overfat "overweight" person. **Obese** is a medical term that refers to the storage of excess body fat. It is generally agreed that men with more than 25% stored fat and women with more than 30% stored fat are considered obese. How much of your body is fat weight and how to measure it is discussed in the next section.

BODY COMPOSITION

Imagine the look of confusion you would receive if you walked up to the counter at a delicatessen and asked for 10 pounds. The store clerk would probably look annoyed and ask, "Ten pounds of what? Ham? Salami? Cheese?" Yet every day, people say they are going to lose (or gain) 10 pounds. And who thinks to ask the same critical question: 10 pounds of what? Would a person claiming to be 10 pounds overweight be satisfied if she or he lost 10 pounds of muscle? Would a person trying to gain weight want to gain 10

pounds of fat? Probably not. It is helpful, then, to differentiate between weight and fat weight.

The body's weight can be broken into two components: fat weight (FW) and lean body mass (LBM). Fat weight is made up of two kinds of fat: subcutaneous fat, which is stored between the skin and the muscles, and intramuscular fat, which is stored between muscle fibers. By pinching yourself, you can feel the subcutaneous fat. To picture intramuscular fat, think of how a prime piece of steak (cow's muscle) is marbled with fat. **Lean body mass (LBM)** is derived from the weight of the skeleton, muscles, water, organs, and connective tissue. It is possible to estimate how much of your body is fat weight and how much is lean body mass. This is called assessing your body composition.

Body composition is usually measured and discussed as the percentage of weight that is fat weight. For example, an individual might be said to be 18% fat. Guidelines for healthy percentages of fat for both men and women are shown in Table 13.1. Note that healthy women have higher levels of fat than healthy men do.

To illustrate the importance of examining body composition, consider the following two women. Both are 5'4" and 120 lb and have a small frame size. Both would be considered at an ideal weight according to a height/weight chart, but as you can see on the next page, their body composition may be very different.

Table 13.1 Percent Body Fat Norms for Men and Women*

AGE	VERY LEAN	EXCELLENT	GOOD	FAIR	POOR	VERY POOR
MEN						
20–29	≤ 6%	7–10%	11–15%	16–19%	20–23%	≥ 24%
30–39	≤ 10%	11–14%	15–18%	19–21%	22–25%	≥ 26%
40–49	≤ 13%	14–17%	18–20%	21–23%	24–27%	≥ 28%
50–59	≤ 14%	15–19%	20–22%	23–24%	25–28%	≥ 29%
WOMEN						
20–29	≤ 13%	14–16%	17–19%	20–23%	24–27%	≥ 28%
30–39	≤ 14%	15–17%	18–21%	22–25%	26–29%	≥ 30%
40–49	≤ 16%	17–20%	21–24%	25–28%	29–32%	≥ 33%
50–59	≤ 17%	18–22%	23–27%	28–30%	31–34%	≥ 35%

*Assumes nonathletes. For athletes, recommended body fat is 5 to 15 percent for men and 12 to 22 percent for women. Note that there are no agreed-upon national standards for recommended body fat percentage.

Source: Based on data from The Cooper Institute, Dallas, TX, www.cooperinstitute.org.

PERSON A		**PERSON B**	
Total weight:	120 lb	Total weight:	120 lb
Fat weight:	24 lb	Fat weight:	38 lb
LBM weight:	96 lb	LBM weight:	82 lb
Percent fat:	20%	Percent fat:	32%
Rating:	**healthy**	Rating:	**obese**

Until groups such as the military, commercial airlines, and cheerleaders realized the difference between overweight and overfat, they were denying valuable, highly fit individuals entry to their programs. Unfortunately, some programs still expect individuals to be at certain weight levels to participate. When a trim, toned individual goes on a crash diet to reach this level, it usually means losing water and muscle to do so. Not only is this highly undesirable, it is also dangerous. People should not be expected to reduce weight levels, they should be expected to attain appropriate body compositions.

The most accurate way to determine the amount of fat a person has is to measure it directly, but unless you are willing to be a cadaver, an indirect and slightly less accurate method is the way to go. There are four common ways to assess body composition. One of the more accurate indirect measures is taken using **hydrostatic** or **underwater weighing.** With this method, a person sits on a platform that is attached to a scale. The platform is lowered into the water until the person is totally submerged. After the person exhales as much air as possible, a weight measurement is taken. Because fat floats, a fatter person will weigh less under water than a lean person. The underwater weight is adjusted to account for any air left in the lungs after full exhalation and any gas trapped in the gastrointestinal tract. Finally, an estimate of fat is computed.

This process is fairly costly in both time and facilities. It requires expensive equipment and well-trained technicians. Although you do not have to be a swimmer to participate, this procedure does not work well with individuals who are uncomfortable under water. If you are comfortable in water and wish to be underwater weighed, check with the physical education department at a university or college or with a local sports medicine center. Most places charge a fee for this service. Sometimes when people are being trained in the procedure, volunteers are weighed at no cost. Be prepared for the process to take at least an hour.

A less expensive, quicker, and more convenient method of assessing body fat is the **skin-fold technique.** It is a little less accurate than underwater weighing, but it still provides a good useful estimate. A caliper is used to measure the thickness of the subcutaneous fat at several sites. The technician uses one hand to pull the skin and subcutaneous fat away from the muscle with his or her thumb and forefinger. With the other hand, she or he uses the caliper to measure the width of the pinched fat (Figure 13.5). The measurements from the different sites are added, and this sum is put into a formula. Some formulas use only one site, some three, and some six or more. Scientists use the multiple-site formulas for accuracy and then recommend the most predictive sites for general use. Some of the most commonly used sites are the back of the arm, just above the hip, the abdomen, just below the shoulder blade, and the front of the thigh. It is easier to train technicians to measure skin folds than to perform underwater weighing. In addition, skin-fold equipment is easily brought to the exercise site. When a fee is charged for this service, it is usually quite small and the test takes only a few minutes.

Another method of analyzing body composition uses what is called a body analyzer or impedance machine. This machine sends a small, harmless electrical impulse through the body. The computer records both the time the impulse takes to travel through the body and the amount of resistance the impulse encounters. The impulse travels quickly and with little resistance through water, which makes up a good portion of muscle. It meets more resistance and travels more slowly through fat, since fat is a poor electrical conductor. The computer uses this data to compute your percentage of body fat. Because this method depends on total body

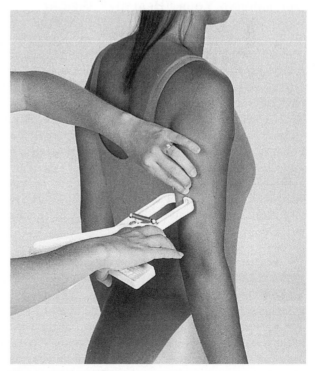

Figure 13.5 Skin-fold measurement.

water values, it is important to be at an appropriate level of hydration each time you are tested. Working out before the test or retaining water due to menstruation can throw off the accuracy of this test. Some universities, hospitals, and health clubs have these machines available but usually charge a fee for their use. The test only takes a few minutes and may be accompanied by a computer printout that includes your percentage of fat, recommended weight, and how to attain your recommended weight. Some professionals still question the accuracy of this test, while others believe it to be as accurate as the skin-fold technique when subsequent tests are performed at a similar hydration level.

The newest method for determining body composition uses air displacement and pressure-volume relationships. In this method, a person sits inside an egg-shaped fiberglass chamber commercially called the Bod Pod. The air inside the unit is measured before and after the person enters. The difference represents the person's body volume. This is then used to calculate body density and percent body fat. One big advantage to this method is that people are much more comfortable sitting in an air-filled chamber than being dunked underwater for hydrostatic weighing. The air displacement plethysmography method is very accurate, but if it is available, a fee is often charged. Tight clothing such as spandex shorts, a stretch cap, and, for women, a sports bra, must be worn to get accurate readings.

DETERMINING YOUR "HEALTHY" WEIGHT

While we do not know for sure what constitutes a healthy weight, we do know enough to make educated guesses. How healthy your weight is depends on how much of it is fat, where on your body extra fat is located, and whether or not you have weight-related medical problems or a high risk of weight-related disease. There are several ways to determine your healthy weight. You can consult a height/weight chart or use BMI to identify a healthy weight, as described in the previous section. The most accurate way is to calculate your healthy weight using your present percentage of body fat. You will need to have your percentage of body fat estimated using one of the techniques described in the body composition section. Using Table 13.1 on page 206 to guide you, determine the body fat percentage you would like to have. The range for good health is 10% to 25% fat for men and 18% to 30% fat for women. (If you are interested in competitive athletics, you may want to select a percentage of fat from the performance range.) Turn to Worksheet 13.1 at the back of the book and online at www.pearsonhighered.com/bishopaerobics, and subtract your desired percentage of fat from your actual percentage of fat. If the result

is a positive number, multiply your present weight by it and subtract the answer from your present weight; if it is a negative number, drop the negative sign, multiply your present weight by it, and then add it to your present weight. Here is an example of the calculation for a woman weighing 160 lb with 32% body fat who wants to drop to 25% body fat. (Remember to convert the percentage to decimal form before multiplying. For example, 6% = 6/100 = 0.06.)

$$32\% - 25\% = 7\% = 0.07$$
$$160 \text{ lb} \times 0.07 = 11.2 \text{ (rounded down to 11)}$$
$$160 - 11 = 149 \text{ lb (healthy weight)}$$

Use your "healthy weight" to determine how much weight you need to lose or gain.

WEIGHT MANAGEMENT

The goal of weight management is to achieve a healthy weight and then maintain it. Diet and exercise can be used to maintain, gain, or lose weight. When the number of calories you consume matches the number of calories you expend, you are in **energy balance.** When you consume more calories than you expend, you create a positive energy balance, and you gain weight. When you consume fewer calories than you expend, you create a negative energy balance and lose weight. To change your energy balance, you can change the number of calories you eat, change the number of calories you burn, or, best of all, combine the effects of both. The next three sections discuss how exercise and diet can be used to achieve a desired weight loss, a healthy weight gain, and weight maintenance. See also the accompanying box, Weight Management.

WEIGHT LOSS

Weight loss should be gradual, about 1–2 lb a week. This gradual weight loss will keep you off the dieting roller coaster and give you the chance to change your lifestyle so that the weight stays off. One pound of fat contains 3,500 calories; to lose it in 1 week you have three choices. You can eat 3,500 fewer calories per week, which is 500 fewer calories per day; you can eat your same diet and exercise off the 500 calories every day; or you can eat 200 fewer calories and exercise off the other 300. The latter is the easiest approach and meets the health recommendation of expending 300 to 500 calories through exercise.

During the first week of a proper diet, you may experience a rapid weight loss. After this initial weight

The more muscle your body has the more it burns

loss, work for a steady 1- to 2-lb loss per week, and don't feel discouraged if your weight remains constant from time to time.

It is a good idea to limit caloric decreases to 500 calories per day or 1,000 calories per day if your diet is above 3,000 calories. Also, women should be sure to consume a minimum of 1,200 calories a day and men a minimum of 1,500 calories a day to maintain the basic nutritional needs of the body. Diets that contain fewer calories should be performed only under the care of a physician.

The following is a short list of helpful hints if you are trying to eat fewer calories.

1. Eat planned meals evenly spaced throughout the day to help keep your level of blood sugar steady.
2. Eat fiber-rich foods, which are bulky and will help make you feel full.
3. Eat baked, broiled, or poached meats and steamed vegetables. Avoid fried or sautéd foods.
4. Eat more slowly so that the meal lasts longer even though you are eating less.
5. Switch to skim milk and low-fat dairy products.
6. Eat low-fat meats whenever possible. Poultry (except duck and goose), especially white meat, and fish are good low-fat choices. Red meat is generally high in saturated fat.
7. Limit the number of times you eat out. This will keep you from eating foods you ordinarily wouldn't cook. And remember, restaurants cook with lots of butter, salt, and fattening sauces.
8. Plan your meals. It's easy to end up eating fat-laden fast foods when you are hungry and there is nothing to eat in the house.
9. Write down everything you eat. Awareness is half the battle.
10. Keep fattening foods out of the house. This helps eliminate temptation.
11. Allow yourself a few sweets during the week, or daily if necessary, so that you aren't tempted to binge on them.
12. Pick one or two areas to improve in at one time. Gradual changes in lifestyle are easier to accept than radically new ones. In other words, don't try to break two favorite habits at the same time, such as drinking too much soda and overeating sweets; take them one at a time.

WEIGHT LOSS AND EXERCISE

There are two really good reasons to combine a healthy weight loss diet with exercise. First is the benefit of changing your body composition – not just losing fat, but also gaining lean body mass (muscle). This will make you look better, give you the muscle fitness to engage in recreational and life activities, and boost metabolism a little bit as muscle burns more calories than fat at rest. A second really important reason to incorporate exercise in your weight management is that exercise is the best predictor of keeping weight off. People who are active 60 – 90 minutes a day are the most successful at keeping lost weight off. So if you are serious about attaining *and* maintaining a healthy body composition, exercise needs to be part of the equation. The exercise guideline previously discussed, 30 minutes of moderately intense physical activity on most or all days of the week, is a good starting place for individuals adding exercise to their weight loss program. If you have not been exercising, you may need to start with fewer days a week, shorter exercise sessions, or both. Consult a fitness specialist. People with excess weight may also need to begin with non-weight bearing activities, such as cycling or aquatic exercises, to prevent overloading the joints. As fitness improves, the frequency of exercise should increase to near daily and the duration and intensity and the duration and intensity should gradually increase as well. For weight loss, The Institute of Medicine of the National Academy of Sciences recommends 60 minutes of moderate-intensity physical activity most days of the week. Data from the National Weight Control Registry (www.nwcr.ws) shows that people who lost at least 30 pounds and were successful keeping it off for 6 years were physically active about 90 minutes a day. This may seem like a lot, but an hour a day (perhaps done in 4 15-minute intervals) to keep weight off is a pretty good trade-off, especially considering all the physical and emotional benefits. If moderate intensity longer duration exercise does not appeal to you, and time in your day is short, read on.

There has been a lot of discussion and misunderstanding concerning the intensity of exercise that is best for burning fat. When you are sitting still, you are actually burning a high percentage of fat. The problem is you are not burning very many overall calories so even though most are fat, you aren't burning very many fat calories. As you increase the intensity of your physical activity, you increase the overall number of calories you are burning. For a while fat dominates but the percentage of fat begins to decrease and the percentage of carbohydrate increases. Intense exercise burns predominantly carbohydrate. The important thing to note however, is that as intensity goes up so does the number of calories burned per minute. So even if you are burning a lower percentage of fat, you may be burning the same or more overall fat calories. Here is an example to make this point more clearly.

If you exercise in the "fat burning zone" indicated on an exercise machine, you are likely exercising at an intensity of about 65% of your maximum heart rate and at this intensity you are burning about an equal number of fat and carbohydrate calories. So if an average person burns 250 calories in 30 minutes at this level, the fat burned would be 50% of 220 or 120 calories. Let's take that person and put them at an intensity closer to 85% (cardio zone) and assume that about 330 calories are burned in 30 minutes. But now only approximately a third of the calories are from fat. Taking 33% of 330 we find that the person has burned 120 calories. So in both cases the person burned the same amount of fat but at the higher intensity an additional 110 calories were burned. Bottom line – most people can go longer and burn more calories at a moderate intensity but for those who can exercise at a higher intensity, this too can be effective. Right now the research leans toward long duration for keeping weight off but the best way to be active is the way that feels good to you and that you are willing to do for the long term.

FUELING YOUR WORKOUT

Fat, carbohydrate, and protein can all be used to fuel movement. The amount of each that is used depends on the intensity and duration of the activity, a person's fitness level, and diet. Fat and carbohydrate are the main sources for movement energy. Protein only contributes about 2% of the fuel for less than an hour of exercise, slightly higher for intense prolonged exercise.[1] At rest, almost all of the body's energy is provided by fat metabolism, but because little energy is being expended, not much fat is burned. Moving at low intensities (less than 30% of VO_2max), energy is still predominantly supplied by fat with carbohydrate supplying the balance. Consider then what happens when the intensity or duration of activity increases.

- If a person increases activity or exercise to a higher intensity (above 30% VO_2max), the percentage of fat burning will decrease and that of carbohydrate increase. The point where carbohydrate exceeds fat is called the "crossover point." As intensity continues to increase the reliance on carbohydrates will grow.
- If a person stays at a relatively low intensity, one where the percentage of fat to carbohydrate is fairly equal, and is active for a prolonged amount

of time (more than 30 minutes), the percentage of fat being burned will slowly increase and the percentage of carbohydrate slowly decrease. In other words, prolonged low intensity exercise results in a higher percentage of fat burning.

These discoveries have led individuals to believe that because exercising longer at low intensities burns more fat, it is the preferable way to approach weight management. This is, however, only partially true. If the individual trying to lose fat is at a low fitness level and low-intensity activity is the healthiest choice, then exercising at a low intensity for longer (building up to 60–90 minutes) is the way to go. If, however, the individual is able to exercise at a higher intensity, shorter duration exercise can actually burn as many or more calories from fat. Less time, more fat burned? How can this be if higher intensity activity favors carbohydrates? The answer has to do with how many calories are being burned. The more vigorous the exercise, the more calories burned. As exercise intensity goes up, the *percentage* of fat being burned goes down, but the actual *number* of fat calories burned will increase because the total number of calories used increases.

Imagine that you are eating at a slow pace. You consume 12 food items: 50% are carrots, 50% are avocado slices. Eating at a faster pace, you consume 24 items: 66.6% are carrots, and 33.3% are avocado slices. Notice that in the first case you ate 6 avocado slices (50% of 12), while in the second case you consumed 8 avocado slices (33.3% of 24). The percentage drops (50% to 33.3%), but the actual number of avocado slices increases.

Now turn it around and think of the avocado as fat being burned. Moderate exercise burns more fat calories than low-intensity exercise if the two are performed for the same amount of time. (*Note:* The percentages used in the avocado/carrot example do not represent the real percentages of fat being burned.)

Increasing the amount of time you exercise at low intensity can offset this difference. Very high intensities burn a lot of calories per minute, but most people find it difficult and uncomfortable to sustain high-intensity exercise. The risk of injury also increases, and mainly carbohydrate is burned. Regardless of how much fat or carbohydrate you are burning at any given time, the key is to burn more calories than you take in over the day.

[1]   S. K. Powers and E.T. Howley. *Exercise Physiology: Theory and Application to Fitness and Performance*. 6th ed. New York: Mcgraw-Hill, 2006, 62–9.

WEIGHT MANAGEMENT

KEY RECOMMENDATIONS

- To maintain body weight in a healthy range, balance calories consumed with calories expended.

- To prevent gradual weight gain over time, make small decreases in caloric intake and increase physical activity.

Fitness professionals recommend that a person expend 300 to 500 calories per exercise session. Individuals at a low fitness level may have to begin with a 200-calorie expenditure, but with gradual overload, they can safely reach a 300-calorie expenditure in about 8 to 12 weeks.

A heavy person will burn more calories than a lighter person doing the same activity because the former must move more weight. Corbin and Lindsey in *Fitness for Life* estimate the following numbers of calories per hour for dance exercise for the body weights listed:

POUNDS	CALORIES/HOUR	CALORIES/MINUTE
100	315	5.25
120	357	5.95
150	420	7.00
180	483	8.05
200	525	8.75

To estimate the number of calories you burn in your class, perform the following easy calculation: Multiply the calories/minute for your weight by the number of minutes in your class.

A 150-pound person would burn 7 calories per minute (420 ÷ 60). In a 50-minute class, this person would burn 350 calories (50 × 7). This class would fulfill the 300- to 500-calorie expenditure requirement for those trying to lose weight. Keep in mind that these are averages (calories/minute). If you are performing an intense version of aerobics, the calorie burn may be higher.

Besides the obvious calorie-burning effect, exercise also provides hidden benefits. Your basal metabolic rate is the rate at which your body uses energy to sustain vital functions when you are at rest. When you exercise, your metabolism increases; therefore, you burn more calories. What you may not be aware of is that your metabolic rate remains raised for a period of time following exercise. Another benefit, albeit a very small one, is that a pound of muscle burns a few more calories per day than a pound of fat. If you gain 5 lb of

muscle, that is about 35 calories a day. This means you are burning more calories without even trying.

A final advantage for adding regular exercise to your diet regimen is that fit people start to burn fat more quickly during exercise than unfit people do. It may seem unfair, but fit people have a definite advantage when it comes to weight control. If it is possible, have your percentage of body fat estimated in about 8-week intervals to see how you are doing. You can also take body measurements to see whether you are slimming down. Inches may come off even when pounds don't. Muscle-weight additions may be counteracting fat-weight losses. Because muscle weighs more than fat, you can actually gain weight, lose fat, and look better all at the same time!

UNBALANCED DIETS, FADS, AND GIMMICKS

Some of the best nonfiction sellers are diet books. An amazing amount of money is spent on diet books, counseling, and products. Many good diet books and diet plans are available, but a tremendous number also violate the most fundamental rules of good nutrition. They are called fad diets because someone makes a lot of money on them when they first come out, and then they pass into anonymity when dieters find out they don't work. Weight-loss fad diets are easy to spot. They promise quick weight losses and advocate unbalanced diets. They depend on your not caring what kind of weight you lose. When you lose more than 1 to 2 lbs a week, you will lose beneficial muscle and water weight to do it. For example, you can wrap yourself in plastic and sweat off pounds of water, pop diet pills that cause food to race through your system without being digested, or drink protein drinks and avoid carbohydrates so that you lose substantial amounts of lean tissue and water. If it is fat you are trying to lose, don't get drawn into a fad diet.

A fad diet that stresses one type of food does so by limiting or excluding intake from one or more of the other food groups. When you don't eat adequate amounts from each food group, you don't obtain all of the essential nutrients. This lack of necessary nutrients can leave you fatigued, depressed, and irritable. Even top athletes who manipulate their diet to carbohydrate load (a process of lowering and raising carbohydrate intake to "trick" the body into storing more glycogen for big events) will tell you that irritability and discomfort often accompany the periods of low carbohydrate consumption.

High-protein diets translate into low-carbohydrate and, often, high-fat diets. When your body does not have sufficient quantities of carbohydrates and fats, it uses protein for energy. Nitrogen is a by-product of the protein energy cycle. Too much nitrogen can be toxic. In an effort to clear the body of excess nitrogen, the kidneys combine it with water to make ammonia. The ammonia is excreted in the urine. (It can also be sweated out in small amounts.) When a lot of protein is consumed, the body has to work very hard to clear the nitrogen. Large quantities of water are needed for this process. High-protein diet plans usually tell you to drink an additional 6 to 8 glasses of water per day. Try drinking 16 glasses of water a day; few people can, and so too often the result is dehydration. If the diet is continued, dehydration can become severe, which can lead to kidney failure and death. Even if you don't dehydrate, the low level of carbohydrates will probably make you feel irritable, sick, and fatigued. High-protein diets often encourage high consumption of meats and dairy foods, which can lead to an unhealthy diet full of saturated fats.

Near-starvation diets, crash diets, and prolonged fasting send signals to your body that food is not available and that your life may be threatened. Sensing starvation, the body conserves the energy it has available. In fact, your body may even begin storing the energy as fat to compensate. Your body actually adjusts itself to survive on fewer calories. Activating this survival instinct makes it more difficult for you to lose fat or, eventually, any form of weight. In fact, some people who are overfat actually eat fewer calories than individuals of normal weight. When you've been on the crash-diet roller coaster, your body needs some time to readjust to a steady caloric diet.

You have already learned how important it is to stay well hydrated. It doesn't make sense, then, to purposely try to lose water. Keeping this in mind, you can avoid some of the diet gimmicks that promise you weight loss and deliver by causing a water-weight loss. For example, rubber suits and plastic wrappings trap in heat so that you sweat out pounds of water. Saunas and whirlpools also sweat out water weight. Some of the diet pills are diuretics that cause you to lose water through frequent urination. Waist and thigh belts temporarily push and sweat water out of targeted areas so

that measurements taken immediately after the belt is removed show lost inches. In a couple of hours, the inches are back. Any program that depends on excessive water loss for weight reduction is dangerous and ineffective. You want to lose fat, not water.

Also watch out for "all you can eat" approaches to dieting. If you eat more calories than you expend, you will gain weight. The origin of the calories doesn't matter; if there are too many, they will be stored as fat. Moreover, if all the calories come from a restricted list of foods, you may miss some essential nutrients.

Perhaps one of the all-time biggest diet and exercise myths is **spot reducing.** You cannot choose where the fat will come off your body. In general, it will come off gradually all over. Genetics plays a role in where you tend to store fat. To eliminate fat, you must first burn more calories than you consume. Don't fall into the trap of thinking that because you use your legs to run, you will get rid of the fat on your thighs more quickly. Running on your hands could be just as effective in removing leg fat. Of course, running on your legs will tone up the leg muscles underneath the fat, and running on your hands would certainly help tone your arms.

Eating Disorders

Some individuals start to diet and then can't stop. They look in the mirror and continue to see a fat person. One such disease, **anorexia nervosa,** is widespread among women. Men can also suffer from it, but the estimated cases of men with anorexia nervosa are thought to be relatively few (about one in ten) at this time. Anorexia nervosa is often associated with life-threatening weight losses and denial of weight loss by the dieter. This disease requires both psychological and medical assistance. If you know anyone suffering from anorexia, do everything possible to get him or her to professional help. Otherwise, your friend may literally starve himself or herself to death.

Bulimia, another eating disorder, is characterized by eating regular-sized or large meals and then intentionally emptying the food out of the stomach by self-induced vomiting or the use of laxatives. The lining of the throat and esophagus can become damaged from repeated contact with stomach acids during regurgitation. People suffering from bulimia look healthy, especially since they try to hide their binge-and-purge behavior. Like people who exhibit anorexia, those who suffer from bulimia need immediate psychological and medical attention.

Binge-eating disorder is characterized by episodes of uncontrolled excessive and rapid overeating. Because there is no purging, theses individuals tend to be overweight or obese. Often ashamed of their eating habits, they dine alone. The cause is not known, but this disorder may be accompanied by feelings of anger, sadness, boredom, or depression. Both women and men suffer from this disorder, approximately two men for every three women. Eating disorder conditions are completely reversible if caught early enough. Help is as close as the health and counseling centers on campus.

WEIGHT GAIN

At first it's hard to imagine that anyone would want to gain weight, but there are actually quite a number of people who need weight-gain diets. Certainly, undernourished individuals and people recovering from illnesses and accidents fall into this category. On a brighter note, so do athletes and body builders who are trying to put on lean body mass and a few, such as sumo wrestlers, who are actually trying to put on fat as well. Of course, pregnant women must be on weight-gain diets.

To gain lean body weight, you increase your calorie consumption so that it exceeds your calorie expenditure and continue to exercise. If you only increase what you eat and don't exercise, you store the extra calories as fat. (Pregnant women are the exception to this rule.) As mentioned previously, you should add the calories in a way that maintains the recommended percentages of carbohydrates, protein, and fat. A common mistake is to increase protein intake without making a corresponding increase in carbohydrate intake. The body ends up with an excess of protein and too few carbohydrates to fuel the exercise workout.

Muscle (lean body mass) is most effectively increased through progressive resistance exercises such as weight training. Participants in group fitness exercise gain lean body mass, depending on their initial strength and whether they use body position and resistance equipment to place a sufficient demand on their muscles. Aerobically trained individuals tend to have lean bodies but not as much muscle mass as those who train more specifically for strength.

A pregnant woman's weight gain is a little different, but it still involves eating more calories than daily activity expends. The extra calories are used to sustain the higher metabolic rate of the mother and for the growth and development of the baby. Roughly speaking, a pregnant woman needs to consume an extra 300 calories per day. If a woman begins an exercise program after getting pregnant, she needs to eat enough extra calories to support the activity as well. Pregnancy weight gains and exercise programs during and after pregnancy should always be done in consultation with a physician.

WEIGHT MAINTENANCE

Maintaining a healthy weight is like standing on your hands. Watch gymnasts carefully and you will see them make slight adjustments with their fingertips and wrists the whole time they are upside down. Balance is dynamic, not static. To keep your weight and body composition in balance, you constantly need to be aware of your body's needs and activity level and adjust your intake accordingly. The first lesson in this adjustment usually occurs in the late teens when you hear yourself remarking, "I haven't changed my diet at all, and suddenly I'm gaining weight." This is probably because you are done growing and don't need as many calories. It may also reflect a change in lifestyle. Whenever you become more or less physically active, whether the activity is job or exercise related, you need to adjust your diet accordingly. Imagine the different caloric needs of a teenager, a nursing mother, a construction worker, a business executive, and an elderly person. Some of the critical adjustment periods occur the first year of college, during and after pregnancy, around middle age, and at retirement. Listening to your body, adjusting your dietary intake, and maintaining a regular exercise regimen can keep you in balance throughout your life.

SUMMARY

Each nutrient plays a special role in your health and well-being, which makes it vital to eat a balanced diet. Being aware of what you are putting in your mouth is the key to eating a balanced, nutritious diet. As an awareness project, record what you eat on a weekday and a weekend day using Worksheets 13.2 and 13.3, available online at www.pearsonhighered.com/bishopaerobics and answer the questions. You may be surprised at what you discover.

The bottom line of weight control is that there are no known quick and easy ways to lose fat. You put it on gradually; it must come off gradually. Exercise makes the process a little easier and a lot more fun.

COMMONLY ASKED QUESTIONS

Will exercise increase my appetite?

Some people worry that exercise will make them hungrier and that they will eat as many or more calories than they exercised off. This does not seem to be the case. Most people who exercise at a moderate intensity eat the same or just slightly more calories—not enough to overtake their increased expenditure. Lean individuals will generally increase their caloric intake to maintain their weight. Moderate exercise one to two hours before a meal may actually decrease appetite, but there is some evidence that hunger returns several hours later. You can take advantage of this if you plan a low-calorie snack for later.

Is yo-yo dieting dangerous to my health?

Yo-yo dieting, losing and gaining back weight repeatedly, also known as weight cycling, was initially reported to be harmful and connected to an increased risk of some diseases. More research on this has not been able to conclusively link yo-yo dieting with greater health risk, other than perhaps depression and loss of self-esteem as a result of repeated failures. Professionals recommend that people who are obese or substantially overweight should try to lose weight even if they tend to put it back on, because any weight loss at this level can have significant health benefits. Just a 10% weight loss greatly reduces disease risk and may improve blood pressure, lipids, and blood glucose.

Should I eat more when I exercise?

If you are trying to maintain or gain weight, yes. If you are trying to lose weight, no. You should, however, maintain at least a 1,200-calorie diet if you are a woman, and 1,500 calories per day if you are a man. Pregnant women who exercise should eat enough additional calories to offset the exercise plus the recommended extra 300 calories a day.

How do I get rid of cellulite?

Cellulite is ordinary fat stored under the skin where it is separated into little compartments by connective fibers. It gets its dimplelike appearance when the fat cells increase in size and bulge out between the connective fibers. The extent to which you develop cellulite is dependent on the amount of fat you store, the strength of the connective fibers, and the thickness of your skin. In women, as compared with men, the fibers tend to be more taut and the skin thinner so that the dimpling is more apparent. Pills, teas, creams, and rolling it under grandmother's rolling pin will not rid you of this fat. Like all fat, it responds to exercise and a balanced low-fat diet. If you have attained a healthy percentage of fat and still have some cellulite, you may have to call a truce.

When should I drink water?

You should stay hydrated at all times. This means that you should drink water about half an hour before class and be sure to replenish your liquids after exercising. Drinking water during class is also a healthy habit. If the class is only an hour long, you probably don't need to stop and get a drink. But if you are thirsty, by all means get one. If you are involved in prolonged exercise, you should drink about half a cup of fluids every half-hour. It is even more critical to drink water on hot days. Thirst is not a good indicator of your need for water during exercise. Drink before you get thirsty.

Will a candy bar before class give me quick energy?

.It will give you a short burst of energy and then actually drop your blood sugar. Whenever the blood glucose level gets too high, the pancreas excretes insulin, which acts to lower the blood sugar. When a lot of sugar is introduced to the system quickly, the pancreas puts out a lot of insulin. That much insulin ends up dropping the blood sugar below the level it was at prior to the candy. Halfway through class, you may suddenly feel very hungry or even sluggish from low blood sugar. Some people are affected more than others. You would be better off eating a few crackers or a piece of fruit before class.

Do I really need to eat breakfast before a morning aerobics class?

Not necessarily. The important thing is that you eat a balanced diet over the course of the day. Many early-morning exercisers eat breakfast after they exercise. However, it would probably be a good idea to hydrate yourself by drinking water or juice before exercising. Other people find they need to eat breakfast to boost their blood sugar before exercising.

Does caffeine improve exercise performance?

Research has shown that caffeine can improve long-distance running performance, but ingesting caffeine has two drawbacks. One is that you end up needing to go to the bathroom in the middle of the race. The other is that since caffeine is a diuretic, you will dehydrate more quickly. There doesn't appear to be any advantage in having caffeine before a typical group exercise class. In fact, in terms of your health, you are better off limiting your caffeine intake, especially if you have high blood pressure.

Can I eat just fruits instead of fruits and vegetables?

A variety of just fruits can provide you with about the same compliment of vitamins and minerals as vegetables but will not provide you with the same richness of phytochemicals and carotenoids needed to help fight heart disease and cancer. There is also still much to understand about how different foods interact. So the healthiest path today is to provide your body with a wide variety of both fruits and vegetables.

Should I change my diet if I start an exercise program?

That depends on what your current diet is and whether you are trying to maintain, lose, or gain weight. If you are eating a healthy, well-balanced diet and are content with your present body composition, you will need to consume more calories to replace the calories you will expend during exercise. For more information, refer to page 211.

If I stop exercising, will my muscle turn to fat?

Not exactly. The muscle does not magically turn into fat. However, when you stop exercising, you will likely lose lean body mass (muscle) from disuse, and, if you do not alter your diet, the calories once expended during exercise will be stored as fat. This is the problem many athletes experience when they graduate and decrease their high levels of training. The key is to keep moving and adjust diet and exercise to your ever-changing life needs.

Are there good carbohydrates and bad carbohydrates?

Yes, there are nutrient-dense and nutrient-empty carbohydrates. See page 194.

Are there good fats and bad fats?

Saturated fats increase the risk of some diseases, whereas unsaturated fats are either neutral or help decrease cholesterol and disease risk. Some, such as omega-3 fatty acids, promote health. See page 196.

Do I need more protein if I am resistance training? Endurance training?

You may need more than the recommended 0.8 g/kg per day, but you will also need more calories overall to sustain your activity. The percentage of protein compared to carbohydrates and fats will not change significantly, but the total amount of calories will. Athletic levels of training may require 1.2 to 1.7 g of protein per kg body weight. Most individuals already consume more protein than they need, even for active exercising regimens.

How can I eat healthy when I'm so busy?

There are a lot of healthy foods that are easy to carry with you. Consider stocking up on these and keeping them handy where you live and in your car if you are a commuter. At first this will take some effort (for example, reading food labels), but when you've become used to doing so, you'll find that it's pretty easy. For example, when you find yourself hungry, avoid the temptation to go for fast food. Instead, eat a handful of nuts. They are better for you and will hold you until you can get to a healthier meal.

KNOWLEDGE TIPS

1. The diet should consist of 45% to 65% carbohydrates, 10% to 35% protein, and 20% to 35% fat.

2. Carbohydrate is the primary source of energy for the body. Fat is used for energy when prolonged periods of activity demand it. Protein is used for energy when there is a shortage of available carbohydrate.

3. Dietary fat from unsaturated fats is healthier than saturated or *trans* fat.

4. A balanced diet should depend primarily on fruits, vegetables, whole-grain breads, cereals, rice, pasta, low-fat milk, yogurt, and cheese, and meats, poultry, fish, dry beans, eggs, and nuts.

5. Vitamins play an essential role in the release of energy from foods.

6. Minerals are inorganic compounds that supply strength and rigidity to body structures and play an important role in the regulation of body processes.

7. Eat fruits and vegetables high in antioxidants and phytochemicals to help reduce risk of cancer and heart disease.

8. Proper hydration is critical to physical health and performance.

9. Plain cool water is the best source of hydration/rehydration for fitness exercisers exercising for one hour or less. Water is absorbed into the body more quickly than sugared drinks.

10. Healthy body composition is characterized by a relatively low percentage of body fat and a relatively high percentage of lean body mass. Healthy women require a higher percentage of fat than do healthy men.

11. During energy balance, caloric intake is equal to caloric expenditure. Weight is gained when intake surpasses expenditure. Weight is lost when expenditure surpasses intake.

12. Genetics, environment, socioeconomic status, gender, and psychological factors all play a role in weight control.

13. High-intensity activity burns more calories per minute than low-intensity activity. Yet, most people are more successful using longer durations at low to moderate intensities than shorter durations at higher intensities to burn the same number of calories.

14. High-intensity work primarily burns carbohydrate. Moderate-intensity work burns carbohydrate and fat.

15. Moderate intensity physical activity most days of the week, for 60 to 90 minutes, is recommended for losing weight and keeping it off.

16. Anorexia nervosa, bulimia, and binge-eating are eating disorders that require immediate medical and psychological attention.

17. Unbalanced and rapid weight-loss diets can be dangerous, even life-threatening.

18. Most weight-loss experts recommend losing about 1 to 2 lb per week.

THINK ABOUT IT

1. Identify the six essential nutrients and explain their key roles.

2. Why do some foods give you more nutrition than others? Give examples.

3. What is the difference between simple and complex carbohydrates?

4. What are "good" fat and "bad" fat?

5. Identify good food sources of fiber.

6. Explain the concept of energy balance and the role exercise can play in it.

7. Describe the role and quantity of protein needed for muscle building.

8. Why is it better to measure body composition than weight?

9. What are some techniques for measuring body composition?

10. What are some good strategies for managing weight?

11. Explain how fat and carbohydrate burning are affected by exercise intensity and duration.

12. What kinds of substitution changes can you make to eat healthier (such as switching to skim milk from whole milk)?

13. How can your diet affect your mood? How can your mood affect your diet?

REFERENCES

Ahrens, J. N., L. K. Lloyd, S. H. Crixell, and J. L. Walker. "The Effects of Caffeine in Women During Aerobic-Dance Bench Stepping." *International Journal of Sport Nutrition and Exercise Metabolism* 17 (No. 1, 2007): 27–34.

American College of Sports Medicine. "Appropriate Intervention Strategies for Weight Loss and Prevention of Weight Regain for Adults." *Medicine and Science in Sports and Exercise* 33 (No. 12, 2001): 2145–56.

American College of Sports Medicine and American Dietetic Association. "Joint Position Statement on Nutrition and Athletic Performance." *Medicine and Science in Sports and Exercise* 41 (No. 3, 2009): 709–31.

American Dietetic Association. "Position Statement on Nutrition and Physical Fitness." *Journal of the American Dietetic Association* 76 (1980): 437–43.

———. "Position of the American Dietetic Association: Nutrition Intervention in the Treatment of Anorexia Nervosa, Bulimia Nervosa, and Binge Eating." *Journal of the American Dietetic Association* 94 (No. 8, 1994): 902–7.

———. "Position of the American Dietetic Association: Vegetarian Diets." *Journal of the American Dietetic Association* 97 (No. 11, 1997): 1317–21.

Blake, J. S. *Nutrition and You*. 2nd ed. San Francisco: Pearson Education, 2012.

Expert Q&A: Getting Started with a Weight Loss Plan. Retrieved on 11/21/12 from http://www.webmd.com/diet/features/expert-qa-starting-weight-loss-plan-james-o-hill?page=3

Food and Nutrition Information Center. *Dietary Guidelines for Americans: A Historical Overview*. Beltsville, MD: National Agricultural Library USDA, 2008.

Foster, C., D. L. Costill, and W. J. Fink. "Effects of Preexercise Feedings on Endurance Performance." *Medicine and Science in Sports* 11 (No. 1, 1979): 1–5.

Hoeger, W.W.K, & S.A. Hoeger. *Principles and Labs for Fitness & Wellness*. 10thed. Belmont: Wadsworth, 2010.

Kirk, E. P., J. E. Donnelly, B. K. Smith, J. Honas, J. D. Lecheminant, B. W. Bailey, D. J. Jacobsen, and R. A. Washburn. "Minimal Resistance Training Improves Daily Energy Expenditure and Fat Oxidation." *Medicine and Science in Sports and Exercise* 41 (No. 5, 2009): 1122–9.

Lee, C. D., A. S. Jackson, and S. N. Blair. "U.S. Weight Guidelines: Is It Also Important to Consider Cardiorespiratory Fitness?" *International Journal of Obesity* 22 (1998, Suppl 2): S2–S7.

Miller, W.C., Koceja, D.M. & E.J. Hamilton. "A Meta-Analysis of the Past 25 Years of Weight Loss Research Using Diet, Exercise, or Diet Plus Exercise Intervention." *International Journal of Obesity* 21(1997): 941–947.

National Dairy Council. "The New Food Guidance System." *Dairy Council Digest* 76 (No. 4, 2005): 19–24.

National Research Council, National Academy of Sciences. *Diet and Health: Implications for Reducing Chronic Disease Risk*. Washington, DC, 1989.

Powers, S. K., and E. T. Howley. *Exercise Physiology: Theory and Application to Fitness and Performance*. 6th ed. New York: McGraw-Hill, 2006, 62–9.

Rixon, K. P., P. R. Rehor, and M. G. Bemben. "Analysis of the Assessment of Caloric Expenditure in Four Modes of Aerobic Dance." *Journal of Strength and Conditioning Research* 20 (No. 3, 2006): 593–6.

The USDA Food Guide in "Preparing Foods and Planning Menus Using the Dietary Guidelines." *HG*, 232–8, 1989.

U.S. Department of Agriculture and U.S. Department of Health and Human Services. *Dietary Guidelines for Americans, 2010*. 7th Edition, Washington, DC: U.S. Government Printing Office, 2010.

14

Prevention and Care

Pain to gain ... you'll wind up lame! No pain,
gradual gain ... win the health fitness game.

- It seems like every time I start exercising I get hurt. How can I avoid this?
- What are the most common injuries in group fitness classes?
- How can I prevent and/or treat shinsplints? Knee pain? Back pain?
- What should I do if I get injured?

IF you are in pursuit of health and fitness, there is no reason to beat your body into the ground. Leave the pain and agony to the professionals who are paid handsomely to put their bodies at risk. Some soreness at the beginning of a program is normal, but if you are hurt, exhausted, and run-down after a workout, something is wrong. You should feel temporarily tired and then actually get a lift of energy from the workout.

Group fitness classes, taught by qualified instructors, are a safe and fun way to exercise. When injuries do occur, they are usually the result of poor exercise technique, trying to do too much too soon, or the result of overuse. It is important to follow the progressive overload principle and also to let your body rest and rebuild between workouts. Injury prevention strategies include wearing the appropriate attire (especially the right

shoes), selecting an overload that matches your present fitness level, and paying close attention to technique throughout the class. This chapter details a number of common injuries which may not seem important to you if you are not presently suffering from them. **However, it is a good idea to read all of the prevention sections so that you can minimize your risk.**

A common mistake is to push through pain. Instead, listen to your body and present it with a workout that matches where you are at that day. This doesn't mean avoiding a hard workout (if that is your goal) but it does mean taking into account previous workouts and activities, allergies, and other issues. It is common to feel some muscle soreness after a new overload and you can warm up and exercise through that, but at the same time, if something is very sore,

---

IS AEROBIC EXERCISE SAFE?

A quick look at the research on aerobic dance injuries can lead you to the wrong conclusions. About 75% of instructors and 45% of students reported having injuries; this percentage might make one think that aerobic dance exercise is a high-risk activity. Examining the research more carefully, however, shows that most of the injuries were not debilitating, did not require medical treatment, and could be remedied without requiring the person to stop exercising. Instructors most likely report more injuries because they spend more time doing the activity. Instructors are often guilty of exceeding the recommended frequency of 3 to 5 times per week and duration of 20 to 30

minutes. This makes them more susceptible to overuse injuries. Participants who get hooked on aerobic dance exercise sometimes become overzealous. It is a good idea to take at least one day off a week and/or use non-weight-bearing aerobic activities such as swimming or bicycling to supplement your aerobic dance exercise. This relieves some of the stress on the lower legs. Not surprisingly, more than half of the reported injuries were below the knee. The most common injuries were shinsplints and tendinitis. In most cases, these are overuse injuries that can be prevented by altering the frequency, intensity, and duration of activity.

it needs time to recover. For example, a student who came back from a big weekend of horseback riding was very stiff through the inner thighs. The adductor muscles are used a great deal in horseback riding. Skipping the adductor exercises for a day, or doing very light loads while the muscles recover, makes good sense.

Another common mistake is to push hard in a workout at the expense of technique. Doing one more repetition but breaking form to do it is a mistake. Continuing with an aerobic activity but losing good foot placement and knee alignment will do more harm than good. If you want to challenge yourself and reach a new fitness level you can train hard, but always stop and take a rest break before good form breaks.

To prevent injury or re-injury, you should also avoid or modify movements that are contraindicated (bad) for your body. For example, someone who gets shinsplints easily can substitute low-impact movements in place of some jumping movements. Someone with knee problems may be able to do straight leg exercises with a band instead of leg curling and leg extension movements and may need to avoid plyometric exercises such as jumping on or off a box. Instructors can help you modify or substitute movements so that your workout is healthy for you.

If an injury does occur it is important to follow good first aid procedures, follow up with a health care professional, and then return to activity gradually. Trying to do too much too soon will result in a frustrating sequence of re-injury. An example of a gradual return for someone who had sprained an ankle or pulled a leg muscle would be to only add weight (resistance) to squats when body weight squats can be performed without pain or hesitation.

When the cause of injury can be identified, the program or facility can be modified to eliminate or minimize the risk of future injury. For example, one major cause of shinsplints is impact stress. Modifications that have been made to minimize shinsplints include the production of better-designed shoes, the installation and use of better floors, and the introduction of nonimpact cardio equipment, such as the elliptical, rowing, and cycling machines.

Participants can also protect themselves against injury by increasing their strength and flexibility. Back pain, for example, can often be prevented or relieved by adopting a good stretching and strengthening program. More group fitness classes are offering ways to increase resistance during muscle-toning exercises. The addition of equipment such as barbells, dumbbells, bands, and stability balls can increase the risk of injury. However, when exercises are done properly and with qualified supervision, the result is a stronger body with a greater resistance to injury. Using the appropriate

overloads and good technique is what makes the difference. Ask your instructor to check your alignment, especially on exercises such as squats and lunges, where proper back, hip, and knee alignment is critical.

People who are beginning a program and those with a history of orthopedic problems run a slightly higher risk of injury. To reduce this elevated risk, they should seek advice from their physician, start slowly, overload gradually, and avoid exercises that hurt.

Unfortunately, there will always be unforeseeable accidents. When an accident occurs, the best thing to do is to have a qualified person administer prompt, proper first aid. Make sure the facility where you exercise is prepared to handle injury and emergency situations.

In the following pages, you will see **RICE** listed as a treatment for some of the injuries. RICE stands for **rest, ice, compression, and elevation.** This is a standard first-aid treatment for injuries such as a muscle strain or sprain. If done soon after the injury, RICE can help cut down on inflammation and swelling and decrease the recovery time. "Rest" means to immediately stop using the injured part. "Ice" means to apply something cold to the injured part. You can use crushed ice in a bag, a cold pack, or, in a pinch, something like a cold drink can until you can find a better source of cold. Ice is usually administered in cycles of 20 minutes on and then 20 minutes off. "Compression" means to apply pressure. This is usually accomplished with an ace bandage. (If there is bleeding, pressure points and more bandaging may be required.) Wetting the bandage on a sprain or strain will help transmit the cold from the ice more effectively. Finally, "elevation" means to put the injured part above the heart. This helps keep the swelling down.

Too often, people who have pulled a muscle or twisted an ankle use heat instead of cold. Heat is therapeutic when the time is right. Check with a health care professional before switching from cold to heat. Another mistake is to avoid performing RICE because you are embarrassed or don't wish to be fussed over. Doing these simple things while the injury is new can make a significant difference to your recovery.

Learn how to put prevention in your program. Listed below are some of the injuries that can occur during group fitness classes. The common causes, preventive actions, and proper first aid for each injury are described.

FOOT INJURIES

BLISTER

DEFINITION Inflammation of the skin that results in a collection of fluid below the skin.

SYMPTOMS Hot and red skin.

CAUSE Friction of the skin against something else.

PREVENTION Wear shoes that fit properly; wear socks. Put bandages or skin tape or rub petroleum jelly over the heel and other high-risk locations before breaking in new shoes or doing a prolonged physical activity.

TREATMENT Apply ice, rest, and put a felt or moleskin donut around the blister so that no further rubbing will occur. If the blister opens, wash with soap and water, dry, apply antibiotic ointment, and cover the area. Do not intentionally pop a blister. If it is in a very uncomfortable location and must be drained, use a sterilized needle to make a small hole in the lower side, drain, use antibiotic ointment, and cover. Do not remove the skin. If the blister develops red streaks or looks infected, see a physician immediately.

BUNION

DEFINITION Irritation of the toe joint (usually the big toe) resulting in a fluid build-up in the capsule surrounding the joint. Toe may turn inward.

SYMPTOMS Burning, tenderness, swelling, redness, pain, and misalignment of toe.

CAUSES Wearing shoes that are too narrow or too short. Individuals with flat feet or who have feet that pronate are more susceptible since their big toe is rolled down and inward which can result in friction.

PREVENTION Wear shoes that fit well and have a sufficient toe box. Orthotics may be needed to correct pronation, flat feet.

TREATMENT Reduce friction by using a felt donut and wearing new shoes with a large enough toe box. Soak your feet in cool water. See a physician. Surgical correction may be necessary.

METATARSALGIA

DEFINITION Irritation of the nerves that lie between the metatarsal bones. (Metatarsals are the bones between the toes and the arch.)

SYMPTOMS Pain under the ball of the foot.

CAUSES Shifting forward of the protective fat pad under the ball of the foot from excessively landing on it; overuse.

PREVENTION An athletic shoe with good metatarsal (forefoot) padding, especially for classes that involve movements that have you land on the ball of the foot (e.g., step aerobics, dance aerobics), good jump-landing technique, and resilient floor. Avoid overuse.

TREATMENT Ice, rest, and cushioned foot pads. If the pain persists, see a physician. You may need metatarsal lifts or orthotics.

PLANTAR FASCIITIS

DEFINITION Strain to the broad sheet of connective tissue that runs from the heel to the metatarsals, which supports the longitudinal arch. When weight is shifted to the ball of the foot, the tension held by this connective tissue equals twice the body's weight. Microtears may occur where the fascia attaches to the heel bone.

SYMPTOMS Pain just in front of the heel where the connective tissue connects to the heel bone. Heel may feel bruised. Pain may also radiate along the arch.

CAUSES A rapid increase in activity that requires pushing off the ball of the foot, particularly on a hard surface; wearing unsupportive shoes.

PREVENTION Work into a new program gradually. Wear shoes that support the arches. Develop calf flexibility. Strengthen the muscles in the foot and ankle.

TREATMENT Rest, soak your feet in cool water, buy new shoes or arch supports. If pain persists, see a physician; you may need orthotics or anti-inflammatory drugs, or surgery.

MORTON'S NEUROMA

DEFINITION Localized swelling of the sensory nerve that lies between the metatarsals (bones in the ball of the foot) and innervates the toes.

SYMPTOMS Pain radiating up between the third and fourth toes.

CAUSES Overuse, too much running on the ball of the foot.

PREVENTION Well-cushioned athletic shoes. Avoid overuse by doing a practical exercise program. Use a metatarsal arch pad (a felt pad that fits under the ball of the foot).

TREATMENT See a physician.

SHIN INJURIES

SHINSPLINTS

DEFINITION This is a general term for pain on the front or side of the lower leg. Some believe the pain comes from minute tearing of the muscle sheath from the shin bone membrane. Others believe the pain comes from damage caused by excessive vibration of the bone.

SYMPTOMS Pain and aching in the shin area after and sometimes during exercise. May be specific areas of tenderness or swelling over the bone.

CAUSES Impact stress from a hard floor, poorly cushioned shoes, too much jumping, poor foot mechanics, poor posture, fallen arches, insufficient warm-up, fatigue, training too fast or too soon, poor exercise technique.

PREVENTION Exercise/dance on a resilient floor with good arch-supporting shoes and use proper footwork. Strengthen the foot muscles and muscles that surround the shin, especially the anterior tibialis. Stretch calves well before and after working out. Also keep shins warm before and during class.

TREATMENT Ice shins for 20 to 30 minutes following exercise. You may want to freeze water in a paper cup and use it to massage your shins. Just peel down the cup as the ice melts.

If any bruising, swelling, or specific point tenderness occurs, stop exercising and rest your legs. If pain persists or worsens, consult a physician. You may need to take an anti-inflammatory drug or be fitted for orthotics.

Some individuals get relief from having their arches, shins, or both taped—consult an athletic trainer or podiatrist. Some people also get relief by running backward.

If your shins start to bother you during a class, try modifying the movements to a low-impact style. If it is a chronic problem, consider a nonimpact style of group exercise (cardio machines, water, etc.)

STRESS FRACTURE

DEFINITION Very thin, undisplaced hairline break in a bone.

SYMPTOMS Pain along the lower leg bones. If you have a stress fracture in the lower leg, it will hurt before, during, and after class and even when you get off your feet. Painful when you touch it, especially in one area.

CAUSES Same as shinsplints.

PREVENTION Wear cushioned, supportive shoes, avoid overuse and nonresilient surfaces.

TREATMENT See a physician. Stress fractures are difficult to diagnose because they don't show up on X-ray images until calcium deposits are made during the healing process. When a stress fracture is diagnosed, activity is restricted and the fractured part of the leg may be immobilized in a cast.

KNEE INJURIES

CHONDROMALACIA PATELLAE

DEFINITION Roughening or softening of the joint surface of the knee cap (patella).

SYMPTOMS Pain when patella is pressed on, maybe creaking and popping noises. May hurt when climbing stairs or kneeling. Knee pain while exercising.

CAUSES Knee cap may be sliding out of alignment and causing irritation. Cartilage may be inflamed or degenerating. May be caused by deep knee bends or other exercises that stress the knee.

PREVENTION Perform a good warm-up. Avoid deep knee bends and knee hyperextension positions. Strengthen the muscles that surround and support the knee, using straight-leg exercises if you already have some knee irritation. Stretch leg muscles, especially the hamstrings and calves.

TREATMENT Ice the knee. See a physician. Strengthen supporting muscles. Avoid kneeling versions of exercises.

MENISCAL INJURIES

DEFINITION Strains or tears of the cartilage that stabilizes the knee joint.

SYMPTOMS Acute pain, popping noise, swelling, knee may "give out" or lock.

CAUSES Rotation or twisting of the knee joint beyond normal limitations. Foot remaining planted when the body turns so that the knee is forced to accept the rotational force. A floor with too much cushion allows the foot to sink into it and remain planted. Sticky floors or treaded shoes on nonslip surfaces may also cause the foot to remain planted. Injury can also be caused by working the knee joint with too much weight.

PREVENTION Select the appropriate shoe for the surface. Select the best possible surface. Use workout routines that don't require sudden pivots or turns, particularly on soft floors. Work with reasonable amounts of weight during leg exercises. Overload gradually and strengthen the supporting muscles.

TREATMENT Support the back of the knee and pack the knee in ice. Move the person only if the knee is supported. Keep injured person warm and call a doctor. Joint may have to be aspirated (excess fluid removed from the joint).

MULTIPLE SITE INJURIES

STRAIN

DEFINITION A **strain** is an injury to a muscle or a tendon. (**Tendons** connect muscles to bone; e.g., the Achilles tendon connects the calf muscle to the heel.)

SYMPTOMS There are three degrees of injury. First-degree symptoms: local pain and tenderness, usually accompanied by swelling and pain. Exercise may be continued when pain and swelling are absent and range of motion is complete. Second-degree symptoms: pain with muscle movement, muscle spasm, increased swelling, and tearing of tissue. Do not continue exercise. Third-degree symptoms: severe pain and disability, severe muscle spasms, and complete tearing of tissue. Do not continue exercise.

CAUSES Pushing a muscle or tendon beyond its normal range, often by a ballistic movement before the body is fully warmed up. May also occur from overuse or flinging the arms, especially when arm weights are used. Older persons are more prone to injury.

PREVENTION Warm up and stretch well before working out. Strengthen both agonists and antagonists.

TREATMENT Rest, ice, compress, and elevate (RICE) the injured muscle or tendon. If pain is acute or persists, see a physician. Do not move anyone who has a third-degree strain. Call a doctor; surgery may be necessary.

SPRAIN

DEFINITION A **sprain** is an injury to a ligament. (Ligaments attach bones to bones.)

SYMPTOMS First-degree symptoms: twinge of discomfort, slight skin discoloration from internal bleeding, some ligament fiber damage. Exercise may be continued when pain and swelling are absent and range of motion is complete. Second-degree symptoms: pain, swelling, loss of function for several minutes, tender to the touch, loss of strength, definite tear of fibers. Do not continue exercise. Third-degree symptoms: severe pain and swelling, discoloration of skin, complete tear of the ligament, loss of function. Do not continue exercise.

CAUSES Any movement that pulls two connected bones apart more than a normal amount.

PREVENTION Warm up and stretch before working out. Exercise regularly so that ligaments are strengthened. Overload gradually and remember that ligament strength gains are usually slower than cardiorespiratory gains. When your heart says keep going, check in with the rest of your body. Strengthen muscles that surround joints so that they can minimize the stress put on the ligaments. Avoid exercises that put pressure on ligaments, and do exercises that strengthen muscles. For example, squats and lunges strengthen the legs as long as you don't bend the knee too much; deep knee bends stress the ligaments, and because the muscles are in a weak mechanical position, they can't help the ligaments.

TREATMENT Rest, ice, compress, and elevate (RICE) the injured part. If pain is acute or persists, consult a physician. If it is a third-degree sprain, do not move the person. Keep the person warm and call a doctor. Surgical repair may be necessary.

TENDINITIS

DEFINITION Chronic inflammation or irritation of a tendon. Microscopic tears in the tendon tissue may be the cause of the inflammation. In aerobics, the most commonly injured tendons are the Achilles, shoulder, and elbow.

SYMPTOMS Area may be painful to the touch, warm, and swollen. Skin may be red.

CAUSES Repeated excessive stretching of a tendon; excessive running or jumping, especially on hard surfaces; flinging of arms, particularly when wrist weights are used.

PREVENTION Use careful, deliberate movements rather than flinging movements. Gradually overload. Warm up and stretch out prior to vigorous activity.

TREATMENT Ice and rest the tendon. If pain is acute or chronic, see a physician. May require anti-inflammatory drugs or surgery.

BURSITIS

DEFINITION Inflammation or irritation of a bursa. bursas are fluid-filled sacks found around the body at sites where friction might occur, such as where muscle tendons and sheaths cross over bones.

SYMPTOMS Localized inflammation, pain, swelling, and heat.

CAUSES Overstretching of the Achilles tendon, direct blow to the elbow or knee, pressure on an area such as the knee, or overuse of a joint, such as the deltoid at the shoulder through unaccustomed overhead arm activity.

PREVENTION Avoid overuse of muscles and joints. Avoid kneeling on a hard floor. Use gradual overloads, especially when adding resistance through weights or exercise bands. Use good exercise technique.

TREATMENT Ice and compress the area. If pain, swelling, or loss of motion persists, consult a physician.

MUSCLE CRAMP

DEFINITION Painful muscle contraction that will not voluntarily release.

SYMPTOMS Acute pain.

CAUSES Fatigue or heat. (Also common among pregnant women, possibly due to chemical changes.)

PREVENTION Warm up well before vigorous exercise. Stretch a muscle following strength and aerobic workouts. Stretch whenever even slight muscle cramping occurs. Wear comfortable, lightweight clothing to prevent heat buildup. Hydrate with water prior to exercise and if cramps develop.

TREATMENT Stretch and massage the muscle. (You can also ice the opposing muscle because its contraction will cause the other muscle to stretch.)

LOW BACK PAIN

Low back pain is actually a symptom and may be the result of a number of underlying causes. For this reason, if you experience back pain you should consult your health care provider. Some of the causes of low back pain include:

- muscle strains or sprains
- disc herniation
- genetic abnormalities
- bony abnormalities
- pregnancy or premenstrual/menstrual symptoms

A normal healthy person may help prevent low back pain by:

1. exercising with good technique and alignment
2. exercising with gradual overloads
3. avoiding positions that put strain on the low back area
4. strengthening and stretching the muscles, especially the core muscles
5. using good postural positions throughout daily life
6. engaging the abdominal muscles when lifting
7. modifying exercises that are too advanced for one's present fitness

Please also refer to Chapter 6 for a discussion on back care and prevention of low back pain.

HEAT-RELATED INJURIES

HEAT CRAMP
See Muscle Cramp.

HEAT EXHAUSTION

DEFINITION Overheating of the body.

SYMPTOMS Muscle spasms or cramping, cold and clammy skin, chills, nausea, dizziness, and profuse sweating.

CAUSES Inability to dissipate heat because the air is too hot or humid for the level of activity. Sometimes workout spaces are not properly ventilated, or the cooling systems are insufficient. Situations can also arise when the exercise room shares air from a pool.

PREVENTION Exercise in a well-ventilated, controlled-temperature environment, or adjust the exercise level so that it is safe for the environment. Keep yourself well hydrated and wear comfortable, lightweight clothing.

TREATMENT Drink water and cool the body by going to a cooler place or using ice. Rest.

HEAT STROKE

DEFINITION Inability of the body to handle heat stress. This is a medical emergency. The core temperature is rising, and brain damage and death can result.

SYMPTOMS Dry and hot skin, pale or flushed skin, nausea, dizziness, faintness, weakness, or exhaustion. Skin may be still sweating if exercise has just stopped.

CAUSES Overexposure to a hot or a hot and humid environment.

PREVENTION Keep yourself well hydrated. Do not exercise in very hot weather or when the heat and humidity combine to cause a hazardous condition. Although these conditions do not occur often in most places, a wise participant will not continue to take a class if the air conditioner fails (or if he or she is attending a class outdoors) on a very hot day. Such a day may be good for water aerobics.

TREATMENT Immediately cool the body. Put person in a cold shower or dump cold water all over him or her. Call an ambulance immediately.

SUMMARY

Many injuries are preventable. Avoid the kinds of exercises that cause injury; you must take responsibility for keeping yourself injury free. If an unforeseen accident does occur, seek proper first aid and then consult a doctor. When you return to class after recovering from an injury, be sure to start out slowly to prevent reinjury.

Much of the fitness information available today is very easy to understand; some of it is very complex; much of it can be misunderstood. Like dieting, exercise information is regularly abused in an attempt to sell quick-fix equipment and programs. The best way to avoid being misinformed is to read exercise literature written by qualified professionals and to ask questions of the experts you have available. Ask your instructors questions—they will welcome the opportunity to enhance your knowledge.

COMMONLY ASKED QUESTIONS

Should I exercise when I'm sick?

No, exercise is a stressor. When your body is trying to fight off infection, it needs rest, not stress.

How can I tell if I am overtraining?

One way to tell is to monitor your resting heart rate first thing in the morning. If it starts to increase, give yourself a day off. Another sign of overtraining is loss of strength. Strength gains are made only when the muscle has enough time to rebuild between exercise bouts. Chronic injury, lethargy, lack of motivation, overuse injuries, and chronic fatigue are all signs of overuse.

Why do I get muscle cramps during class?

Most cramps occur when a muscle is fatigued. If you experience cramping, warm up well, lower your exercise intensity, and stretch the muscle more often during class. Sometimes poor choreography overworks one set of muscles. This can make you stiff and sore or make you cramp. The best choreography works both muscles in a muscle pair. If you know that you worked one muscle harder than another, do a set of exercises to balance the workout.

Other causes for cramping include overheated muscles, dehydration, and electrolyte imbalance. Drinking water prevents heat cramps. Taking salt pills to prevent heat cramps is not a good idea. The salt can upset your stomach during exercise; furthermore, most American diets contain more salt than is recommended. Only in rare cases is a salt supplement required. Some people find that eating a banana (a good source of potassium) and calcium-rich foods helps prevent cramping. Consult your physician if cramping is persistent.

Sometimes I feel dizzy during class. Can I prevent that?

Dizziness can be caused by a number of things. It may be brought on by low blood sugar. This is often the case when people take a morning class without eating anything for breakfast or skip lunch and take a late afternoon class. Another cause can be heat stress. Wear loose, comfortable clothing and drink water. Dizziness may also be a sign of illness. Medications, both over-the-counter and prescription, can also be the reason. If dizziness occurs, stop exercising. If you feel as though you are going to faint, lie down and elevate your feet. If dizziness persists, check with a doctor.

I get a side ache (stitch) when I exercise. Why does this happen, and what should I do?

NOT ASTHMA

A side-stitch, a pain just under the ribs, can be caused by a poorly conditioned diaphragm muscle, a food allergy (usually to milk), gas, or exercising too soon after eating. To relieve a side-stitch brought on by gas, try stretching up with the arm on the side giving distress. If it continues, slow down your activity and try doing some side and waist stretches. The diaphragm is a muscle that separates the chest and abdomen. It moves down when you inhale and up when you exhale. When you exercise more, or faster than usual, this muscle can cramp. Try starting more slowly and performing a more gradual overload. Belly breathing (allowing the abdominal muscles to relax and push out as you inhale and contract slightly when you exhale) may help. Belly breathing in combination with exhalations through pursed lips may also help. Strengthening the abdominal muscles by performing curl-ups may help prevent side stitches.

KNOWLEDGE TIPS

1. You can prevent injuries by wearing good shoes, exercising on a resilient surface, using good exercise technique, maintaining proper alignment throughout the class, and modifying exercises to suit your ability.

2. Listen to your body, and adjust your workout accordingly.

3. When well instructed, group fitness classes are a safe way to exercise.

4. Instructors receive more injuries than do students, probably because instructors spend more time doing aerobics and strength-training classes and are therefore more susceptible to overuse injuries.

5. The immediate first aid for a sprain or strain is RICE: rest, ice, compression, and elevation.

6. Aerobic dance exercise is one of the safest activities available.

THINK ABOUT IT

1. What are the most common injuries in group fitness exercise?

2. What is the first aid for injuries? (*Hint:* RICE)

3. What are some strategies for preventing injury?

4. If you are experiencing pain during an exercise, what should you do?

5. What are some specific strategies you can use to prevent shinsplints?

6. What are the symptoms of heat exhaustion? heat stroke?

7. What is the difference between a muscle sprain and a muscle?strain?

8. How are the shoes you wear related to injury prevention?

REFERENCES

Belt, C. R. "Injuries Associated with Aerobic Dance." *American Family Physician* 41 (June 1990): 1769–72.

Bishop, J. G., and D. Booth. "Injury Prevention and Care of Aerobic Dance-Exercise Injuries." *National Aerobics Training Association Manual.* Mesa, AZ: National Aerobics Training Association, 1986.

Burkett, L. "Causative Factors in Hamstring Strains." *Medicine and Science in Sports* 2 (1970): 39–42.

Clement, D. B., W. Ammann, J. E. Taunton, R. Lloyd-Smith, D. Jesperson, H. McKay, J. Goldring, and G. O. Matteson. "Exercise-Induced Stress Injuries to the Femur." *International Journal of Sports Medicine* 14 (No. 6, 1993): 347–52.

Clippinger, K. S. *Dance Anatomy and Kinesiology.* Champaign, IL: Human Kinetics, 2007.

du Toit, V., and R. Smith. "Survey of the Effects of Aerobic Dance on the Lower Extremity in Aerobic Instructors." *Journal of the American Podiatric Medical Association* 91 (No. 10, 2001): 528–32.

Fardy, P. S. "Isometric Exercise and the Cardiovascular System." *The Physician and Sportsmedicine* 9 (No. 9, 1981): 42.

Garrick, J. G., D. M. Gillien, and P. Whiteside. "The Epidemiology of Aerobic Dance Injuries." *The American Journal of Sports Medicine* 14 (1986): 67–72.

Hickey, M., and C. A. Hager. "Aerobic Dance Injuries." *Orthopedic Nursing Journal* 13 (No. 5, Sept.–Oct. 1994): 9–12.

Janis, L. R. "Aerobic Dance Survey. A Study of High-Impact Versus Low-Impact Injuries." *Journal of the American Podiatric Medical Association* 80 (No. 8, August 1990): 419–23.

Liemohn, W. "Factors Related to Hamstring Strains." *American Journal of Sports Medicine* 18 (1978): 71–6.

Martin, K. "Soft Aerobics: Gain Without Pain?" *Ms* 14 (May 1986): 52, 54, 113.

Michaud, T. J., J. Rodrigues-Zayas, C. Armstrong, and M. Hartnig. "Ground Reaction Forces in High Impact and Low Impact Aerobic Dance." *Journal of Sports Medicine and Physical Fitness* 33 (No. 4, 1993); 359–66.

Pollock, M. L., L. Gettman, C. Mileses, M. Bah, J. Durstine, and R. Johnson. "Effects of Frequency and Duration of Training on Attrition and Incidence of Injury." *Medicine and Science in Sports* 9 (No. 1, 1977): 31–6.

Richie, D. H., S. F. Kelso, and P. A. Bellucci. "Aerobic Dance Injuries: A Retrospective Study of Instructors and Participants." *The Physician and Sportsmedicine* 13 (No. 2, 1985): 134–5.

Vetter, W. L., D. L. Helfet, K. Spear, and L. S. Matthews. "Aerobic Dance Injuries." *The Physician and Sportsmedicine* 13 (No. 2, 1985): 114–20.

15

A Lifetime of Aerobics ...

"Light tomorrow with today."

ELIZABETH BARRETT BROWNING

- How do I find a good place to work out during vacation or after I graduate?
- I find health clubs intimidating. Are there alternatives? Or, how do I get past this feeling?
- What should I expect when I visit an exercise facility?
- What questions should I ask before joining a program?

HEALTH-RELATED physical fitness is a lifetime endeavor. It is relatively easy to exercise in a collegiate setting since you are surrounded by other exercisers, recreational facilities, and qualified instructors. After you leave school, your surroundings will change; hopefully your exercise habits will not. To help you take the first step toward continuing your commitment to a lifetime of physical activity, this chapter offers a few suggestions on how to find group fitness classes outside the college setting.

SELECTING A FACILITY

Exercise programs are offered at a variety of places ranging from town recreation offerings to health clubs. If you are only interested in a group fitness class, a health club may be an unnecessary expense. Quality instructors can be found teaching in places such as churches, town halls, schools, hospitals, and town recreation facilities. Some programs let you pay as you go; others will ask you to sign up and pay for a period of weeks. The fees for programs will vary depending on their overhead costs. The four most important things to investigate concerning these classes are the quality of instruction, the type of floor on which you will be exercising, the quality and quantity of equipment available, and how convenient the time and location are for you.

If you are looking for more, such as a weight room, aerobic machines, a pool, or a nursery, check out your local health clubs, employee (corporate wellness) programs, YMCA/YWCA, town recreation programs, and large churches. Knowing some of the characteristics of good programs can help you formulate questions and make decisions as you look at the possibilities in your area.

When you visit a fitness facility, you should receive a full tour and a thorough explanation of the classes that are offered, available equipment, daily hours, and fee structure. Take time to really look around. Bring a friend along if you can so that you feel more relaxed during the tour and can take in more information. Compare notes when you leave. It is easy to feel intimidated when you first visit a facility. A trial membership (2 to 4 weeks) is often available. This gives you a chance to try out equipment, take classes, and see whether you like the instructors. After a few classes and as the staff and other members begin to know you, you should feel more comfortable. Surveying the new scene from a cardio-machine or from a mat where you can stretch are a couple of other ways you can ease yourself into life at a club. Over time, you will become more aware of what a program/facility offers . . . or lacks. Check the equipment you plan to use, and make sure that it is available in sizes and weights that fit you and is clean and well maintained. Attending the facility during the time you plan to use it gives you a chance to see how crowded it is, the level of cleanliness, staff availability, and the type of classes offered. If after several visits you don't feel positive when you walk in the door, keep looking. It has to be a good match, or you won't go.

Figure 15.1 A lifetime of fitness. Resistance and encouragement come in many forms!

When you join a fitness program, you should receive an orientation to the facility and programs. This orientation should include an introduction to the facility and equipment, a medical history, a fitness evaluation, and exercise prescription. A member of the staff should show you the entire facility and teach you how to use available equipment. A good program will always have someone to help you with exercise questions, equipment, and fitness testing. Sometimes this person is the fitness instructor, sometimes an additional staff person.

The medical history you complete allows the instructor to work in an informed environment, to decide whether certain exercises should be modified. Find out if the instructor reviews your medical questionnaire or whether it is just filed away.

The fitness evaluation provides baseline data about your personal fitness level. Based on this information, goals and a plan of action can and should be formulated. The program should offer periodic testing to measure improvement, provide motivation, and evaluate the effectiveness of your exercise program. The fitness evaluation should offer measures of cardiorespiratory endurance, muscular strength and endurance, body composition, and flexibility. The person conducting these tests should be knowledgeable and, preferably, have a college degree and/or certification in fitness testing and exercise prescription.

Watch the group fitness class you want to join from beginning to end. See whether it includes a good warm-up and cool-down and the kind of workout you want. If the class uses equipment, check to make sure there is plenty available in a variety of sizes. Listen for heart rate or other intensity checks during the class. Check the starting and finishing times for promptness. Make sure you like the instructor's style, and make sure there is room for you in the class. Check to see if enrollment is limited and if it guarantees you space on the floor. If the class runs on a first-come, first-served basis, be sure you will have enough time to arrive early.

Program variety allows you to select a class that most closely fits your fitness goals and interests. Many programs now offer a variety of workout levels. Check with the instructor to find out what constitutes a beginning, intermediate, and advanced class. Different programs use different criteria for establishing class levels.

As a guideline, beginning aerobic exercise classes usually have a 15- to 20-minute standing aerobics section, work at near-threshold intensities, and include shorter sections of resistance exercises. Intermediate classes work aerobically for a minimum of 20 minutes and include fairly demanding resistance exercises, possibly using weights, bands, or balls. Advanced classes work at high intensities and may include workouts with more difficult regimens of weights, bands, or balls. The aerobic section is often 30 minutes or longer.

Low-impact and step classes are offered in both low and high intensities. Find out when each kind meets and whether equipment like weights and bands are used and supplied. Group fitness resistance training classes will range in style and level, as well. They are also often combined with an aerobic workout in the form of a fusion class. See whether there is a convenient class that matches your fitness level and preferred style of exercise.

Special classes may be taught for children, elderly persons, pregnant women (pre/postnatal), people with disabilities, and people who are overweight (overfat). Each class should use music and techniques appropriate to the people involved. Instructors should be qualified to teach these specialty classes.

Select a program that can meet your needs now and in the future. For instance, if you are very active now and are considering becoming pregnant, select a program that has both an advanced class and a pre/postnatal class. That makes it easy to switch from one to the other at the appropriate time. If you can attend only one time of day and one class, look for an instructor who has experience working at different intensities of classes and who is capable of effectively handling people of different fitness levels within one class.

Although major injuries are rare in group fitness classes, it is always comforting to know that the program or facility has an emergency procedure. Check for easy exits, sprinklers, and an available telephone. In addition, the instructors and staff should be educated and certified in cardiopulmonary resuscitation (CPR) and standard first aid. Ice should be readily available in the event of a strain or sprain.

The following is a quick checklist of items to look for as you select an exercise facility. The perfect facility is difficult to find and may be expensive to join, so decide which items are most important to you.

1. The facility should be in a convenient location near home or work.
2. The building should be well ventilated and the temperature set at a comfortable exercise temperature.
3. The lighting should be good quality and non-glare.
4. The whole facility, including locker rooms, should be clean and well supplied even at peak hours.
5. The water in pools and whirlpools should be clear and clean.
6. Mirrors should be strategically placed so that you can check your alignment during exercise.
7. The best aerobics floor is a wooden floor with air space underneath it so that it "gives." Carpet over cement is very hard on shins. Heavy padding can have a tendency to grab your shoe and make changes of direction hazardous.
8. There should be 25 square feet (sft) of space available for each person on the exercise floor. (The absolute minimum is 9 sft.)
9. The stereo equipment and facility acoustics should project music with a quality sound. The instructor should also be easily heard—many now wear wireless microphones.
10. For larger classes, the instructor should stand on a platform for easy visibility. Mirrors also enhance visibility for both the instructor and the participant.

Selecting a facility is similar to buying a car. Shop around and visit last the place you think you'll like the most. Clubs may offer a first visit (or initial visit) discount. If you have shopped the competition and like what you see, you'll be able to take advantage of the discount. However, the initial visit discount should not pressure you into buying. Clubs often offer a membership plan on your second visit that is similar to the offer on your first visit.

When you enter into a contract with a health club, it is good to know your consumer rights. Start by checking to see if the club is listed with the Better Business Bureau and then check with your state's Consumer Protection Agency to find out what regulations health clubs must meet. Don't feel pressured to sign a contract; take it home and read it over carefully. Make sure that it includes all the services you want and that all the promises made to you verbally are written in the contract. Look for cancellation policies including the ability to cancel penalty-free within 3 days of signing and cancellation terms if you move a distance away from the club and/or the club goes out of business. In the case of the latter, check the state regulations for terminating the contract. If your club is bought out by another and you want to continue to attend, see if you have the right to continue your original contract, as it may have better rates and services than a contract with the new owner. If you opt for direct deposit payments, be sure to cancel them if the club goes out of business as the club may continue to collect from you. Long-term memberships are often less expensive, but before choosing this option check the track record of the club for longevity and ask for monthly payments instead of a one time up-front payment.

Many clubs will not disclose their membership costs over the telephone. Most recreation, school, or church groups will tell you the cost of the program, if any, over the telephone.

In all cases, the facility should be well staffed with friendly, qualified people. Some locations include a juice bar, weights, a pool, a sauna, a hairdresser, a nursery, and other amenities. Determine what is important to you before you look, so that you won't be distracted by things you don't need and won't use. Find the best facility for you at the most affordable price.

SELECTING AN INSTRUCTOR

As you move away from the college or university setting where group exercise and fitness/wellness classes are offered by physical fitness educators and recreation professionals, it is helpful to know how to select a qualified instructor in a club, dance studio, or recreational setting. Some program directors and club owners carefully screen their fitness instructors and only hire qualified individuals; some unfortunately are not as careful. The private sector also has to handle staffing demands for trends that gain popularity quickly. It can be difficult to find enough qualified instructors for what is often part-time work.

To help you be a good consumer, here are some ways you can determine the qualifications and traits of a good instructor:

- *Meet the instructor.* Ask the person how he or she feels about lifetime fitness and how he or she can help you toward your goals.
- *Watch and listen to the instructor in action.* Qualified instructors will constantly demonstrate different levels of intensity, offer tips on positioning and

alignment, provide safety guidelines, and move around the room to assist individuals as needed.

- *Check the instructor's training and experience.* Find out if the instructor has a fitness education or is certified by a reputable fitness certification program. There are a number of groups that certify aerobics instructors and still more that offer certifications for personal training and fitness education. Some training programs are more comprehensive than others. The strongest preparation is through a higher education program (such as an exercise science, physical education, or health promotion major in college) or through a specific course of study through a trade school. Other programs offer training ranging from a weekend up to several weeks. There are no rules governing certification of an aerobics instructor, so the quality of the programs varies. In the United States the two most recognized certifying bodies for aerobics instructors are the American Council for Exercise (ACE) and the Aerobics and Fitness Association of America (AFAA). Other, broader and often more in-depth certifications include, but are not limited to, ones through the American College of Sports Medicine (ACSM), the National Academy of Sports Medicine (NASM), and the National Strength and Conditioning Association (NSCA). There are also a number of regional certification programs, and the quality of these programs depends on the expertise of the individuals doing the training and the rigor of the certification testing.

  At this time, there are no national or state mandates for certification or strict controls over what such a program offers. Therefore, certification alone does not ensure a good instructor, but it does demonstrate a certain commitment toward learning and attaining basic knowledge. In addition to his or her training, find out how much experience the instructor has teaching a particular type and level of course.

- *Determine whether the instructor is up-to-date.* Information changes, and instructors need to stay updated. Find out how the instructor is staying current. You may want to ask a question about something you've read recently to see if the instructor can speak about current issues in fitness and wellness.

- *Find out the procedure for new people joining a class.* When new people join an exercise class, they should have to fill out a medical form, and the instructor should speak with them concerning their exercise background, level of fitness, and how to monitor their exercise intensity.

- *Determine whether the instructor is "onstage" or focused on participants.* Look for an instructor who is clearly watching the class and adjusting the pace and exercises to match the class's needs.

- *Check the instructor's attendance record.* Instructor consistency means that the instructor has a chance to get to know you, identify your needs, and guide your progression. When you keep getting different instructors (substitutes) you lose this personalization.

- *Talk to other members or previous members of the class.* Participants can give you a sense of whether the instructor is prepared for class, personable, and motivating.

FITNESS TRENDS—MORE OPTIONS

Fitness opportunities have expanded, and cross-training (using a variety of fitness modes) is a great way to keep things interesting. You may want to try one or more of the following.

- Dancing is getting some wonderful television press and dance studios and dance clubs are growing in popularity, offering lessons in hip-hop, Latin dancing, line dancing, ballroom, and other styles.
- Some boxing clubs now offer a wider variety of programs including some group fitness classes.
- You can join a walking or running club or take friends or family on a town- or state-managed trail.
- Par courses are located in many parks; these are trails with embedded exercise stations.
- You can hire a personal trainer or join a group training for a charity event.
- In winter climates, consider snowshoeing or cross-country skiing.
- In summer (or indoors), experiment with water aerobics, water polo, canoeing/kayaking, or a nice long swim.

Indoor and outdoor rock climbing is a great way to challenge your muscles and build confidence. Bike trails are expanding—some use old railroad track beds, which allow for good riding without traffic concerns. More programs are offering functional fitness—building your fitness in a way that helps you meet daily activity. Balance and coordination and core training are often at the center of these workouts. Other approaches use these ideas (and more) with the intent of building sport-specific fitness and skill. Wellness centers, hospitals, and universities offer programs that combine healthy habits, good nutrition, and physical activity. If you are seeking the mind-body connection, there are studios and clubs and recreation departments offering yoga, pilates, and the martial arts. Or perhaps you'd enjoy tapping into technology using a pedometer or a heart-rate monitor, tune into a workout via your ear buds, or pop in a DVD or use a game console and exercise at home. The options are many and new ideas develop everyday—all you have to do is put on your exercise clothes and jump into activity.

SUMMARY

Make finding a place to continue your exercise program a priority. In addition to staying fit, going to exercise class is a great way to meet other people who, like you, enjoy an active, healthy lifestyle.

KNOWLEDGE TIPS

1. Before looking for a fitness facility, make a prioritized list of features to look for.

2. Visit a facility at the time of day you will be most likely to use it.

3. Look for a fitness facility that will take you on a complete tour, have you complete a medical/health questionnaire, give you a fitness evaluation, explain how to use the equipment, help you get started in an exercise program, and have someone available for consultation on an ongoing basis.

4. Look over the whole facility. Check for cleanliness, ventilation, good lighting, sound acoustics, well-maintained equipment, and a good exercise floor.

5. Find out how qualified the instructor is in terms of education, certification, and experience.

6. Check the instructors' educational backgrounds to see whether they are certified in CPR, first aid, aerobic dance exercise, or other group fitness specialties.

7. A quality instructor is a good role model, knowledgeable, experienced, up to date, well prepared, places students' needs first, can individualize the lesson, has regular attendance, and is personable and motivating.

8. Observe, from start to finish, the classes you want to join.

9. Consider the financial commitment carefully. Be sure to ask about all the plans.

10. Join and have fun!

THINK ABOUT IT

1. Where are exercise programs available?

2. What types of services do clubs offer?

3. What are desirable qualifications for an instructor?

4. Identify the qualities of a facility/program (i.e., location, cost, etc.) that are most likely to keep you coming back long term.

5. What time of day are you most likely to exercise and what implications does the time of day you are most likely to exercise have on selecting a program and facility?

6. What are some ways that you can find out if the instructor and program you are interested in are of good quality?

7. Where can you obtain consumer information on health clubs?

REFERENCES

American Council on Exercise. *Aerobics Instructor Manual: ACE's Guide for Fitness Professionals.* San Diego, CA: American Council on Exercise, 2000.

Champion, N., and G. Hurst. *Aerobics Instructor's Handbook.* Sydney: Kangaroo Press, 2000.

Kernodle, R. G. "Space: The Unexplored Frontier of Aerobic Dance." *Journal of Physical Education, Recreation, and Dance* 63 (May–June 1992): 65–9.

Muscles of the Body

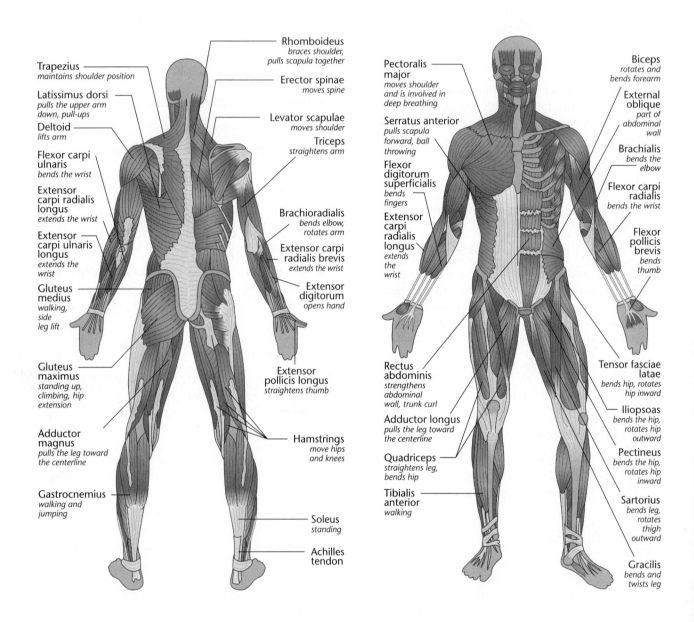

Rhomboideus
braces shoulder, pulls scapula together

Trapezius
maintains shoulder position

Erector spinae
moves spine

Latissimus dorsi
pulls the upper arm down, pull-ups

Levator scapulae
moves shoulder

Deltoid
lifts arm

Triceps
straightens arm

Flexor carpi ulnaris
bends the wrist

Extensor carpi radialis longus
extends the wrist

Brachioradialis
bends elbow, rotates arm

Extensor carpi ulnaris longus
extends the wrist

Extensor carpi radialis brevis
extends the wrist

Gluteus medius
walking, side leg lift

Extensor digitorum
opens hand

Gluteus maximus
standing up, climbing, hip extension

Extensor pollicis longus
straightens thumb

Adductor magnus
pulls the leg toward the centerline

Hamstrings
move hips and knees

Gastrocnemius
walking and jumping

Soleus
standing

Achilles tendon

Pectoralis major
moves shoulder and is involved in deep breathing

Biceps
rotates and bends forearm

Serratus anterior
pulls scapula forward, ball throwing

External oblique
part of abdominal wall

Flexor digitorum superficialis
bends fingers

Brachialis
bends the elbow

Flexor carpi radialis
bends the wrist

Extensor carpi radialis longus
extends the wrist

Flexor pollicis brevis
bends thumb

Rectus abdominis
strengthens abdominal wall, trunk curl

Tensor fasciae latae
bends hip, rotates hip inward

Adductor longus
pulls the leg toward the centerline

Iliopsoas
bends the hip, rotates hip outward

Quadriceps
straightens leg, bends hip

Pectineus
bends the hip, rotates hip inward

Tibialis anterior
walking

Sartorius
bends leg, rotates thigh outward

Gracilis
bends and twists leg

Fitness Clothes, Shoes, and Equipment

ALTHOUGH group fitness exercise has introduced a style of dress all its own, to get started all you really need are shoes that provide good support, flexibility, and cushioning, and clothes that allow you to move, breathe, and sweat freely.

Avoid materials such as nylon that trap heat and moisture. Stick with cotton, which absorbs moisture, or one of the newer materials that wick away moisture. Loose clothing allows for freedom of movement, but a baggy outfit can make it difficult for an instructor to see your body alignment and can keep you from getting the most out of your exercises. Wear layers if you are in a cooler environment so that you can strip off outer garments as you warm up. A sweatband or rolled and tied bandanna can be worn around your forehead to absorb perspiration and keep it out of your eyes. Wrist sweatbands can be worn as well to absorb arm sweat or to wipe your brow.

TRAINING SHOES

Now that group fitness means a wide variety of activities, shoe designs are changing to match the needs of participants. To select a pair of training shoes, or perhaps more than one pair, the most important thing is to identify what activities you will be doing in the shoes. If you plan on doing a variety of activities at a relatively casual level, a cross trainer will likely meet your needs. These are designed with forefoot and heel padding, lateral support, midsole cushioning, and relatively flexible outer soles. These can handle a typical group fitness class, court game activity, and short runs. If you participate in a particular sport such as running

or basketball more than 2 times per week, the American Academy of Podiatric Sports Medicine recommends investing in a sport-specific shoe. If you cross train at a high level, you may also want a pair of shoes specifically designed for that. Training shoes come in many forms. General features will be discussed next, followed by key features by activity.

GENERAL FEATURES

Most aerobic/cross-trainer shoes have similar features. The bottom of the shoe is called the outersole. Select tread to coincide with the surface on which you will be exercising. Smoother treads help you pivot more easily on wooden floors and carpeted surfaces. The outersole may be cut away under the arch to save on materials and weight, and many of the new shoes also have a shank made up of supportive material running across the midfoot section of the outersole to provide lateral stability. Most companies also design the outersole to promote flexibility. Try bending the shoe to see if it flexes easily. The outersole should also have flex points so that the shoe bends easily. Test the flex point locations by standing on the balls of your feet; see if the bend of the shoe agrees with the bend in your foot.

The midsole rests on top of the outersole and supplies most of the shock absorption. Many aerobic dance exercise steps involve landing on the ball of the foot first; therefore, forefoot padding is crucial. A good shoe will have shock absorption under both the ball of the foot and the heel. Manufacturers are using three shock-absorbing materials for midsole construction: EVA (ethyl vinyl acetate), compressed molded

SHOE FEATURES AND FUNCTIONS

OUTERSOLE

- Traction—match grid to surface and movement (pivots, etc.).
- Durability—less toughness is needed for indoor sports. Save your soles by wearing your shoes only for class.
- Flexibility—bend the shoe. Look for outersole designs that allow it to flex.

INSOLE

- Arch support—the arch cookie (bump in the insole) supports the arch.
- Cushioning—the insole provides some, but most comes from the midsole; can supplement with upgraded insoles.

MIDSOLE

- Cushioning—needed to offset impact stress; more cushioning is needed for high-impact exercise than for low-impact exercise.

- Flexibility—needed for stepping off steps, landing on ball of foot, etc.
- Motion control and support—needed to keep foot in control during lateral and twisting movements as well as forward and back motions.

UPPER

- Motion control and support—strong, well-designed lateral straps, heel support, etc., prevent pronation or supination of the feet.
- Durability—not as big an issue; usually cushioning wears out first.
- Fit—should be snug and comfortable.
- Heat dissipation—shoes need ventilation, especially if your feet sweat a lot.

EVA, and polyurethane. The compressed molded EVA is an improved version of EVA and is therefore preferable. Polyurethane provides the best shock absorption but is slightly heavier and is thus not used or used only sparingly. In addition to these effective synthetic foams, manufacturers have designed unique shock-absorption systems using midsoles filled with gels, Freon, or air, and springs. For example, Avia uses a cantilever system, Nike an encapsulated air system, Asic an encapsulated gel, Ryka encapsulated nitrogen, and Reebok a honeycombed inset called Hexalite. All of them are effective. Check for midsole flexibility by performing toe raises while wearing the shoes. Check for shock absorbency by jumping up and down and performing aerobic steps. See the box, Shoe Shopping Checklist.

Your feet rest on insoles inside the shoe; along with the midsoles, insoles provide arch support and cushioning. Look for insoles that pull out so they can be aired between classes and replaced when worn out. You can purchase insoles made of compressed molded EVA, polyurethane, or neoprene at stores that sell athletic shoes. If you plan on using one of these insoles, try on the shoe with the insole. You may need a half-size larger shoe. Regularly washing the insoles

will allow them to breathe better and keep your feet cooler. You will be unclogging their pores, so to speak.

Materials that provide lateral support help stabilize your foot during side-to-side movements and keep it from twisting when you place your weight on the ball of your foot. The previously mentioned midfoot shank, as well as reinforcement in the heel cup and, in some cases, thermoplastic urethane supports in the midsole, help stabilize the foot. Leather straps that run from the midsole up to the lacing provide lateral support; some lacing systems run on the sides of shoes to add support. Other sources of lateral support include outersoles that wrap up the sides of the shoe and insoles and midsoles that curve up on the inside edges of the shoe to cradle the foot. Beware of cosmetic stitching that looks like lateral reinforcement.

To prevent side-to-side slippage in the heel, the shoe should have a firm, reinforced heel counter. The sole beneath the heel should extend out a little wider than the upper but should not have the flare of a running shoe. The heel should also be well padded and notched to support but not irritate the Achilles tendon during jumping and stepping.

Both leather and synthetic leather are good materials. Firm leather provides support, and soft leather

Aerobics shoe.

Source: "Aerobics Shoe" by Melissa Galen Benine. Reprinted by permission.

stretches out and allows the feet to roll out over the soles. Synthetic leather tends to stretch less than natural leather, but it may also be hotter. Usually, additional mesh areas are built in to provide the necessary breathability.

Feet with significant mechanical or structural abnormalities, such as very high arches, flat feet, or feet that tend to pronate (roll in) or supinate (roll out), often need more support than ordinary shoes can provide. In addition to making your feet ache, these abnormalities can cause impact vibrations to be sent up the legs on an angle. Vibrations repeatedly striking the knee at an angle can cause irritation on the inside or outside of the knee. Shinsplints, hip pain, and even lower back pain can originate from problems with the feet.

If you think your feet need extra support, consult a podiatrist. You may need orthotics—custom-made plastic insoles that slip inside your shoe to provide form-fitting support. If you are being fit for orthotics, be sure to tell the podiatrist you intend to use them for exercise, because sports orthotics are more flexible than others. Orthotics are relatively expensive, but they are as indispensable to bad feet as eyeglasses are to bad eyes.

Finally, be sure to replace your shoes when they start to wear out. Simply because a shoe *looks* like it is still good does not guarantee that it has not worn out. See the When to Replace Your Training Shoes box for tips on when it's time to get new training shoes.

ACTIVITY-SPECIFIC FEATURES

DANCE-EXERCISE ACTIVITY

For dance-exercise or step aerobics, lateral support, cushioning, and flexibility are key features. You will want to select a shoe that has good forefoot padding as you are often required to land on the ball of the foot. Each time you jump, your feet absorb the impact of 3 to 6 times your body weight. The impact vibrations (shock) that cannot be absorbed by your arches are transmitted up your ankles, shins, knees, thighbones, hips, and spine and are eventually dissipated in the soft viscera (organs) in your trunk. With normal, routine activity, this system works beautifully, but when you add repetitive high-impact jumping, your body's shock-dissipating system may need help. Shoes with good support and cushioning help absorb impact shock and are believed to prevent chronic stress injuries. Aerobic/fitness shoes are designed to be lightweight, flexible, and shock-absorbing. If you are a big person bringing a lot of weight down on the shoe, a slightly heavier, sturdier shoe may be better than a light shoe that compresses too easily.

The most common mistake beginning students make is to wear a running shoe for dance-exercise. Here are some good reasons not to do that:

- You want a relatively smooth tread for easy pivoting, NOT the heavy tread of a running shoe made for road and track use.
- You want lateral support and a sole designed for multidirectional use, NOT a sole designed to push off in one direction. Runners typically move in a relatively straight line.
- You want a moderate cut-out in the arch with midfoot lateral support, NOT a high arch cut-out that makes a running shoe lighter and more flexible but less stable during side-to-side motions.
- You want forefoot padding for landing on the ball of the foot, NOT heel strike cushioning for heel-toe action.
- You want a shoe with a stable base (sole) to prevent ankle injuries during multidirectional movement, NOT one with a narrower base that allows slippage during lateral movements.

SHOE SHOPPING CHECKLIST

- Shop late in the day, when your feet are their largest. Feet tend to swell as the day progresses.
- Let the salesclerk know what type of activity you will be performing, such as step aerobics or kickboxing.
- Try the shoes on with the socks, inserts, or orthotics you intend to wear when using the shoes. See whether the insole will pull out for easy washing, airing or replacement.
- Try on several different brands. Different brands use different lasts. A last is the mold from which the shoe is constructed. Some lasts are more curved than others. Find the one that fits your foot. The shoe should be comfortable right away—there is no need for a "break-in" period.
- Ask what materials are used for cushioning and shock absorption. Are they quality materials, such as molded compressed EVA, dual density EVA, etc.?
- Relace the shoes starting at the farthest eyelets. Use the lacing system that is appropriate for your feet.
- Wiggle your toes while standing still—all your toes should be free to wiggle if the toe box is high and wide enough.
- Perform a variety of movements, and see whether the shock absorption system feels natural to you as you move.
- Perform some forward and backward jumping motions to make sure your toes do not hit the end of the shoes.

- Check the heel counter by moving side to side and see whether the shoe continues to fit snugly. Your heel should not slide.
- Check to see whether the heel is padded and notched and fits comfortably.
- Stand on your toes and twist or swivel side to side. Make sure the lateral support holds your feet in position.
- Jump from side to side and see whether the lateral support (straps, shanks, wrapped outsole, etc.) holds your feet in position. You should not feel as though you are rolling out over the side of the shoe or sliding from side to side.
- Check for arch support. The arch cookie should be in contact with your arch.
- Check for flexibility by walking normally, standing on the balls of your feet, and jumping up and down on the balls of your feet. The shoe should "break" at the same point as your foot bends. You should also be able to bend the shoe easily so that you can roll down from the balls of your feet. Look for outsole grooves and flex points.
- Make sure there is adequate ventilation for your feet. Mesh breathes more than leather. Look for air holes.
- Check the price. Quality shoes will cost more, but they last longer. Ask about the difference between last year's model and this year—you may be able to save money buying last year's model if the changes are primarily cosmetic.

CROSS TRAINING ACTIVITY

As cross training fitness activities (i.e. Crossfit, bootcamp) have gained in popularity, participants are looking for a shoe that will allow them to do everything from agility runs, plyometrics such as box jumping, to rope climbing, to weight lifting. A shoe that will do all this needs an outsole that will hold up on concrete and asphalt and that is designed to move in multiple directions, a midsole with enough cushion to handle the jumps, and enough lateral support for weightlifting and agility movements. It also needs to breathe well and be relatively light. To offer the stable platform for weightlifting, the sole of the shoe needs to be more flat as opposed to shoes with outer sole cut-away arches. High-end shoes provide a more durable sole (carbon rubber), a side sole design that allows you to better grip a rope, a midsole that you can heat and form to your foot, and a highly breathable upper.

WEIGHT TRAINING/LIFTING

The key feature here is a stable platform. The shoe should have a minimal arch cut out and solid outsole to provide the stable platform during lifts. It should also have lateral support and good flexibility. The heavier the load, the less compressible the sole should be, as you don't want the shoe to "give way." Heavy loads will likely require a specific weightlifting shoe rather than a cross trainer.

WHEN TO REPLACE YOUR TRAINING SHOES

It's time to replace your shoes when:

- you have worn them for 3–6 months, depending on how often you exercise in them and how sturdy their construction is
- you experience any foot pain or chronic injury symptoms that you don't normally experience, such as shinsplints, knee soreness, etc.

- the shoe has stretched and become loose on your foot
- the heels are rolling over
- the shoe allows you to pronate (roll your ankle inward)
- the tread has become too smooth

RUNNING

A cross trainer can be used for short running distance such as might be involved in some cross training regimens, but it should not be used for long distance training. A running shoe is designed for unilateral movement and therefore does not need the lateral support typical of a cross trainer. The tread is also generally heavier and made to grip the surface so that a good push-off can be obtained. These shoes are light to save on metabolic cost (energy to move them) and breathe well to dissipate heat. The heel cup is reinforced and the outer heel is built up to provide heel strike shock absorption.

OTHER ACTIVITIES

Cycling shoes are quite different as they need to have a stiff sole so they don't "give" each time you pedal. Cardio kickboxing can be done barefoot or in a cross trainer with good traction, flexibility, and lateral support. For yoga and Pilates, bare feet or socks that don't slip are preferred.

THE SHOE–BAREFOOT DEBATE

The debate as to whether it is better to run in supportive cushioned shoes or run barefoot has received a lot of attention in the last few years. The question centers around whether the foot and leg perform better when the mechanics are left to what mother nature has provided than when the motion is influenced by technologically advanced shoes. Barefoot runners tend to land more forward on their feet, and take shorter and more frequent strides than runners in shoes. The research that has been done is fascinating but leaves us with no conclusive evidence that the heel strike pattern of the shod runner results in any more injury than the barefoot technique. The only documented benefit to barefoot running is a metabolic cost savings (less energy) which is probably due to the fact that moving the weight of shoes takes energy. While the idea is that barefoot running is the most natural technique and allows the muscles to absorb more shock, the vast majority of elite athletes are still training and winning races in shoes, albeit light weight racing shoes. In the past couple of years, more people have tried a minimalist shoe that is one step above barefoot. Minimalist shoes have enough sole to protect the foot from harmful surfaces, allow more foot movement, have less of a rise in heel height compared to the forefoot (heel drop), provide some heel strike protection, and may have a little bit of cushion. Some allow the toes their own separate toe box, while others look more shoe-like. An important note of caution – the research that has been done centers around running and does not address the mechanics and impact shock that arises from sustained vertical exercise steps like those common to aerobic dance-exercise. We need more research!

OTHER CLOTHING

SOCKS AND FOOT CARE

Socks prevent blisters and calluses by reducing the friction between your shoes and the skin on your feet. To prevent soreness when you are breaking in a new pair of shoes, place bandages or tape over sensitive areas such as the back of your heels and the outside of your little toes. If you have sensitive feet or are planning a long day at a workshop or competition, you can further reduce friction by wearing double-layer socks or two pairs of socks (the inner pair should be thinner), putting baby powder between your pairs of socks, or applying petroleum jelly to your feet.

Socks also absorb perspiration, thus keeping your feet dry and helping to prevent itching, cracking, and athlete's foot. Basic cotton socks absorb moisture well but do not wick it away. The newer blend socks effectively wick moisture away from the skin, which keeps your feet dryer and cooler. White socks are recommended over colored socks because the dye in the latter may irritate the skin when sweat-soaked. People with diabetes should take extra good care of their feet and see a physician immediately if problems occur.

DANGEROUS CLOTHING

Rubber or plastic suits (or regular sweats worn in warm/hot conditions) prevent normal body cooling; dehydration and dangerous heat stress may result. The large weight losses observed after exercising in this type of outfit can be attributed to large fluid losses. As soon as the body is properly rehydrated, the weight will return. No positive health benefits are achieved by the use of these suits. Plastic wraps (cellophane) trap heat the same way rubber suits do and should be avoided for the same reasons. Warm clothing should be removed following the warm-up.

Avoid restrictive clothing that interferes with breathing. Exercise demands oxygen and causes deeper, faster breathing. Tight belts, tight-fitting shorts, or other tight clothing may result in shallow, inadequate breathing and can lead to fainting. Restrictive clothing also limits your ability to perform an exercise through its full range of motion; this will limit the benefits you will achieve from your exercise.

EQUIPMENT

Equipment will generally be provided for you. Different types of classes use different equipment. Mats and positional aids will be described here; other equipment, including pedometers, heart-rate monitors, exercise bands, stability balls, weights, and step benches, are described within the appropriate chapters.

MATS

Exercise mats come in a variety of thicknesses. Pilates and yoga mats are generally $\frac{1}{8}$- or $\frac{1}{4}$- inch thick. You can also purchase thicker mats so that you "feel the floor" less. Most mats roll or fold up for easy carrying. Some people prefer to bring their own mat or a towel to place on top of a mat to ensure cleanliness.

POSITIONAL AIDS

When you are performing certain stretches, you may need to extend your reach. Special yoga/pilates straps or a simple towel can be wrapped around a limb and then pulled to create the desired stretch. For some examples of positional aids, see Chapter 7. Pillows, wedges, blocks, bolsters, and towels are also used to add comfort during exercise positions. The most commonly used are foam or wooden blocks in yoga and a step bench during a step class. For example, persons who are too inflexible to place their hands on the floor during a standing forward lunge can place their hands on the blocks or straddle the step bench and place hands on top of the step (Figure 7.25c).

Internet Resources

Health and Wellness

American Medical Association
www.ama-assn.org

Centers for Disease Control and Prevention
www.cdc.gov

CNN Health
www.cnn.com/HEALTH

Go Ask Alice! Columbia University's Health Q & A
Internet Service
http://goaskalice.columbia.edu

Healthfinder
www.healthfinder.gov

Healthy People 2020
www.healthypeople.gov

Mayo Clinic
www.mayoclinic.com

National Center for Chronic Disease Prevention and
Health Promotion
www.cdc.gov/nccdphp

National Health Information Center (NHIC)
www.health.gov/nhic

National Women's Health Information Center
www.womenshealth.gov

New York Online Access to Health (bilingual Spanish
and English site)
www.noah-health.org

Physical Fitness

Aerobics and Fitness Association of America (AFAA)
www.afaa.com

American Alliance for Health, Physical Education,
Recreation, and Dance (AAHPERD)
www.aahperd.org

American College of Sports Medicine (ACSM)
www.acsm.org

American Council on Exercise (ACE)
www.acefitness.org

American Diabetes Association
www.diabetes.org/exercise

Internet Fitness Resource
www.netsweat.com

The Fitness Partner Connection Jumpsite
http://primusweb.com/fitnesspartner

Aerobic (Cardiorespiratory) Endurance

American Heart Association
www.heart.org

National Heart, Lung, and Blood Institute
www.nhlbi.nih.gov

Muscular Strength and Endurance

Human Anatomy On-line
www.innerbody.com/htm/body.html

National Academy of Sports Medicine (NASM)
www.nasm.org

National Strength and Conditioning Association
www.nsca-cc.org

Flexibility

NIH Back Pain Fact Sheet
www.ninds.nih.gov/health_and_medical/
disorders/backpain_doc.htm

Southern California Orthopedic Institute
www.scoi.com

Nutrition, Weight Control, and Body Composition

Academy of Nutrition and Dietetics
www.eatright.org

American Heart Association: Delicious Decisions
www.deliciousdecisions.org

Arbor Nutrition Guide
http://arborcom.com

Calorie Control Council
www.caloriecontrol.org

Cancer Information Service
www.cancer.gov/aboutnci/cis

Center for Nutrition Policy and Promotion, USDA
www.usda.gov/cnpp

Fast Food Facts—Interactive Food Finder
www.foodfacts.info

Food and Drug Administration
www.fda.gov

National Osteoporosis Foundation
www.nof.org

USDA MyPlate
www.ChooseMyPlate.gov

Veggies Unite!
www.vegweb.com

Injury Prevention and Care

National Athletic Trainers' Association
www.nata.org

Indoor Cycling

Fly Wheel
www.flywheelsports.com

Indoor Cycling 2.0
www.indoorcycleinstructor.com

Keiser
www.keiser.com

Training Tips
www.spinning.com/en/training_tips

Kickboxing

Kickboxing Technique Video: Back Kick
www.ehow.com/video_2368162_kickboxing-
technique-back-kick.html

Kickboxing Technique Video: Cross
www.ehow.com/video_2368152_kickboxing-
technique-cross.html

Kickboxing Technique Video: Front Kick
www.ehow.com/video_2368158_kickboxing-
technique-front-kick.html

Kickboxing Technique Video: Hook
www.ehow.com/video_2368153_kickboxing-
technique-hook.html

Kickboxing Technique Video: Jab
www.ehow.com/video_2368151_kickboxing-
technique-jab.html

Kickboxing Technique Video: Round Kick
www.ehow.com/video_2368159_kickboxing-
technique-round-kick.html

Kickboxing Technique Video: Stance
www.ehow.com/video_2368150_kickboxing-
technique-stance.html

Kickboxing Technique Video: Uppercut
www.ehow.com/video_2368154_kickboxing-
technique-uppercut.html

Water Exercise

Aquajogger
www.aquajogger.com

Aquatherapeutics
www.aquatherapeutics.com

Aquatic Exercise Association
www.aeawave.com

Poolates
www.poolates.com

U.S Synchronized Swimming Association
www.usasynchro.org

WaterArt Fitness International
www.waterart.org

WaterFit
www.waterfit.com

Military/Cross Fitness

Beachbody Fitness Programs
www.beachbody.com

British Military Fitness
www.britmilfit.com/why-bmf/

CrossFit Games
http://games.crossfit.com/workouts

Functional Training

Function Follows Fitness
www.acefitness.org/getfit/studies/functionfitness
.pdf

Functional Training: Is It Right for You?
www.mayoclinic.com/health/functional-fitness/
MY01378

What Is Functional Training?
www.humankinetics.com/excerpts/excerpts/
what-is-functional-training-

Working Out for Real-life Fitness
www.webmd.com/fitness-exercise/features/
working-out-for-real-life-functions

Yoga

Anusara Yoga
www.anusara.com

Ashtanga Yoga
www.ashtanga.net

Bikram Yoga
www.bikramyoga.com

Iyengar Yoga
www.iynaus.org

Kripalu Center for Yoga and Health
www.kripalu.org

Sivananda Yoga
www.sivananda.org

Yoga
www.yoga.about.com

Yoga Alliance
www.yogaalliance.org

Yoga Fit
www.yogafit.com

Yoga Journal
www.yogajournal.com

Yogilates
www.yogilates.com

WORKSHEET 4.1: CALCULATING YOUR TARGET HEART RATE RANGE

Maximum Heart-Rate Formula (Zero to Peak Formula)

Refer to Chapter 4, pages 39–40 and Table 4.2. The target heart rate range (target heart rate zone) you select to calculate depends on your fitness level. The example provided here uses a range of 70%–85% of HRmax. This range runs from the midpoint of moderately intense to the midpoint of vigorously intense exercise. **To adjust this range, multiply by different percentages in Steps two and three.**

STEP ONE
Find your maximum heart rate (HRmax).

$-$ ☐   (0.7 × age)

☐   (HRmax)

EXAMPLE:
The HRmax of a 20-year-old.

$$\begin{array}{r} 207 \\ -14 \quad (0.7 \times 20) \\ \hline 193 \end{array}$$

STEP TWO
Find the lower end of your THR in beats/minute.

☐   (HRmax)

× _____ 0.7   (you can adjust this percentage if desired)

☐   (beats/minute)

EXAMPLE:

$$\begin{array}{r} 193 \\ \times 0.7 \\ \hline 135.10 \end{array}$$

STEP THREE
Find the upper end of your THR in beats/minute.

☐   (HRmax)

× _____ 0.85   (you can adjust this percentage if desired)

☐   (beats/minute)

EXAMPLE:

$$\begin{array}{r} 193 \\ \times 0.85 \\ \hline 965 \\ 15440 \\ \hline 165.05 \end{array}$$

My target heart-rate range is $\overline{\quad\text{(lower)}\quad}$ to $\overline{\quad\text{(upper)}\quad}$ beats/minute.

EXAMPLE: My THR is 135 to 165 beats/minute.

Continued on next page

STEP FOUR

Find the lower end of your THR in beats/10 seconds.

6 ⟌ [_____] = _____ beats/10 seconds
    Step 2 Answer

EXAMPLE:

```
     22.5
6 ) 135
    12
    ───
    15
    12
    ───
    30
    30
    ───
     0
```

STEP FIVE

Find the upper end of your THR in beats/10 seconds.

6 ⟌ [_____] = _____ beats/10 seconds
    Step 3 Answer

EXAMPLE:

```
     27.58
6 ) 165
    12
    ───
    45
    42
    ───
    35
    30
    ───
    50
    48
    ───
     2
```

My target heart-rate range is $\frac{\quad}{\text{(lower)}}$ to $\frac{\quad}{\text{(upper)}}$ beats/10 seconds.

EXAMPLE: My THR is 23 to 28 beats/10 seconds.

242

WORKSHEET 4.2: CALCULATING YOUR TARGET HEART RATE RANGE

Karvonen Formula

Refer to Chapter 4, pages 39–40 and Table 4.2. The target heart rate range (target heart rate zone) you select to calculate depends on your fitness level. The example provided here uses a range of 60%–80% of HRR. This range represents a commonly used range for vigorous intensity exercise. **To adjust this range, multiply by different percentages in steps three and five.**

First find your average resting heart rate by counting your pulse for 1 minute while you are still lying in bed. Do this on three consecutive mornings.

Resting heart rate on the first morning: _____ beats/minute
Resting heart rate on the second morning: _____ beats/minute
Resting heart rate on the third morning: _____ beats/minute
Average Resting Heart Rate (RHR): _____ beats/minute

STEPS ONE AND TWO

Find your maximum heart rate and heart-rate reserve.

$$207$$

$-$ ☐ (0.7 × age)

☐ (HRmax)

$-$ ☐ (RHR)

☐ (HRR)

EXAMPLE:

A 20-year-old with an RHR of 75.

$$
\begin{array}{ll}
207 & \\
- 14 & (0.7 \times 20) \\
\hline
193 & \\
- 75 & (RHR) \\
\hline
118 & (HRR)
\end{array}
$$

STEPS THREE AND FOUR

For the lower limit of the THR, calculate 60% of the HRR and add the RHR to the answer.

☐ (HRR)

× _____ 0.6 (you can adjust this percentage if desired)

☐

+ ☐ (RHR)

☐ Lower end of THR in beats/minute

EXAMPLE:

$$
\begin{array}{ll}
118 & (HRR) \\
\times\, 0.6 & \\
\hline
70.8 & \\
+75.0 & (RHR) \\
\hline
145.8 &
\end{array}
$$

Continued on next page

STEPS FIVE AND SIX

For the upper limit of the THR, calculate 80% of the HRR and add the RHR to the answer.

	(HRR)

$\times$ _____ 0.8 (you can adjust this percentage if desired)

$+$ _____ (RHR)

	Upper end of THR in beats/minute

My target heart-rate range is $\dfrac{\quad\quad}{\text{(lower)}}$ to $\dfrac{\quad\quad}{\text{(upper)}}$ beats/minute.

EXAMPLE:

118	(HRR)
$\times\ 0.8$	
94.4	
$+75.0$	(RHR)
169.4	

EXAMPLE: My THR is 146 to 169 beats/minute.

STEPS SEVEN AND EIGHT

Divide both ends of the THR in beats/minute by 6 to obtain a THR in beats per 10 seconds.

$6\overline{\big)\;\boxed{}\;} = \boxed{}$

(lower limit)

$6\overline{\big)\;\boxed{}\;} = \boxed{}$

(upper limit)

My target heart-rate range isis $\dfrac{\quad\quad}{\text{(lower)}}$ to $\dfrac{\quad\quad}{\text{(upper)}}$ beats/10 seconds.

EXAMPLE:

```
      24.3
  6 ) 146
      12
      ---
      26
      24
      ---
       20
       18
       ---
        2
```

EXAMPLE:

```
      28.1
  6 ) 169
      12
      ---
      49
      48
      ---
      10
       6
```

EXAMPLE: My THR is 24 to 28 beats/10 seconds.

WORKSHEET 5.4: CARDIORESPIRATORY FITNESS

YMCA Step Test (12-inch)

EQUIPMENT:

1. bench 12' high—a step aerobics bench will work (a bleacher 16¼" high can be substituted, and the norms will still be reasonably accurate)

2. stopwatch

3. metronome or other means of establishing the cadence

4. pencil or pen

DIRECTIONS:

1. Practice taking your heart rate. If you will be working with a partner, practice taking your partner's heart rate.

2. Warm up and stretch.

3. Face the bench and practice the stepping pattern: Up, Up, Down, Down.

   Up—step up on the bench with your right foot.

   Up—bring your left foot up on the bench.

   Down—step down to the floor with your right foot.

   Down—step down to the floor with your left foot.

4. Rest until your breathing is back to normal.

5. Set the cadence (rate at which you will step) to 96 beats/minute (24 step/cycles per minute).

6. With the start of the stopwatch, begin the stepping pattern and continue stepping for 3 minutes. If you cannot complete the whole 3 minutes (too tired to keep cadence), stop and record the amount of time you were able to complete: _____ minutes _____ seconds.

7. Stop and find your pulse. Begin counting the pulse within 5 seconds after you stop stepping. Count for an *entire minute*.

   _____ recovery heart rate (RecHR) in beats/minute

8. Look at the chart on the following page to determine your fitness rating.

   My fitness rating is _____.

9. Stretch your legs to prevent muscle soreness.

Continued on next page

Fitness ratings for a 3-minute step test.

| | | 1-MINUTE POST-EXERCISE HEART RATE | | | | | | | |
| | | 18–25 YEARS OLD | | 26–35 YEARS OLD | | 36–45 YEARS OLD | | 46–55 YEARS OLD | |
FITNESS RATING	% RANKING	M	F	M	F	M	F	M	F
	100	50	52	51	58	49	51	56	63
	95	71	75	70	74	70	77	77	85
Excellent	90	76	81	76	80	76	84	82	91
	85	79	85	79	85	80	89	87	95
	80	82	89	83	89	84	92	89	98
Good	75	84	93	85	92	88	96	93	101
	70	88	96	88	95	92	100	95	104
	65	90	98	91	98	95	102	99	107
Above Average	60	93	102	94	101	98	104	101	110
	55	95	104	96	104	100	107	103	113
	50	97	108	100	107	101	109	107	115
Average	45	100	110	102	110	105	112	111	118
	40	102	113	104	113	108	115	113	120
	35	105	116	108	116	111	118	117	121
Below Average	30	107	120	110	119	113	120	119	124
	25	111	122	114	122	116	124	121	126
	20	114	126	118	126	119	128	124	128
Poor	15	119	131	121	129	124	132	126	132
	10	124	135	126	134	130	137	131	137
	5	132	143	134	141	138	142	139	143
Very Poor	0	157	169	161	171	163	169	159	171

Note: This test presents fitness ratings based on percentiles. If you are in the 95th percentile, you are more fit than 95 out of 100 people. Another way to say this would be to say you are in the top 5%. For basic health-fitness, you do not need to be in the highest categories. If you score in the poor or fair category, you may want to begin with a walking program or equivalent. Those who score as average or higher should have sufficient cardiorespiratory capacity to start out in a regular beginner's program or, if in the higher categories, work out using a program commensurate with their fitness rating.

Source: Adapted from "YMCA of the USA Physical Fitness Evaluation Profile," from the *YMCA Fitness Testing and Assessment Manual,* 4th ed., 2000, 200–11.

WORKSHEET 5.5: CARDIORESPIRATORY FITNESS

12-Minute Walk/Run Test

Note: This is a maximum-effort test. It is recommended that you exercise regularly for 6 to 8 weeks prior to taking this test.

EQUIPMENT:

1. stopwatch
2. track or other measured course
3. pencil or pen

DIRECTIONS:

1. Warm up with light jogging and stretching.
2. Run/walk as far as possible in 12 minutes. This is best achieved by maintaining a steady pace. Be sure to keep track of how far you run. You may want to do this with a partner so that you can count laps for each other.
3. Record the distance you covered: _____miles.
4. Cool down with light jogging and stretching.
5. Consult the chart below to determine your fitness rating. My fitness rating is _____.

Distance (miles) covered in 12-minute walk/run test.

FITNESS CATEGORY		AGE (YEARS)					
		13–19	20–29	30–39	40–49	50–59	60+
I. Very Poor	(men)	<1.30*	<1.22	<1.18	<1.14	<1.03	<.87
	(women)	<1.0	<.96	<.94	<.88	<.84	<.78
II. Poor	(men)	1.30–1.37	1.22–1.31	1.18–1.30	1.14–1.24	1.03–1.16	.87–1.02
	(women)	1.00–1.18	.96–1.11	.95–1.05	.88–.98	.84–.93	.78–.86
III. Fair	(men)	1.38–1.56	1.32–1.49	1.31–1.45	1.25–1.39	1.17–1.30	1.03–1.20
	(women)	1.19–1.29	1.12–1.22	1.06–1.18	.99–1.11	.94–1.05	.87–.98
IV. Good	(men)	1.57–1.72	1.50–1.64	1.46–1.56	1.40–1.53	1.31–1.44	1.21–1.32
	(women)	1.30–1.43	1.23–1.34	1.19–1.29	1.12–1.24	1.06–1.18	.99–1.09
V. Excellent	(men)	1.73–1.86	1.65–1.76	1.57–1.69	1.54–1.65	1.45–1.58	1.33–1.55
	(women)	1.44–1.51	1.35–1.45	1.30–1.39	1.25–1.34	1.19–1.30	1.10–1.18
VI. Superior	(men)	>1.87	>1.77	>1.70	>1.66	>1.59	>1.56
	(women)	>1.52	>1.46	>1.40	>1.35	>1.31	>1.19

*< means "less than"; > means "more than."
Source: "1.5 Mile Run Tests" and "12-Minute Walk/Run Test" from *The Aerobics Program for Total Well-Being* by Kenneth H. Cooper, M.D., M.P.H. Copyright © 1982 by Kenneth H. Cooper. Used by permission of Random House, Inc.

Continued on next page

WORKSHEET 5.6: CARDIORESPIRATORY FITNESS

1.5-Mile Timed Run Test

Note: This is a maximum-effort test. It is recommended that you exercise regularly for 6 to 8 weeks prior to taking this test.

EQUIPMENT:

1. stopwatch
2. measured course
3. pencil or pen

DIRECTIONS:

1. Warm up and stretch.
2. On the start signal, run/walk the 1.5-mile course as quickly as possible. (An even pace throughout the course is recommended.)
3. Check your time at the end of the course: _____ minutes.
4. Consult the chart below to find your fitness rating. My fitness rating is _____.

Time in minutes for 1.5-mile run test.

FITNESS CATEGORY		AGE (YEARS)					
		13–19	20–29	30–39	40–49	50–59	60+
I. Very Poor	(men)	>15:31*	>16:01	>16:31	>17:31	>19:01	>20:01
	(women)	>18:31	>19:01	>19:31	>20:01	>20:31	>21:01
II. Poor	(men)	12:11–15:30	14:01–16:00	14:44–16:30	15:36–17:30	17:01–19:00	19:01–20:00
	(women)	16:55–18:30	18:31–19:00	19:01–19:30	19:31–20:00	20:01–20:30	20:31–21:00
III. Fair	(men)	10:49–12:10	12:01–14:00	12:31–14:45	13:01–15:35	14:31–17:00	16:16–19:00
	(women)	14:31–16:54	15:55–18:30	16:31–19:00	17:31–19:30	19:01–20:00	19:31–20:30
IV. Good	(men)	9:41–10:48	10:46–12:00	11:01–12:30	11:31–13:00	12:31–14:30	14:00–16:15
	(women)	12:30–14:30	13:31–15:54	14:31–16:30	15:56–17:30	16:31–19:00	17:31–19:30
V. Excellent	(men)	8:37–9:40	9:45–10:45	10:00–11:00	10:30–11:30	11:00–12:30	11:15–13:59
	(women)	11:50–12:29	12:30–13:30	13:00–14:30	13:45–15:55	14:30–16:30	16:30–17:30
VI. Superior	(men)	<8:37	<9:45	<10:00	<10:30	<11:00	<11:15
	(women)	<11:50	<12:30	<13:00	<13:45	<14:30	<16:30

*< means "less than"; > means "more than."
Source: "1.5 Mile Run Tests" and "12-Minute Walk/Run Test" from *The Aerobics Program for Total Well-Being* by Kenneth H. Cooper, M.D., M.P.H. Copyright © 1982 by Kenneth H. Cooper. Used by permission of Random House, Inc.

Continued on next page

WORKSHEET 7.1: FLEXIBILITY

Trunk Forward Flexion Tests

EQUIPMENT:

1. flexometer (Modified Wells and Dillon)[1]
2. partner
3. pencil or pen

Note: Be sure to take this test under the same conditions each time you take it. For example, if you take the test before working out in the afternoon, take it again at the same time of day, after you warm up, but before you exercise.

DIRECTIONS:

1. Perform a warm-up that includes slow static stretching of the lower back and posterior thighs prior to taking this test (modified hurdle stretch held for 20 seconds repeated twice on each leg).
2. Remove your shoes and sit on the floor with your legs fully extended and the soles of your feet placed flat against the flexometer. Have your partner adjust the flexometer so that the balls of your feet rest against the upper crossboards. Place the inner edge of the soles of your feet 2 centimeters (cm) from the edge of the scale.
3. Keeping your knees fully extended, your arms evenly stretched, and your palms down, bend and reach forward (without jerking), pushing the sliding marker along the scale with your fingertips as far forward as possible. **Note:** Lowering your head will help you reach farther.
4. Hold the position of maximum flexion (stretch) for approximately 2 seconds.
5. DO NOT count the attempt if the knees bend. Your partner should watch for knee bend, but not try to hold your knees down.
6. Take the test twice. Record your scores to the nearest 0.5 cm.
7. Record your maximum score: _____ cm.*
8. Consult the chart below to determine your fitness rating. My fitness rating is: _____.

Norms by age groups and gender for trunk forward flexion (cm).*

| | AGE (YEARS) | | | | | | | | | | | |
| | 15–19 | | 20–29 | | 30–39 | | 40–49 | | 50–59 | | 60–69 | |
FITNESS RATING	M	F	M	F	M	F	M	F	M	F	M	F
Excellent	≥39	≥43	≥40	≥41	≥38	≥41	≥35	≥38	≥35	≥39	≥33	≥35
Very Good	34–38	38–42	34–39	37–40	33–37	36–40	29–34	34–37	28–34	33–38	25–32	31–34
Good	29–33	34–37	30–33	33–36	28–32	32–35	24–28	30–33	24–27	30–32	20–24	27–30
Fair	24–28	29–33	25–29	28–32	23–27	27–31	18–23	25–29	16–23	25–29	15–19	23–26
Needs Improvement	≤23	≤28	≤24	≤27	≤22	≤26	≤17	≤24	≤15	≤24	≤14	≤23

*Based on data from the Canada Fitness Survey, 1981.
Source: The Canadian Physical Activity, Fitness and Lifestyle Appraisal: CSEP's Plan for Healthy Active Living. 2nd ed.
© 1998. Reprinted by permission from the Canadian Society for Exercise Physiology.

---

* Note: This test was designed to test both legs at the same time. Other tests evaluate one leg at a time in order to identify asymmetry. You can adjust this test by bending one leg so that the sole of the foot is on the ground one fist-width from the knee of the extended leg with the knee pointing to the ceiling (FITNESSGRAM) or assume a modified hurdler's position (Figure B next page). Record scores for each leg.

Right leg extended: _____cm _____fitness rating
Left leg extended: _____ cm _____fitness rating

---

1. For directions on how to construct a Modified Wells and Dillon flexometer, along with a drawing showing how to use it, please refer to the instructor's manual.

Continued on next page

MODIFIED TRUNK FORWARD FLEXION TEST

Note 1: This test can be performed without a flexometer. It may be a little less accurate, but, if done carefully, will still supply a good working estimate of flexibility. Please note that the fitness ratings on the previous page were developed using a Modified Wells and Dillon flexometer. Use of those ratings with this test may not be fully accurate. Following the directions carefully each time you take this test will help ensure a good estimate of flexibility.

Note 2: Be sure to take this test under the same conditions each time you take it. For example, if you take the test before working out in the afternoon, take it again at the same time of day, after you warm up, but before you exercise.

EQUIPMENT:

1. meterstick
2. two partners
3. pencil or pen

DIRECTIONS:

1. Perform a warm-up that includes slow static stretching of the lower back and posterior thighs prior to taking this test (modified hurdle stretch held for 20 seconds, repeated twice on each leg).
2. Remove your shoes and sit on the floor with your legs fully extended. Have another person sit opposite you in the same position so that the soles of your feet are against those of the other person. All toes should point directly toward the ceiling throughout the test (Figure A). A one-legged version can also be performed (Figure B). An imbalance in hamstring flexibility can be noted this way.
3. The measurer (third person) holds the meterstick just above your toes with the number 26 cm even with the bottom of the soles of your feet. If you wish to keep your shoes on, place the 26-cm mark where the soles of your feet would be, rather than at the bottom of the soles of the shoes. The number 1 on the meterstick should be close to you, number 39 away from you.
4. Place one hand over the other, palms down, so that your fingertips are even. Then with your knees fully extended, and your arms evenly stretched, slide your fingers as far down the meterstick as possible. Use a smooth, sustained motion. **Note:** Lowering your head will help you reach farther.
5. Hold the position of maximum flexion (stretch) for approximately two seconds.
6. DO NOT count the attempt if the knees bend. Your partner should watch for knee bend, but should not try to hold your knees down.

Figure A

Figure B

7. Take the test twice. Record your scores to the nearest 0.5 cm.
8. Record your maximum scores: Two legs: _____ cm
   R: _____ cm L: _____cm.
9. Consult the chart on the previous page for an approximate fitness rating. My fitness rating is
   _____.

TRUNK FLEXION WALL TEST

Note: This is a quick and easy check for flexibility that you can perform anywhere there is a wall with sitting space in front of it.

DIRECTIONS:

1. Warm up with 5 to 10 minutes of light cardio work followed by some static stretches of the lower back and posterior thighs.
2. Place your feet flat against a wall.
3. Reach forward with both hands and try to touch the wall.

FITNESS CATEGORY:

Poor	Can't touch the wall.
Good	Can touch the wall with your fingertips.
Very Good	Can touch the walls with your knuckles (hands in fists).
Excellent	Can place both palms flat on the wall.

WORKSHEET 7.2: QUICK CHECK FLEXIBILITY TESTS

The following 12 tests are pass/fail. They are quick and easy to perform and require only a yardstick and a partner. Because flexibility is joint specific, a variety of tests is provided. Check for imbalances from one side of the body to the other and between paired muscles or muscle groups.

If you would like to keep a record of your flexibility and then check for improvement in 6 to 8 weeks, draw a stick figure indicating the angle of your joint for each test on the record sheets on pages 243–244. If you have a protractor you can measure and record the angle. Another way to measure the angle is to use a simple tool you can create by fastening together two straightedges (for example, plastic rulers or pieces of stiff cardboard) at one end using a paper fastener. Hold your tool near or against your partner's body and open or close the straightedges until the angle of the tool matches the angle of the joint you are measuring. Then move the tool to your record sheet and trace the angle. Be sure to measure both limbs or sides of the body as appropriate.

Neck Test

Stand or sit with your back straight and your face looking forward. Drop your chin to your chest. If you are able to press your chin against an open hand placed on your chest, give yourself a passing grade. If not, measure and record the distance between your chin and hand.

Shoulder Test I

Stand up straight with your arms at your side, palms touching your leg. Raise one arm *forward* and up overhead. If you reach 180 degrees (directly overhead) or more give yourself a passing grade. If not, measure and record the angle between your body and your raised arm.

Shoulder Test II

Stand up straight with your arms at your side, palms touching your leg. Raise one arm *out to the side* and up overhead. If you reach 180 degrees (by your ear), give yourself a passing grade. If not, measure and record the angle between the side of your body and your arm.

Shoulder Test III

Stand up straight and attempt to touch your fingertips by reaching one arm over the shoulder and one arm up the middle of your back. If you can touch your hands, give yourself a passing grade. If not, have a partner measure and record the distance between your fingertips.

Trunk Test

Sit in a chair with your feet flat on the floor. Turn your upper body while keeping your hips square to the front. If you are able to twist 90 degrees or more (shoulders will be square to the side) give yourself a passing grade. If not, have a partner measure and record the angle of rotation. (If you are turning right, measure the angle your left shoulder moved away from dead front.) It will be easier to see whether you have succeeded if you place your hands on your shoulders while you twist.

Lower Back Test

Lie on your back with both knees bent, feet off the floor, and head and lower back touching the floor. Grasp your legs underneath your knees and pull gently toward your shoulders (if you have to pull hard you fail the test). To pass, touch both knees to their respective shoulders or lay your thighs flat along your torso with your lower back and head still touching the floor. If you are unable to, measure the angle between your thighs and your torso.

Hip Flexor Test

Lie on your back on the floor with both legs straight. Keeping one leg straight and along the ground, draw the knee of the other leg up toward your chest. Place your hand on the back of your thigh underneath your knee and pull gently. Give yourself a passing grade if your thigh touches your torso and your other leg remains straight. If not, have your partner measure and record the angle between your torso and thigh.

ALTERNATE TEST:

Lie on your back on a knee-high firm surface, such as a folded mat, bleacher, or table. Bend your knees over

Continued on next page

the edge and put your feet flat on the floor. Draw one knee to your chest while trying to keep the opposite foot flat on the floor. If you can do this comfortably, give yourself a passing grade. If your heel lifts up, have your partner measure and record the distance between your heel and the floor.

Hip Abduction Test

Either standing straight or lying on the ground, move one leg sideways as far from the other leg as possible. If the angle between the legs measures 45 degrees or more, give yourself a passing grade. If not, have your partner measure and record the angle.

Hamstring Test

Lie on your back with both legs straight. Keeping both legs straight, lift the one up and as far toward your head as possible. Give yourself a passing grade if you were able to reach a 90-degree angle (straight up) or more. If not, have your partner measure and record the angle between the floor and your raised leg.

Quadriceps Test

Lie prone on the floor with your head turned to one side. Bend one knee and grasp the ankle. Without forcing it, draw your ankle toward your buttocks. Give yourself a passing grade if your heel touches your buttocks or your lower leg rests against your upper leg. If not, have your partner measure and record the angle behind your knee made by your lower and upper leg.

Calf Test

Sit on the floor with your legs extended straight in front of you. Flex one ankle as much as you can. Give yourself a passing grade if the angle between the sole of your shoe and your shin is 80 to 90 degrees or less. If not, have a partner measure and record the angle.

ALTERNATE POSITION:

Stand with your weight on one foot and the heel of the other foot on the ground. Dorsiflex the ankle of the unweighted foot by drawing the toes toward the shin. Measure the angle created between the floor and the sole of the foot. A passing score is a 10- to 20-degree angle.

Important Notes:

Asymmetry in flexibility is one of the most common causes for muscular pain and/or injury. An asymmetry is when one side of the body is more flexible than the other. When an asymmetry exists, you will accommodate this lack of flexibility by making compensations in your movement pattern. Unfortunately these compensations create movement patterns that aren't healthy. If you find you test better on one side than the other, work first to balance the two sides and then if you are still not "passing," increase the flexibility in both sides together.

In Shoulder Test III, if your two hands are within one hand's length (base of the hand to tip of middle finger) this would be considered good functional movement. It is very common to see an asymmetry in shoulder flexibility. Improve the "weak" side first, and then both together.

Quick Flexibility Test Record

Test	Passing	Your Results			
		Date:	Date:	Date:	Date:
Neck Test	0 inches	___ inches between hand and chin	___ inches between hand and chin	___ inches between hand and chin	___ inches between hand and chin
Shoulder Test I	180 degrees	Left arm Right arm __ deg. __ deg.	Left arm Right arm __ deg. __ deg.	Left arm Right arm __ deg. __ deg.	Left arm Right arm __ deg. __ deg.
Shoulder Test II	180 degrees	Left arm Right arm __ deg. __ deg.	Left arm Right arm __ deg. __ deg.	Left arm Right arm __ deg. __ deg.	Left arm Right arm __ deg. __ deg.
Shoulder Test III	0 inches (fingers touching)	Right arm up: ___ inches between fingertips Left arm up: ___ inches between fingertips	Right arm up: ___ inches between fingertips Left arm up: ___ inches between fingertips	Right arm up: ___ inches between fingertips Left arm up: ___ inches between fingertips	Right arm up: ___ inches between fingertips Left arm up: ___ inches between fingertips
Trunk Test	90 degrees*	___ degrees of rotation	___ degrees of rotation	___ degrees of rotation	___ degrees of rotation
Lower Back Test	Thighs touching chest (0 degrees)	___ deg.	___ deg.	___ deg.	___ deg.

* For clarity, only 45 degrees is shown. Continue to 90 degrees.

Continued on next page

Test	Passing	Your Results			
		Date:	Date:	Date:	Date:
Hip Flexor Test	Thigh touching chest (0 degrees)	left leg: ___ deg. right leg: ___ deg.	left leg: ___ deg. right leg: ___ deg.	left leg: ___ deg. right leg: ___ deg.	left leg: ___ deg. right leg: ___ deg.
Alternate Hip Flexor Test	0 inches	right leg ___ inches between heel and floor left leg ___ inches between heel and floor	right leg ___ inches between heel and floor left leg ___ inches between heel and floor	right leg ___ inches between heel and floor left leg ___ inches between heel and floor	right leg ___ inches between heel and floor left leg ___ inches between heel and floor
Hip Abduction Test	45 degrees	left leg: ___ deg. right leg: ___ deg.	left leg: ___ deg. right leg: ___ deg.	left leg: ___ deg. right leg: ___ deg.	left leg: ___ deg. right leg: ___ deg.
Hamstring Test	90 degrees	left leg: ___ deg. right leg: ___ deg.	left leg: ___ deg. right leg: ___ deg.	left leg: ___ deg. right leg: ___ deg.	left leg: ___ deg. right leg: ___ deg.
Quadriceps Test	Heel touching buttocks (0 degrees)	left leg: ___ deg. right leg: ___ deg.	left leg: ___ deg. right leg: ___ deg.	left leg: ___ deg. right leg: ___ deg.	left leg: ___ deg. right leg: ___ deg.
Calf Test	80 to 90 degrees	left ankle: ___ deg. right ankle: ___ deg.	left ankle: ___ deg. right ankle: ___ deg.	left ankle: ___ deg. right ankle: ___ deg.	left ankle: ___ deg. right ankle: ___ deg.

256

WORKSHEET 10.1: MUSCULAR ENDURANCE

Partial Curl-Up Test

Note: A person who suffers from lower back or neck ailments should not perform this test.

EQUIPMENT:

1. gym mat with tape, string, wire, or Velcro markers as indicated below
2. metronome or cassette player and tape with a recorded beat
3. metric ruler
4. pen or pencil
5. carpenter's square, or book, or piece of paper
6. partner

MAT SETUP:

On a gym mat use tape, string, wire, or strips of Velcro and a metric ruler to lay out the diagram below. You can also set this up so that the edge of the mat is the 10-centimeter (cm) mark.

Guidelines for tape and string/Velcro placement on gym mat

DIRECTIONS:

1. Lie on your back with your head on the mat, arms straight and parallel to your trunk, palms flat on the mat, and the middle fingertip of both hands at the zero mark.

   With the soles of your feet touching the mat, bend your knees at a 90-degree angle. Your partner can use the corner of a textbook or standard piece of paper to check your knee angle.

   Have your partner place a strip of tape under your heels to mark where your heels are to stay in contact with the mat.

2. Turn on the metronome to 50 beats per minute (or cassette tape recording of the same). You will be curling up on one beat and down on the next at a rate of 25 curl-ups per minute.

Continued on next page

3. Curl up by first flattening out your lower back region (pelvic tilt) and then slowly curling up your upper spine. Slide your palms in contact with the mat along the tape until they touch the string or Velcro at the 10-cm mark. During the curl-up, the palms and heels must remain in contact with the mat. Anchoring of the feet is not permitted. Breathe normally throughout, exhaling as you curl up.

4. Return to your starting position—lying flat, head down, fingertips at the zero mark on the string or Velcro. Practice twice, making sure that you take an equal amount of time to curl in each direction. Use continuous and well-controlled movements.

5. Perform continuous curl-ups until you reach a maximum of 25. Stop sooner if you experience severe discomfort or pain, if you fall 2 repetitions behind cadence, or if your partner indicates that you have lost proper technique over 2 consecutive repetitions as outlined below:
- moving your seat (changing your knee angle)
- lifting or sliding your heels
- bending your elbows or lifting your palms off the mat
- sliding your fingers short of, or beyond, the 10-cm mark
- pausing between movements at either the top or bottom of the curl-up
- getting ahead of or behind the cadence

6. Stretch your abdominal and leg muscles.

7. Record the number of curl-ups you completed: _____

8. Consult the chart below and determine your fitness level. Be sure to look under the appropriate age and gender.

My fitness rating is: _____.

Norms and health benefits by age groups and gender for partial curl-up.

	AGE (YEARS)											
	15–19		20–29		30–39		40–49		50–59		60–69	
FITNESS RATING	M	F	M	F	M	F	M	F	M	F	M	F
Excellent	25	25	25	25	25	25	25	25	25	25	25	≥18
Very Good	23–24	23–24	23–24	23–24	23–24	23–24	22–24	21–24	20–24	16–24	16–24	11–17
Good	21–22	21–22	21–22	19–22	21–22	16–21	16–21	13–20	20–24	16–24	16–24	11–17
Fair	16–20	16–20	13–20	13–18	13–20	11–15	11–15	6–12	9–13	4–8	4–9	2–5
Needs Improvement	≤15	≤15	≤12	≤12	≤12	≤10	≤10	≤5	≤8	≤2	≤3	≤1

Source: The Canadian Physical Activity, Fitness and Lifestyle Appraisal: CSEP's Plan for Healthy Active Living. 2nd ed.
© 1998. Reprinted by permission from the Canadian Society for Exercise Physiology.

WORKSHEET 10.2: MUSCULAR ENDURANCE

Push-Up Test

EQUIPMENT:

1. partner
2. mat or towel (for knees during modified push-ups)
3. pencil or pen

IMPORTANT NOTES:

1. A person who suffers from any lower back ailment should not perform this test.
2. The norms for this test are based on women performing modified push-ups and men performing regular push-ups. If, however, a woman wishes to perform regular push-ups, she can with the understanding that the norms are based on men. Similarly, men who lack the upper-body strength to do regular push-ups can begin with modified push-ups and record their progress.

DIRECTIONS FOR THE MODIFIED PUSH-UP:

1. Warm up and stretch, especially your arms and chest.
2. Lie on your stomach, legs together. Position your hands under your shoulders with fingers pointing forward. Push up from the mat by fully extending your elbows and using your knees as the pivot point. The upper body must be kept in a straight line. Return to the starting point, chin to the mat. The stomach should not touch the mat. The lower legs remain in contact with the mat, ankles plantar-flexed (extended), and feet in contact with the mat. Exhale when you push up and inhale as you lower down.
3. Perform as many consecutive push-ups as you are able. There is no time limit. The test stops when you have to strain forcibly or are unable to maintain the proper push-up technique over 2 consecutive repetitions.

4. Record the number of correct push-ups you completed: _____.
5. Consult the normative chart and determine your fitness level: _____. (Fill in an "x" if there are no gender-appropriate norms for the test you performed.)
6. Stretch your arms and chest muscles to prevent soreness.

DIRECTIONS FOR THE REGULAR PUSH-UP:

1. Warm up and stretch, especially your arms and chest.
2. Lie on your stomach, legs together. Position your hands under your shoulders with fingers pointing forward. Push up from the mat by fully extending your elbows and using your toes as the pivot point. The upper body must be kept in a straight line. Return to the starting point touching only the chin, not the stomach or the thighs. Exhale when you push up, and inhale as you lower down.
3. Perform as many consecutive push-ups as you are able. There is no time limit. The test stops when you have to strain forcibly or are unable to maintain the proper push-up technique over 2 consecutive repetitions.
4. Record the number of correct push-ups you completed: _____.
5. Consult the normative chart and determine your fitness level: _____. (Fill in an "x" if there are no gender-appropriate norms for the test you performed.)
6. Stretch your arms and chest muscles to prevent soreness.

Continued on next page

Norms by age groups and gender for push-ups.*

	AGE (YEARS)											
	15–19		20–29		30–39		40–49		50–59		60–69	
FITNESS RATING	M	F	M	F	M	F	M	F	M	F	M	F
Excellent	≥39	≥33	≥36	≥30	≥30	≥27	≥22	≥24	≥21	≥21	≥18	≥17
Above Average	29–38	25–32	29–35	21–29	22–29	20–26	17–21	15–23	13–20	11–20	11–17	12–16
Average	23–28	18–24	22–28	15–20	17–21	13–19	13–16	11–14	10–12	7–10	8–10	5–11
Below Average	18–22	12–17	17–21	10–14	12–16	8–12	10–12	5–10	7–9	2–6	5–7	1–4
Poor	≤17	≤11	≤16	≤9	≤11	≤7	≤9	≤4	≤6	≤1	≤4	≤1

*Based on data from the Canada Fitness Survey, 1981.
Source: The Canadian Physical Activity, Fitness and Lifestyle Appraisal: CSEP's Plan for Healthy Active Living. 2nd ed.
© 1998. Reprinted by permission from the Canadian Society for Exercise Physiology.

WORKSHEET 13.1: HEALTHY WEIGHT

WAIST/HIP RATIO

1. Measure, or have a partner measure, your waist at the point of noticeable waist narrowing (approximately at your navel). If there is no noticeable narrowing, feel for the twelfth (bottom or floating) rib and take the measurement just below it. Pull the tape enough to maintain its position but not so much that it indents the skin. Be sure the tape is horizontal all the way around your body. Record the measurement to the nearest eighth of an inch ($\frac{1}{8} = .13$, $\frac{2}{8} = .25$, $\frac{3}{8} = .38$, $\frac{4}{8} = .50$, $\frac{5}{8} = .63$, $\frac{6}{8} = .75$, $\frac{7}{8} = .88$).
Waist measurement: _____ inches

2. Measure, or have a partner measure, your hips at the greatest circumference to the nearest eighth of an inch.
Hip measurement: _____ inches

3. Calculate the waist/hip ratio:

$$\frac{\rule{1cm}{0.4pt}}{\text{waist}} \div \frac{\rule{0.6cm}{0.4pt}}{\text{hip}} = \frac{\rule{0.8cm}{0.4pt}}{\text{ratio}}$$

4. A waist-to-hip ratio greater than 1.0 for men and 0.8 for women indicates an increased cardiac risk.
___ I **do not** have an increased risk.
___ I **do** have an increased risk.

BODY MASS INDEX (BMI)

Note: Be sure to read the discussion in the text about BMI. Muscular individuals can be incorrectly classified.

1. Weigh yourself without shoes. If your weight is in pounds, convert it to kilograms.
_____ (pounds) ÷ 2.2 = _____ kilograms

2. Determine your height. If your height is in inches, convert it to meters.
_____ inches ÷ 39 = _____ meters

3. Calculate BMI:

$$\frac{\text{weight}}{\text{height} \times \text{height}} = \underline{\hspace{2cm}} \text{ BMI}$$

OR

1. Multiply your weight in pounds (no shoes) by 703.

2. Divide the answer by your height (in inches, no shoes).

3. Divide the answer again by your height (in inches, no shoes).

_____ I am normal weight.	BMI = 18.5–24.9
_____ I am overweight.	BMI = 25–29.9*
_____ I am obese.	BMI = 30 or greater

*Individuals who are overweight should try not to gain weight. Individuals who are overweight and have two or more risk factors for heart disease and/or have a high waist measurement should try to lose weight. Individuals who are obese should try to lose weight gradually with a ½- to 2-pound loss per week.

Source: Clinical Guidelines on the Identification, Evaluation, and Treatment of Overweight and Obesity in Adults, National Heart, Lung, and Blood Institute, in cooperation with the National Institute of Diabetes and Digestive and Kidney Diseases, National Institutes of Health, June 1998.

Continued on next page

Healthy Weight Calculated Using Known Percent Fat

(See page 193, Chapter 13.)

☐	Present % fat

−

☐	Ideal % fat

☐	Difference in % fat

÷   100

☐	Decimal form of % fat difference

☐	Present weight in pounds

×

☐	Decimal form of % fat difference

☐	Pounds to be lost

☐	Present weight in pounds

−

☐	Pounds to be lost

☐	Healthy weight

Glossary

active stretching A flexibility exercise in which the muscle or muscle groups that oppose the target muscle(s) (one being stretched) are contracted with the effect of relaxing the target muscle(s). Also known as antagonist stretching.

adenosine triphosphate (ATP) The high-energy phosphate molecule used to make cellular energy. Muscle cells use ATP to fuel contraction.

aerobic Living, active, or occurring only in the presence of oxygen.

aerobic exercise Exercise that demands a large and continuous supply of oxygen and that ultimately results in the improvement of the oxygen carrying and delivery systems. Exercise that involves continuous rhythmic large-muscle movements.

aerobic glycolysis The metabolic process of breaking down carbohydrate in the presence of oxygen.

aerobic target zone The fitness target zone for aerobic activity. *See* fitness target zone.

aerobics Any physical activity that requires oxygen for a prolonged amount of time.

agonist A muscle that is undergoing contraction.

anaerobic Without or in the absence of oxygen.

anaerobic glycolysis *See* glycolytic system.

anaerobic system The metabolic processes that produce energy (ATP) in the absence of oxygen. *See* phosphagen system *and* lactic acid system.

anorexia nervosa An eating disorder characterized by a continual desire to lose weight because of fear of being fat. Unless treated, individuals suffering from this disease can starve themselves to death.

antagonist A muscle working in opposition to the agonist. When the agonist contracts, the antagonist relaxes.

antagonist stretching A type of stretching in which the agonist is contracted to aid the stretch and relaxation of the antagonist. Works on the principle of reciprocal innervation. Also known as active stretching.

antioxidants Chemical compounds that neutralize cell-damaging free radicals that are created when oxygen is used inside the body's cells.

aqua aerobics A low-impact form of aerobic conditioning performed in water using water resistance to enhance training. (*Synonym:* water aerobics)

arteriosclerosis Hardening of the arteries. *See* atherosclerosis.

artery A vessel that carries blood away from the heart.

assisted stretching *See* passive stretching.

atherosclerosis A specific form of arteriosclerosis characterized by the formation of fatty deposits (plaque) along the walls of the arteries.

ATP *See* adenosine triphosphate.

autogenic training A psychophysiological technique of using visual metaphors to relax the body.

ballistic stretching A technique used to develop flexibility. It is characterized by a series of bouncing or pulsing movements that alternately stretch and then relax the muscle. These movements may elicit the stretch reflex. (Opposite of static stretching.)

beta oxidation The process of producing energy from fatty acids stored in muscles.

binge-eating disorder A type of eating disorder characterized by episodes of uncontrolled excessive and rapid overeating without purging.

blood pressure The amount of pressure the blood exerts against the walls of the arteries during ventricular contraction (systolic pressure) and ventricular relaxation (diastolic pressure). It is generally represented as a fraction: systolic/diastolic pressure.

body alignment The positioning of the body's segments in relationship to each other.

body composition The relative amounts of lean body mass and fat in the body.

body mass index (BMI) A measure of weight in relation to height which is used to estimate healthy weight and determine health risk.

body posture The position of the body in space (e.g., sitting, standing, lying down).

bulimia An eating disorder characterized by binge-and-purge behavior. Purging may be accomplished through self-induced vomiting or use of diuretics or laxatives.

CAD *See* coronary artery disease.

calorie Common usage form of the word *kilocalorie*. A measure of the value of foods to produce heat and energy in the human body. One calorie is equal to the amount of heat required to raise the temperature of 1 gram of water 1°C.

capillaries The smallest blood vessels in the body. They supply blood (oxygen) to the tissues.

carbohydrates Compounds such as sugars and starches that are made up of carbon, hydrogen, and oxygen. Carbohydrates serve as the primary source of energy for the body. They are broken down and transported in the blood as glucose and stored in the liver and muscles as glycogen. Dietary sources include complex carbohydrates (e.g., grains and beans) and simple carbohydrates (e.g., refined sugars and natural sugars).

cardiac output The amount of blood pumped by the heart in 1 minute.

cardiorespiratory endurance The ability to perform large-muscle movements over a sustained period of time. Also, the ability of the lung-heart system to deliver oxygen for sustained energy production. (*Synonyms:* cardiovascular fitness *or* endurance; cardiorespiratory fitness)

carotid artery An artery that runs close to the surface of the skin just to either side of the larynx. This artery is commonly used for counting the pulse.

cellulite Fat stored under the skin where it is separated into little compartments by connective fibers.

CHD *See* coronary heart disease.

cholesterol A fatty substance in the blood and body tissues that is naturally synthesized by the body and is also contained in certain foods. High levels of cholesterol in the blood are associated with atherosclerosis.

CIA *See* combination high-/low-impact aerobics.

circuit training A method of aerobic or resistance training that involves moving through a series of exercise stations with short or no breaks between stations.

combination high-/low-impact aerobics (CIA) A form of aerobic dance exercise that uses both low- and high-impact movements in one class. (*Synonyms:* hi-/lo-impact, combo-impact)

combo-impact *See* combination high-/low-impact aerobics.

concentric contraction A muscle contraction during which the muscle is shortening.

cool-down Movements performed after the aerobic workout that systematically decrease in intensity so that the body can return to a near resting level.

core training The use of resistance exercises to develop the muscles that support the middle of the body, especially the spine.

core warm-up *See* general warm-up.

coronary arteries The arteries that supply the heart with oxygen.

coronary artery disease (CAD) Narrowing or blockage of the coronary arteries resulting in reduced blood supply, and therefore, reduced oxygen supply to the heart muscle.

coronary heart disease (CHD) The major form of cardiovascular disease, or a disease of the heart or blood vessels. It is the single largest leading cause of death in the United States.

cross training 1) The use of two or more activities (modes of training) to achieve the same goal, i.e., a specific component of fitness. 2) The use of a variety of activities (modes of training) to achieve overall fitness.

diabetes mellitus A group of metabolic diseases in which the body is unable to produce sufficient insulin (type I), or effectively use the insulin it does produce (type II).

diastolic pressure The pressure exerted by the blood in the arteries when the ventricles are filling. Diastolic pressure is represented by the denominator in the blood pressure fraction.

duration The length of a single exercise session.

dynamic contraction A muscle contraction taken over a range of motion. It is used to increase strength throughout a movement. Also known as isotonic contraction. Also known as isotonic contraction.

dynamic flexibility Ranges of motion achieved with exercises that use the speed of the movement to assist in stretching muscles through a range of motion; smooth controlled movements are used, rather than ballistic ones.

dynamic stretching A type of stretching that uses the pull of a muscle or group of muscles and the body's momentum to move through a full range of motion.

dynamic warm-up A series of exercises that include general mobility exercises, dynamic stretching, and balance and coordination movements.

eccentric contraction A muscle contraction during which the muscle is lengthening.

energy balance A state in which caloric intake is equal to caloric expenditure. No weight change occurs during energy balance.

exercise ball *See* stability ball.

exercise band A form of resistance training equipment that consists of a band of stretchable material. This may be a stretch cable, specialized exercise/therapeutic band, surgical tubing, or heavy duty rubber band.

extrinsic motivation Motivation that has its source outside the individual.

failure The point during a resistance exercise when proper technique is lost or when an additional repetition of the exercise cannot be performed.

fat One of the six essential nutrients. This energy-rich compound made up of glycerol and fatty acids serves as a source of energy for the body, particularly during aerobic activity. It is stored as adipose tissue.

fatty acid oxidation An aerobic metabolic process that produces energy (ATP) through the breakdown of fatty acids.

fiber A general term for food substances that the body can't fully digest. (*Synonym:* roughage)

fitness target zone The optimal range of exercise, defined by frequency, intensity, and time (duration) and performed with the purpose of maintaining or improving physical fitness. The lower limit of the zone is called the threshold of training. The upper limit is the maximum amount of exercise that is beneficial.

FITT An acronym for the four variables involved in overload: frequency, intensity, time, and type of activity.

FITT principle An exercise principle describing the frequency, intensity, time, and type of activity.

flexibility The ability to move a joint or series of joints through its full range of motion.

free weights Resistance equipment that is not part of a machine, for example, dumbbells, barbells, and medicine balls.

frequency The number of times a person exercises per week.

functional fitness A workout used to develop strength and flexibility in movements that are used every day.

general warm-up A series of easy, active large muscle movements that increase blood circulation and raise the core temperature 1 to 2 degrees.

glucose The simplest form of sugar. Carbohydrate is broken down into glucose before being absorbed into the bloodstream and taken to the cell for energy production.

glycogen A form of carbohydrate stored in the muscle.

glycolytic system Produces ATP by breaking down carbohydrate (glucose) without oxygen. Also known as anaerobic glycolysis.

group fitness The popular term for exercise classes, such as aerobic dance and group cycling, that emphasize working out as a group, usually to highly motivating music.

hatha yoga The physical aspect of yoga; what most Americans call yoga. Uses a variety of poses, breathing techniques, and meditation. *See also* yoga.

HDL *See* high-density lipoprotein.

heart rate (HR) The number of times the heart beats per minute.

heart-rate reserve (HRR) The maximum heart rate minus the resting heart rate.

HIA *See* high-impact aerobics.

hi-/lo-impact aerobics *See* combination high-/low-impact aerobics.

high-density lipoprotein (HDL) A complex of lipids (fat) and proteins that picks up cholesterol in the blood and carries it to the liver. (Often called HDL-C when carrying cholesterol.) Exercise increases the amount of HDL in the blood.

high-impact aerobics (HIA) A style of aerobics in which both feet may temporarily leave the floor at the same time when performing moves such as jogging, jumping, and hopping.

High-Intensity Training (HIT) Bouts of exercise performed at high percentages of maximal exertion for a particular type of training, i.e., high intensity aerobics or high intensity anaerobics. Sometimes used interchangeably with HITT.

High-Intensity Interval Training (HIIT) Repeated bouts of exercise (intervals) performed at near maximal levels of exertion separated by short breaks or lower intensity bouts of exercise. Cycles of high and low intensity may be maintained for several minutes up to about 20 minutes. There is no set formula.

homeostasis State of balance or dynamic equilibrium. The energy demand is being met by energy production.

HRmax *See* maximum heart rate formula

HRR *See* heart-rate reserve.

hydrostatic weighing A method of estimating body fat. (*Synonym:* underwater weighing)

hypertension A higher than normal blood pressure.

hypertrophy An increase in size. In exercise this usually refers to an increase in muscle size.

intensity The level of exertion during exercise.

interval training A method of conditioning that alternates short, high-intensity exercise bouts with short rest periods or lower-intensity bouts.

intrinsic motivation Motivation that arises from within a person; self-motivation.

isokinetic contractions A muscle contraction in which the speed of movement is controlled and the force applied is met with an equal resistance. Especially good for rehabilitation.

isometric contraction A muscle contraction in which there is tension but no movement. It is used to increase strength in one position. Also known as a static contraction.

isotonic contraction Muscular strength and endurance exercises in which the tension of the muscle remains the same throughout the range of the motion. Also known as dynamic contraction.

Karvonen formula A method of calculating the intensity target range for aerobic work using a percentage of the heart-rate reserve.

lactic acid A by-product of high-intensity anaerobic exercise. Accumulation of lactic acid is associated with muscle fatigue and "burn."

LBM *See* lean body mass.

LDL *See* low-density lipoprotein.

lean body mass (LBM) All the tissues of the body except fat. LBM includes bone, muscle, water, organs, connective tissue, etc., and is used to determine body composition.

LIA *See* low-impact aerobics.

ligament The fibrous tissue that connects bones to bones.

low-density lipoprotein (LDL) A complex of lipids and proteins that carries cholesterol and deposits it along the walls of the arteries. (Often called LDL-C when carrying cholesterol.) High concentrations of LDL are associated with an increased risk of heart disease.

low-impact aerobics (LIA) A type of aerobics in which the participant keeps one foot on the floor at all times. It is often characterized by moderately paced movements involving a full range of motion with a lot of upper-body work.

maximum heart rate (HRmax) The highest heart rate obtainable with exertion.

maximum heart-rate formula A method of estimating the intensity range for an aerobic workout using a percentage (70 to 85%) of the maximum heart rate. (*Synonym:* zero to peak formula)

mental imagery A cognitive (thought-based) technique to enhance task performance. Uses mental rehearsal/practice.

MIA *See* moderate-impact aerobics.

minerals Inorganic compounds that are essential to normal body function.

moderate-impact aerobics (MIA) A form of aerobic dance in which the center of gravity is raised and lowered (all the way up on and off the balls of the feet) while using steps that keep one foot on the floor at all times.

muscular endurance The ability of a muscle, or group of muscles, to apply force repeatedly or to sustain a muscular contraction for a period of time.

muscular strength The maximum force a muscle, or group of muscles, can exert against a resistance.

obese Being more than 30% fat for women and 25% fat for men.

one repetition maximum (1 RM) To exert one maximal force.

overfat A condition in which the percentage of body weight that is fat weight is too high.

overweight An amount of weight above the average as determined by a standard height/weight chart or body mass index.

oxidative system: A metabolic system that uses oxygen to produce energy (ATP) from carbohydrates and fatty acids.

oxygen consumption The rate at which oxygen is used to produce energy, measured in liters per minute or milliliters per kilogram of body weight per minute. (*Synonym:* oxygen uptake)

passive stretching Flexibility exercise in which the stretch (lengthening) of the muscle is created by an outside source such as a partner, gravity, or body part not involved in the stretch.

phosphagen (ATP-PCr) system An anaerobic system that rapidly produces energy through the breakdown and resynthesis of high-energy phosphagens (not carbohydrate). This system can supply only a few seconds of energy.

physical fitness The physical aspects of a person's well-being that enable a person to function at an optimal level.

physioball *See* stability ball.

phytochemicals Food components, "plant chemicals," that ward off cancer, cardiovascular diseases, diabetes, and hypertension.

pilates A method of mental and physical conditioning that aims to develop strength balanced with flexibility.

PNF stretching A method of stretching that uses proprioceptive neuromuscular facilitation (PNF). First the muscle is isometrically contracted, and then it is stretched.

pre-exercise heart rate (PreHR) The rate at which the heart is beating prior to exercise.

PreHR *See* pre-exercise heart rate.

principle of individuality An exercise principle that states that any two people can react differently to the same exercise.

principle of overload An exercise principle stating that a physiological system or organ of the body repeatedly subjected to greater than normal stress will adapt to the stress. A proper amount of overload will result in positive adaptations.

principle of overuse An exercise principle that states that too much stress over a period of time can result in fatigue and injury.

principle of progression An exercise principle that states that the gradual increase (or overload) of the intensity, frequency, or duration of exercise will improve physical fitness.

principle of regularity An exercise principle stating that a physiological system or organ that is not repeatedly stressed but is instead subjected to less than normal amounts of stress will adapt by deconditioning. (*Synonyms:* use/disuse principle; principle of reversability)

principle of reversability *See* principle of regularity.

principle of specificity An exercise principle stating that physiological adaptations are specific to the systems that are overloaded through exercise.

progressive relaxation A physiolgoical method of systematically relaxing skeletal muscles with the belief that this will reduce tension throughout the body. Muscles are alternately contracted and relaxed.

proprioceptive neuromuscular facilitation stretching *See* PNF stretching.

protein A compound made up of amino acids that is found in certain foods. It is primarily used to build and repair body tissues but may also serve as a source of energy.

psychoneuroimmunology An area of neurology that studies how the psyche (brain) influences the immune system.

pulse The wave of pressure felt in the arteries when the heart beats.

radial artery An artery that runs close to the surface of the skin on the inside of the wrist. This artery is commonly used for counting the pulse.

ratings of perceived exertion (RPE) A method of estimating the intensity of an exercise session that uses a scale of numbers with brief qualifiers developed by Gunnar Borg.

RecHR *See* recovery heart rate.

recovery heart rate (RecHR) The rate at which the heart beats following exercise. Usually counted 1 or 2 minutes after exercise is stopped.

repetitions A resistance training term that refers to the number of times an exercise is executed.

repetition maximum To exert a maximal force over 1 repetition (1 RM).

resistance ball *See* stability ball.

rhabdomyolysis The rapid destruction of skeletal muscle resulting in leakage of myoglobin (muscle protein) into the urine.

RICE An acronym for immediate first aid for injuries such as sprains, strains, and contusions: rest, ice, compression, elevation.

RPE *See* ratings of perceived exertion.

set A resistance training term that refers to one group of consecutive repetitions.

set point theory A genetic-based theory that asserts that the body seeks to maintain a preset level of fat.

shinsplints A general term for pain on the front or side of the shin. A common overuse injury in aerobic activity.

skin-fold technique A method of estimating a person's percentage of body fat. Subcutaneous fat is measured using a skin-fold caliper.

spot reducing One of the all-time greatest myths that states an individual can take fat off a specific part of the body by exercising that specific part. A person actually can lose fat throughout the body only by exercising aerobically and eating a proper diet.

sprain Overstretching or tearing a ligament or joint capsule resulting in swelling, discoloration, and pain.

stability ball A large inflated rubber, vinyl, or solid foam ball used to perform resistance and/or core training exercises using an unstable environment.

static contraction *See* isometric contraction.

static stretching A technique of developing flexibility that places the muscle in a stretch position and then holds that stretch without moving. (Opposite of *ballistic stretching.*)

step aerobics A form of aerobic dance exercise in which you step up and down on a bench to the beat of the music at a rate of 118 to 122 bpm (beginners), maximum 128 bpm (advanced).

strain Overstretching or tearing a muscle or tendon, resulting in swelling, discoloration, and pain.

strength *See* muscular strength.

stretch reflex The automatic muscular contraction that occurs when a muscle is suddenly stretched.

stroke volume The amount of blood the heart pumps in 1 beat.

supersetting A method of resistance training in which an exercise for one muscle is immediately followed by an exercise for the opposing muscle. (Sometimes the definition also includes performing two exercises for the same muscle group one immediately after another.)

Swiss ball *See* stability ball.

systolic pressure The pressure exerted by the blood in the arteries when the ventricles are contracting. Systolic pressure is represented by the numerator in the blood pressure fraction.

tapless step A type of step aerobics that makes transitions from one lead leg to another without using a tap change.

target heart-rate zone (THZ) *See* training heart-rate range.

TC *See* total cholesterol.

tendinitis Inflammation of a tendon. This is a common overuse injury.

tendon Fibrous tissue that connects muscle to bone.

THR *See* training heart-rate range.

threshold of aerobic training The lower limit of the aerobic target zone. It is usually described by a percentage of the maximum volume of oxygen consumed, the maximum heart rate, or the heart-rate reserve. *See* threshold of training.

threshold of training The minimum amount and intensity of exercise that must be performed for an individual to make physical fitness gains.

THZ *See* target heart-rate zone.

time The length of a single exercise session. Also sometimes referred to as duration.

total cholesterol The sum of HDL and LDL.

training heart-rate range (THR) The optimum intensity range for aerobic exercise using the exercise heart rate as the indicator of intensity. Training within the range improves cardiorespiratory endurance. (*Synonym:* target heart-rate zone (THZ))

trans **fats** Fats artificially produced from liquid unsaturated fats into solid fats. Linked to higher cholesterol levels and greater risk of coronary heart disease.

type of exercise The activity in which a person chooses to engage; it represents the second "T" in the FITT Principle.

underwater weighing *See* hydrostatic weighing.

use/disuse principle *See* principle of regularity.

vein A vessel that carries blood toward the heart.

venous pump Action of the muscles that helps to massage blood up the veins against gravity.

vitamins Organic compounds that help release energy from food and act as metabolic regulators. Vitamins A, D, E, and K are fat soluble; the rest are water soluble.

VO$_2$max The largest amount of oxygen the body can consume in 1 minute, measured in liters per minute or milliliters per kilogram of body weight per minute. (*Synonym:* maximum oxygen uptake *or* MOU)

warm-up The period of time in which individuals prepare the body for vigorous activity by performing easy movements through a range of motion, thus raising the core temperature of the body and stretching out and lubricating muscles and joints. Leading into the aerobic workout, it is a gradual increase in activity level that allows the heart and lungs to make a smooth transition into exercise.

water aerobics A low-impact form of aerobic conditioning performed in water using water resistance to enhance training. (*Synonym:* aqua aerobics)

wellness A way of being that involves taking responsibility for one's own well-being and practicing lifestyle habits that promote physical, social, emotional, mental, and spiritual health.

yoga An ancient Eastern Indian philosophy with an ultimate goal of reaching self-realization. Embraces living in harmony and achieving an inner peace. *See also* hatha yoga.

zero to peak formula *See* maximum heart-rate formula.

Index

Page references followed by *f* indicate figure; by *t* indicate table; by *b* indicate box.